Self-Assessment of Current Knowledge in Otolaryngology

SECOND EDITION

1,500 Multiple Choice Questions and Referenced Answers

Edited by

GEORGE I. UHDE, M.D.
Professor of Otolaryngology
Chief, Otolaryngology Section
University of Louisville Medical School
Consultant,
Veteran's Administration Hospital
Founder, Otology Clinics,
Kentucky Commission
Handicapped Children
Fellow,
American College of Surgeons and
American Trilogical Society

MEDICAL EXAMINATION PUBLISHING COMPANY, INC.
65-36 Fresh Meado~~ Lane
Flushing, N.Y.

Library of Congress Card Number
74-28667

ISBN 0-87488-270-2

November, 1976

Printed in the United States of America

PREFACE

Learning, by whatever media, is eventually self-instruction by problems in patient care, response to medical and surgical treatment, reinforcement by medical student and resident questions, and media for learning – in this instance, an otolaryngology review book of recent advances in otolaryngology.

This book has an alphabetical subject and author index to question numbers and references about the most recent advances in diagnosis and treatment. Coordination of this book's contents index with self-evaluation and patient care has proved more useful than the usual examination book to medical students, residents and practicing-teaching otolaryngologists.

The author acknowledges the sympathetic understanding and many hours of additional work by his secretary, Mrs. Joyce Guderian.

Constructive or critical comments by colleagues would be appreciated to improve any future publication.

SELF-ASSESSMENT
OF
CURRENT KNOWLEDGE
IN
OTOLARYNGOLOGY

SECOND EDITION

CONTENTS

SELECT ONE OR MORE APPROPRIATE ANSWERS

1. The medial wall of the protympanum (bony portion of the eustachian tube) may be dehiscent and in curettement of this area during surgery which of the following structures may be injured?
   A. middle meningeal artery
   B. tensor tympani muscle
   C. mandibular branch of trigeminal nerve
   D. chorda tympani nerve in the canal of Huguier
   E. internal carotid artery and/or caroticotympanic vessels
   REF. Proctor B: Arch Otolaryng, 97:2, Jan '73

2. Of the following muscles concerned with function of the eustachian tube, which has the greatest influence?
   A. tensor veli palatini
   B. levator veli palatini
   C. superior pharyngeal constrictor
   D. salpingopharyngeal
   E. tensor tympani
   REF. Proctor B: Arch Otolaryng, 97:2, Jan '73

3. An anatomical variation of the eustachian tube which can cause malleus fixation and conductive deafness is:
   A. intertympanosquamosal crest of the petrosa
   B. squamosa
   C. processus cochleariformis
   D. crista tegmentalis
   E. overriding squamosa posteriorly by the petrosquamosal crest
   REF. Proctor B: Arch Otolarying, 97:2, Jan '73 (See Fig. 1)

4. On ascent a sensation of fullness and a slight bulge of the tympanic membrane results at a level of:
   A. 33 ft.
   B. 110 - 180 ft.
   C. 2300 - 3100 ft.
   D. 4100 - 7500 ft.
   E. 10,000 - 12,000 ft.
   REF. Donaldson JA: Arch Otolaryng, 97:9, Jan '73

5. On ascent after the first 500 feet (200 mm H_2O) a click may be heard as the eustachian tube opens and the tympanic membrane snaps back lowering the intratympanic pressure to 50 mm H_2O. Thereafter the eustachian tube opens at approximately which of the following foot-intervals?
   A. 150
   B. 375
   C. 425
   D. 500
   E. 650
   REF. Donaldson JA: Arch Otolaryng, 97:9, Jan '73

6. The problem of aerotitis media usually occurs during descent when swallowing is deferred and the pressure holding the fibrocartilaginous portion of the tube collapsed cannot be overcome and the tube cannot be opened. Aerotitis media results when there is a negative intratympanic pressure of mm H_2O of:
   A. 250 to 300
   B. 550 to 575
   C. 725 to 800
   D. 1,100 to 1,250
   E. 1,375 to 1,450
   REF. Donaldson JA: Arch Otolaryng, 97:9, Jan '73, Holmquist J: Acta Otolaryngol (Stockholm) 66:289, Oct. '68

7. Results of tubal function tests are useful in predicting success in myringoplasty surgery. Unfortunately, few studies have been reported. Of the following methods devised to test eustachian tube function, which is probably the least accurate?
   A. transport of sound
   B. transport of air
   C. radiopaque media

D. fluorescein
E. solution of sulfisoxazole diolamine (Gantrisin)
REF. Donaldson JA: Arch Otolaryng, 97:9, Jan '73

8. Tympanostomy tubes are useful in which of the following conditions?
A. chronic nonsuppurative otitis media
B. ventilating and reversing the atelectatic ear
C. tympanoplasty in a patient with persistent eustachian tube malfunction
D. acute suppurative otitis media
E. recurrent ear disease without eliminating contributing disease (enlarged adenoids, allergy, and sinusitis)
REF. Armstrong BW: Arch Otolaryng, 97:13, Jan '73 (See Fig. 2)

9. Middle fossa eustachian tuboplasty is a procedure for correction of bony or fibrous closure of the osseous (static) segment of the tube. The three most dependable tests for preoperative evaluation of the tube are:
A. Miller gas transducer
B. Toynbee test
C. Madsen impedance bridge
D. politzerization
E. Compere x-ray clearance study
REF. Glasscock III ME: Arch Otolaryng, 97:15, Jan '73

10. The eustachian tube has a dynamic (cartilaginous) and a static (osseous) portion and the vast majority of problems arise from:
A. fibrous overgrowth of the osseous portion
B. bony overgrowth of the osseous portion
C. nasopharyngeal disease
D. sinus disease
E. allergy
REF. Glasscock III ME: Arch Otolaryng, 97:15, Jan '73

11. Basically all techniques for tympanometry for eustachian tube evaluation fall into which of the following categories?
A. transmission of sound through the eustachian tube
B. fluoroscopy or clearance tests
C. radiographic examination
D. equilibration of negative or positive air pressure introduced to the middle ear
E. impedance measurements
REF. Harford ER: Arch Otolaryng, 97:17, Jan '73

12. Air pressure in the middle ear should equal the atmospheric level. A simple quantitative technique for measurement of air pressure in the middle ear is important because:
A. diagnosis of eustachian tube insufficiency
B. prognosis for medical treatment (allergy, sinusitis)
C. prognosis for surgical treatment (tympanoplasty with or without mastoidectomy)
D. evaluation of effectiveness of medical treatment
E. evaluation of effectiveness of surgical treatment
REF. Harford ER: Arch Otolaryng, 97:17, Jan '73

13. Tympanometry is an objective, practical measurement of Van Dishoeck's subjective pneumophone test which is based on the principle that a tone fed into the ear canal will be heard most distinctly when the air pressure on both surfaces of the tympanic membrane is:
A. equal
B. less on the middle ear side
C. greater on the middle ear side
D. less on the external auditory canal side
E. greater on the external auditory canal side
REF. Harford ER: Arch Otolaryng, 97:17, Jan '73

14. Which of the following statements is correct?
    A. impedance audiometry can be measured by the electro-acoustic impedance meter (Madsen, model ZO 70)
    B. the electromechanical bridge of Zwislocki uses the same approach as A above
    REF. Harford ER: Arch Otolaryng, 97:17, Jan '73 (See Fig. 3)

15. Type A (normal) tympanogram is observed in patients with:
    A. normal ear
    B. sensorineural damage without tubal inefficiency
    C. stapedial otosclerosis without tubal inefficiency
    D. sensorineural damage with tubal inefficiency
    E. stapedial otosclerosis with tubal inefficiency
    REF. Harford ER: Arch Otolaryng, 97:17, Jan '73

16. Type B (flat, somewhat depressed) tympanogram is observed in patients with:
    A. stapedial otosclerosis without eustachian tube blockage
    B. middle ear fluid
    C. negative middle ear pressure
    D. ossicular discontinuity
    E. massive ossicular fixation
    REF. Harford ER: Arch Otolaryng, 97:17, Jan '73

17. Type C (deepest portion of the notch located in the negative range) tympanogram is observed in patients with:
    A. abnormal, negative middle ear pressure
    B. ossicular discontinuity
    C. middle ear fluid
    D. stapedial otosclerosis
    E. sensorineural hearing loss without tubal insufficiency
    REF. Harford ER: Arch Otolaryng, 97:17, Jan '73

18. Type D (large curve undulations) tympanogram is observed in patients with:
    A. middle ear fluid
    B. negative middle ear pressure
    C. stapedial otosclerosis
    D. ossicular discontinuity
    E. massive ossicular fixation
    REF. Harford ER: Arch Otolaryng, 97:17, Jan '73

19. Tympanomaxillary shunt (TMS) establishes a permanent communication between the middle ear and the maxillary sinus by way of a silicone-rubber tube and is a method for obtaining permanent ventilation of the middle ear in cases with long-term obstruction of the eustachian tube. The advantages of a TMS shunt are:
    A. permanent ventilation of the middle ear including positive pressure by Valsalva maneuver
    B. provides for drainage of the middle ear
    C. tympanic membrane remains intact (patient may go swimming without danger of infection)
    D. auditory canal intact
    E. may be used in growing children before adolescence
    REF. Ekvall L, Drettner B: Arch Otolaryng, 97:21, Jan '73 (See Fig. 4)

20. The disadvantages of a tympanomaxillary shunt (TMS) are:
    A. does not provide drainage of the middle ear
    B. not as simple a surgical technique as a tubomyringotomy
    C. more risk of surgical complications than a direct surgical attack on the obstructed eustachian tube, e.g., internal carotid artery or intracranial structures
    D. not advisable in children
    E. applicable to only a few patients since permanent closure of the bony eustachian tube in adults is a very rare condition
    REF. Ekvall L, Drettner, B: Arch Otolayrng, 97:21, Jan' 73

21. The bony portion of the eustachian tube (protympanum) measures:
A. 1.0 cm long and 2.0 mm wide
B. 0.5 cm long and 1.0 mm wide
C. 2.0 cm long and 2.0 mm wide
D. 0.5 cm long and 2.0 mm wide
E. 2.0 cm long and 1.0 mm wide
REF. Proctor B: Arch Otolaryng, 97:2, Jan '73

22. The cartilaginous portion of the eustachian tube measures in mm in length:
A. 10
B. 15
C. 25
D. 30
E. 35
REF. Proctor B: Arch Otolaryng, 97:2, Jan '73

23. Ankylosis of the stapes in the oval window as a cause of deafness was first described macroscopically in the early 18th century by:
A. Von Troelth
B. Politzer
C. Bezold
D. Siebenmann
E. Valsalva
REF. Lindsay JR: Arch Otolaryng, 97:24, Jan '73

24. In 1894, ankylosis of the stapes in the oval window was for the first time considered a "primary disease of the bony labyrinthine capsule" and the term "otosclerosis" was first used by:
A. Valsalva
B. Politzer
C. Von Troelth
D. Bezold
E. Wittmack
REF. Lindsay JR: Arch Otolaryng, 97:24, Jan '73

25. Clinical otosclerosis (impairment of hearing due to otosclerosis) usually becomes evident in the following decades of life:
A. first
B. second
C. third
D. fourth
E. fifth
REF. Lindsay JR: Arch Otolaryng, 97:24, Jan '73

26. The incidence of clinical otosclerosis is most common in:
A. black women
B. white men
C. white women
D. mongoloids
E. white children
REF. Lindsay JR: Arch Otolaryng, 97:24, Jan '73

27. Which of the following statements is/are correct?
Available information on genetics of otosclerosis favors a:
A. recessive autosomal type
B. dominant type
REF. Lindsay JR: Arch Otolaryng, 97:24, Jan '73

28. Otosclerosis is found most frequently in one or more localized foci. The most common site is:
A. posterior to the oval window
B. middle of oval window
C. outer attachment of the round window membrane
D. region anterior to the oval window
E. anterior inferior border of the internal meatus at the junction of the enchondral and periosteal layers of the capsule
REF. Lindsay JR: Arch Otolaryng, 97:24, Jan '73 (See Fig. 5)

29. Multiple foci of otosclerosis are:
A. relatively common in older age groups
B. sometimes associated with severe or profound sensorineural deafness
C. sometimes associated with stapes ankylosis

D. sometimes associated with round window blockage
E. may be separate foci in cochlear capsule, apart from the oval window region
REF. Lindsay JR: Arch Otolaryng, 97:24, Jan '73 (See Fig. 6)

30. Otosclerotic foci in the vicinity of the semicircular canals occur:
A. as single discrete focus alone
B. as multiple discrete foci alone
C. as single discrete focus but always in association with one or more foci at usual areas of predilection
D. as multiple discrete foci but always in association with one or more foci at usual areas of predilection
E. never
REF. Lindsay JR: Arch Otolaryng, 97:24, Jan '73

31. Which of the following statements is/are correct?
A. blockage of the round window may occur without oval window involvement
B. blockage of the round window may occur with stapes ankylosis
REF. Lindsay JR: Arch Otolaryng, 97:24, Jan '73 (See Fig. 7)

32. Blue mantles:
A. are common findings in temporal bones with otosclerosis
B. are clearly distinguished from lamellar bone found around vascular channels in the physiologic process of resorption and deposition of bone
C. occur in periosteal layers
D. occur in enchondral layers
E. are seen but only rarely in the absence of otosclerosis
REF. Lindsay JR: Arch Otolaryng, 97:24, Jan '73

33. The pathophysiology of otosclerosis is based on the following etiology:
A. unsolved
B. abnormalities in calcium-phosphorus metabolism
C. abnormality in the lipoproteins
D. abnormality in the acid and alkaline phosphatase activity
E. lysosomes in osteocytes is the source of the enzymes involved in the destructive phase
REF. Lindsay JR: Arch Otolaryng, 97:24, Jan '73

34. Otosclerosis is:
A. a misnomer
B. loss of density of bone of the labyrinthine capsule
C. sclerosis of the labyrinthine capsule
D. otospongiosis (Siebenmann)
E. localized otoporosis
REF. Shambaugh Jr. GE, Daniel III HJ, Linthicum FH, Lindsay J, Schuknecht HE, Valvassori GE: Arch Otolaryng, 97:30, Jan '73

35. Pure cochlear otosclerosis is:
A. vestibular otosclerosis
B. labyrinthine otosclerosis
C. otosclerosis involving the endosteum of the cochlea without stapes fixation
D. evidence of otosclerosis by polytomography
E. progressive sensorineural loss of 40 db or more with a characteristic flat audiometric configuration, type II Bekesy, very high short increment sensitivity index score, and a low-tone decay
REF. Shambaugh Jr. GE, Daniel III HJ, Linthicum FH, Lindsay J, Schuknecht HF, Valvassori GE: Arch Otolaryng, 97:30, Jan '73

36. Which one of the following diseases alone has the peculiar characteristic of attacking the endochondral layer of the otic capsule and invading the annular ligament?
    A. osteoporosis
    B. osteomalacia
    C. osteitis fibrosa
    D. Recklinghausen's disease
    E. Paget's disease
    F. otosclerosis
    REF. Shambaugh Jr. GE, Daniel III HJ, Linthicum FH, Lindsay J, Schuknecht HF, Valvassori GE: Arch Otolaryng, 97:30, Jan '73

37. In reference to so-called pure cochlear otosclerosis, which of the following statements may be considered applicable?
    A. large otosclerotic foci of the bony labyrinth causing sensorineural hearing loss without stapes fixation is debatable
    B. relationship between otosclerosis and osteoporosis appear unrelated
    C. clinical otosclerosis frequently becomes manifest during pregnancy (or hearing loss becomes accelerated) so birth-control pills must remain suspect in young women with rapidly progressive hearing loss and with x-ray evidence of otosclerosis
    D. dominant type of hereditary characteristic is unknown
    E. autosomal recessive type of hereditary characteristic is unknown
    REF. Shambaugh Jr. GE, Daniel III HJ, Linthicum FH, Lindsay J, Schuknecht HF, Valvassori GE: Arch Otolaryng, 97:30, Jan '73

38. The goal of stapedectomy may be considered which of the following (and this must be made clear to the patient)?
    A. complete closure of the air-bone gap with a hearing level above the 25-30 decibel line
    B. better hearing with a body aid
    C. getting rid of body aid so patient can wear an ear-level aid
    D. may need aid for distant conversation only
    E. may be able to disregard aid completely
    REF. House HP, Farrior JB, Goodhill V, Harrison,WH, Shea JJ, Portmann M, Schuknecht, HF: Arch Otolaryng, 97:35, Jan '73

39. What complications may arise from stapedectomy and the surgeon should so advise the patient?
    A. eight or nine out of ten are improved with conductive deafness
    B. one or two out of 100 are worse with conductive deafness
    C. sensation of taste on that side of the tongue may be damaged
    D. facial paralysis may result
    E. in mixed deafness only the conductive portion of the hearing loss may be expected to improve
    REF. House HP, Farrior JB, Goodhill V, Harrison WH, Shea JJ, Portmann M, Schuknecht HF: Arch Otolaryng, 97:35, Jan '73

40. What is the age category in years (lower and upper limits) for stapes surgery in persons with good health?
    A. no limit
    B. not under 20
    C. not over 60
    D. 25 - 55
    E. 20 - 60
    REF. House HP, Farrior JB, Goodhill V, Harrison WH, Shea JJ, Portmann M, Schuknecht HF: Arch Otolaryng, 97:35, Jan '73

41. Who in age in years are unexpectedly most pleased with stapes surgery even though a hearing aid provides hearing?
    A. 20 - 39
    B. 40 - 49
    C. 50 - 69
    D. 70 - 79
    E. 80 and over
    REF. House HP, Farrior JB, Goodhill V, Harrison WH, Shea JJ, Portmann M, Schuknecht, HF: Arch Otolaryng, 97:35, Jan '73

42. A patient with progressive otosclerosis with cochlear hydrops or cochlear Ménière's disease (constantly unsteady or episodic vertigo with fluctuant hearing loss) but no Ménière's symptoms for several years should have:
    A. mobilization
    B. no form of stapes surgery
    C. stapedectomy
    D. treatment for Ménière's and then stapes surgery
    E. concomitant Ménière's treatment and stapes surgery
    REF. House HP, Farrior JB, Goodhill V, Harrison WH, Shea JJ, Portmann M, Schuknecht HF: Arch Otolaryng, 97:35, Jan '73

43. A patient with progressive otosclerosis with vestibular hydrops or vestibular Ménière's disease (constantly unsteady or episodic vertigo without fluctuant hearing loss) but no symptoms for several years should have:
    A. mobilization
    B. no form of stapes surgery
    C. stapedectomy
    D. treatment for possible recurrence of vertigo and then stapes surgery
    E. concomitant treatment for possible vertigo and stapes surgery
    REF. House HP, Farrior JB, Goodhill V, Harrison WH, Shea JJ, Portmann, M, Schuknecht HF: Arch Otolaryng, 97:35, Jan '73

44. In this day of excellent audiology being generally available are tuning forks really necessary?
    A. always
    B. occasionally
    C. never
    REF. House HP, Farrior JB, Goodhill V, Harrison WH, Shea JJ, Portmann M, Schuknecht HF: Arch Otolaryng, 97:35, Jan '73

45. In this day of excellent audiology being generally available are tuning forks' lateralization of value to the surgeon in any of the following conditions?
    A. acoustic tumor
    B. completely deaf ear due to viral diseases
    C. otosclerosis
    D. otitis media
    E. simulation or in the malingerer
    REF. House HP, Farrior JB, Goodhill V, Harrison WH, Shea JJ, Portmann M, Schuknecht HF: Arch Otolaryng, 97:35, Jan '73

46. Preparation of the patient for stapes surgery should include which of the following?
    A. tetracycline one gram 24 hours before operation and a gram daily for five days after operation
    B. no prophylactic antibiotics
    C. cleaning ear canal day before surgery (nurse) and dropping antiseptic gtts (nurse) into the canal morning of surgery and before starting the operative procedure; the surgeon or resident cleans the ear canal with suction, antiseptic gtts and then discards the instrument used for cleaning
    D. ampicillin unless patient is allergic
    E. culture with sensitivity tests of ear canal prior to stapes surgery because of high incidence of otitis media
    REF. House HP, Farrior JB, Goodhill V, Harrison WH, Shea JJ, Portmann M, Schuknecht HF: Arch Otolaryng, 97:35, Jan '73

47. What type of anesthesia is best for stapes surgery?
    A. none, depends on experience and use of by the individual surgeon
    B. lidocain hydrochloride (xylocainc hydrochloride) 2% with patient under drugs ("Balfium") under control of anesthetist (Portmann method)
    C. preoperative droperidol 2 ml intramuscularly with 0.6 mg atropine and Innovar (1 ml/11.3 kg body weight) or about 6 ml. (Shea method)

D. local with Demerol or phenobarbital sodium or diazepam (Valium) as needed (Goodhill method)
E. general with minimal injection to control hemorrhage
REF. House, HP, Farrior JB, Goodhill V, Harrison WH, Shea JJ, Portmann M, Schuknecht HF: Arch Otolaryng, 97:35, Jan '73

48. In performing stapes surgery the chorda tympani nerve must be cut in the following percent of patients depending on the surgeon?
A. 10
B. 20 - 30
C. 40 - 50
D. 60 - 70
E. 80 - 90
REF. House HP, Farrior JB, Goodhill V, Harrison WH, Shea JJ, Portmann M, Schuknecht HF: Arch Otolaryng, 97:35, Jan '73

49. If the chorda tympani nerve obstructs the operative view during stapes surgery, is it better to?
A. move the nerve without overstretching gently against the bony overhang (portion of bone remaining after removal of annulus tympanicus above the emergence of the chorda tympani)
B. move the nerve laterally without overstretching
C. overstretch the nerve as needed
D. cut the nerve
E. A or B with draping absorbable gelatine sponge (gelfoam) across the nerve to prevent drying from exposure and intense light
REF. House HP, Farrior JB, Goodhill V, Harrison WH, Shea JJ, Portmann M, Schuknecht HF: Arch Otolaryng, 97:35, Jan '73

50. If the chorda tympani nerve must be sacrificed to ensure adequate safe exposure during stapes surgery, which of the following is the procedure of choice?
A. simply cut the nerve
B. cut the nerve but approximate loosely the ends after surgery
C. overstretch the nerve medially as needed
D. overstretch the nerve laterally as needed
E. cut and suture the ends of the nerve
REF. House HP, Farrior JB, Goodhill V, Harrison HW, Shea JJ, Portmann M, Schuknecht HF: Arch Otolaryng, 97:35, Jan '73

51. If the chorda tympani nerve is overstretched or sacrificed completely especially in both ears during stapes surgery, which of the following age groups in years appear to have the most distressing symptoms of a dry mouth and taste disturbance?
A. 20 - 25
B. 26 - 29
C. 30 - 35
D. 36 - 45
E. postmenopausal group
REF. House HP, Farrior JB, Goodhill V, Harrison WH, Shea JJ, Portmann M, Schuknecht HF: Arch Otolaryng, 97:35 , Jan '73

52. In obliterative otosclerosis the best procedure for treatment of the footplate appears to be:
A. Harrison scrape knife technique
B. very slowly rotating cutting burr (not diamond) with Kerr drill with twisted wire inserted into a perforating hole (Goodhill)
C. drill to create a wide blue area and then enter the inner ear with an oval window excavator to enlarge the perforating hole to about 0. 8 mm in diameter and then inserting a polytef wire piston (Farrior)

D. slowly running Kerr drill with 1 mm cutting burr down to a blue line and then make a small fenestra and insert a 0. 6 mm polytef (teflon) cup prosthesis piston
E. no surgery - use hearing aid
REF. House HP, Farrior JB, Goodhill V, Harrison WH, Shea JJ, Portmann M, Schuknecht HF: Arch Otolaryng, 97:35, Jan '73

53. Which of the following foot-plates is most likely to end up as a floater unless special precautions are taken?
A. thin
B. moderately thick
C. thick
D. obliterative without any marginal edges
E. thick foot-plate of a biscuit type with an annulus all the way around, with a little bit of foot-plate showing and a lot more in the inner ear
REF. House HP, Farrior JB, Goodhill V, Harrison WH, Shea JJ, Portmann M, Schuknecht HF: Arch Otolaryng, 97:35, Jan '73

54. In obliterative otosclerosis which of the following techniques appears to help prevent a floater?
A. drill directly on the foot-plate with a slowly rotating cutting burr (Kerr drill creating a wide area)
B. scrap technique directly on the foot-plate
C. drill on the foot-plate and inferior margin simultaneously until a thin blue-line appears and then move onto the foot-plate
D. use a diamond burr with a Kerr drill
E. perforate the foot-plate with 1mm cutting burr
REF. House HP, Farrior JB, Goodhill V, Harrison WH, Shea JJ, Portmann M, Schuknecht HF: Arch Otolaryng, 97:35, Jan '73

55. Which of the following techniques for stapes surgery appears to be developing less enthusiasm among otologic surgeons?
A. wire-gelfoam prosthesis after total removal of the foot-plate (House)
B. push posterior crus forward, remove posterior two-thirds foot-plate and place vein or human amniotic membrane over the opening and replace posterior crus (Portmann)
C. piston on vein (Shea)
D. wire-fat prosthesis after total removal of the foot-plate (Schuknecht)
E. wire prosthesis with single (usually double) loop with fascia graft after total removal of the foot-plate
REF. House HP, Farrior JB, Goodhill V, Harrison WH, Shea JJ, Portmann M, Schuknecht HF: Arch Otolaryng, 97:35, Jan '73

56. What can the surgeon do when he cannot use the incus as a supporter device for the stapes prosthesis (short incus, necrotic incus, overhanging facial nerve, bad angle to the incus)?
A. polytef piston from malleus handle
B. routine stapedectomy with short process of incus onto a flat graft in oval window
C. sculpture long process incus or short process and place the incus against the promontory
D. fenestration
E. type III tympanoplasty
REF. House HP, Farrior JB, Goodhill V, Harrison WH, Shea JJ, Portmann, M, Schuknecht HF: Arch Otolaryng, 97:35, Jan '73

57. Tympanic fibrosis is one of the most defeating postoperative complications but can be treated by:
A. steroids in the middle ear
B. revision of surgery with radical removal of all adhesions

C. preoperative steroids and continued during postoperative period
D. discontinuance of use of polyethylene prosthesis
E. no known effective treatment
REF. House HP, Farrior JB, Goodhill V, Harrison WH, Shea JJ, Portmann M, Schuknecht HF: Arch Otolaryng, 97:35, Jan '73

58. What is the average hospitalization period in days following total stapedectomy?
A. one
B. two
C. three
D. four
E. five or more
REF. House HP, Farrior JB, Goodhill V, Harrison WH, Shea JJ, Portmann M, Schuknecht HF: Arch Otolaryng, 97:35, Jan '73

59. For what period should patients be quiet (no active exercise) following stapes surgery?
A. one week
B. two weeks
C. three weeks
D. four weeks
E. two months
REF. House HP, Farrior JB, Goodhill V, Harrison WH, Shea JJ, Portmann M, Schuknecht HF: Arch Otolaryng, 97:35, Jan '73

60. What forms of predisposing circumstances must be avoided for at least one month following stapes surgery because sensorineural deafness appears sometimes during the third postoperative week?
A. exertion in any form, such as lifting
B. nice dinner with two wines
C. sexual contact
D. athletic activities
E. upper and lower respiratory infections with coughing, eustachian tube blockage, nasopharyngitis and middle ear infection
REF. House HP, Farrior JB, Goodhill V, Harrison WH, Shea JJ, Portmann M, Schuknecht HF: Arch Otolaryng, 97:35, Jan '73

61. Ears with moderate and severe grades of acute diffuse external otitis showed which of the following organisms?
A. pseudomonas
B. proteus mirabilis
C. klebsiella pneumoniae
D. beta hemolytic streptococci
E. staphylococcus epidermidis
REF. Senturia BH: Ann Otol, 82:Supp. No. 8, Sept - Oct '73

62. When may a patient use an elevator especially in high buildings following stapedectomy?
A. anytime after present day surgery
B. always dangerous, even for years, after the polyethylene on vein prosthesis
C. same as B after polyethylene against absorbable gelatin sponge
D. not for one month under any circumstances
E. with acute respiratory infections immediately after surgery
REF. House HP, Farrior JB, Goodhill V, Harrison WH, Shea JJ, Portmann M, Schuknecht HF: Arch Otolaryng, 97:35, Jan '73

63. The incidence of granuloma of the inner ear is one to three percent following stapedectomy. The etiology of granuloma is due to:
A. fat graft
B. absorbable gelatin sponge
C. perilymph fistula
D. middle ear mucosa pushed into the inner ear vestibule
E. unknown
REF. House HP, Farrior JB, Goodhill V, Harrison WH, Shea JJ, Portmann M, Schuknecht HF: Arch Otolaryng, 97:35, Jan '73

64. The incidence of fistulization of the oval window following stapedectomy (characterized by a little unsteadiness with or without fluctuation in hearing) with excellent hearing is around:
   A. 0.0% (Portmann-posterior crus on vein or thick membrane)
   B. 2.0% (Harrison-wire-gelfoam)
   C. 7.0% (Harrison -wire-connective tissue plug)
   D. exact incidence unknown and probably higher than realized
   E. two fistulas in 350 patients with wire-fascia
   REF. House HP, Farrior JB, Goodhill V, Harrison WH, Shea JJ, Portmann M, Schuknecht HF: Arch Otolaryng, 97:35, Jan '73

65. How can an otologist suspect or diagnose fistulization of the oval window following stapes surgery?
   A. mimic hydrops - fullness or pressure
   B. conductive deafness
   C. vertigo
   D. sudden hearing loss primarily sensorineural with fluctuating discrimination
   E. use of pneumatic otoscope with electronystagmograph
   F. no true diagnostic key
   REF. House HP, Farrior JB, Goodhill V, Harrison WH, Shea JJ, Portmann M, Schuknecht HF: Arch Otolaryng, 97:35, Jan '73

66. Fistulization of the oval window following stapedectomy is best treated by:
   A. freshen the edge of fistula usually at the distal part of prosthesis, clip the wire, put new fascia against oval window membrane and insert a new prosthesis
   B. remove entire foot-plate membrane and start over again with a new membrane and prosthesis
   C. remove mucosa lining fistula and closing gap with piece of viable tissue
   D. antibiotic therapy
   E. reduction of cerebrospinal fluid pressure
   REF. House HP, Farrior JB, Goodhill V, Harrison WH, Shea JJ, Portmann M, Schuknecht HF: Arch Otolaryng, 97:35, Jan '73

67. The commonest site of origin of squamous carcinoma of the ear is:
   A. pinna due to keratosis, frostbite, and actinic rays
   B. auditory canal with associated chronic otitis externa and otorrhea
   C. middle ear superimposed on cholesteatoma
   D. mastoid superimposed on cholesteatoma
   E. no specific site of most common origin
   REF. Lewis JS: Arch Otolaryng, 97:41, Jan '73

68. The period of time from the initial symptoms to the diagnosis of squamous carcinoma of the ear is:
   A. 2 weeks
   B. 1 month
   C. 3 months
   D. 6 months
   E. 1 year
   REF. Lewis JS: Arch Otolaryng, 97:41, Jan '73

69. The earliest symptom of squamous carcinoma of the ear is:
   A. bleeding
   B. pain
   C. hearing loss with otorrhea
   D. vertigo
   E. facial parlysis
   REF. Lewis JS: Arch Otolaryng, 97:41, Jan '73

70. Symptoms indicative of advanced squamous carcinoma of the ear are:
   A. bleeding
   B. pain (x-ray evidence of bone erosion)
   C. hearing loss with otorrhea
   D. vertigo
   E. facial paralysis
   REF. Lewis JS: Arch Otolaryng, 97:41, Jan '73

71. Glomus jugulare tumors are considered inoperable by many surgeons and treated by radiation therapy alone when:
A. tumor limited to the middle ear but attached to the adventitia of the dome of the jugular bulb
B. tumor limited to the middle ear and mastoid
C. bone involvement by x-ray
D. paralysis involving ninth, tenth, eleventh, and even the twelfth cranial nerves
E. within the cranial cavity as a cerebellopontine angle tumor or outside the cranial cavity as a nasopharyngeal or upper cervical mass
REF. Silverstone SM: Arch Otolaryng, 97:43, Jan '73

72. Radiation therapy is effective in the control of glomus jugulare tumors with improvement in symptoms (bleeding, otorrhea, tinnitus and vertigo) and even some cranial nerve palsies. Dosage in the range of 5,500 to 7,000 rads is very effective but incurs serious adverse effects such as:
A. brain necrosis
B. death
C. chrondritis of the auricle
D. secondary neoplastic changes
E. bone necrosis
REF. Silverstone SM: Arch Otolaryng, 97:43, Jan '73

73. The optimum dose for treatment of glomus jugulare tumors must be effective but safe. Consensus of many radiotherapists places this dosage in the 4,000 - to 5,000 - rad range over a period of four to six weeks. The source of this radiation should be:
A. 200 to 250 kv radiation
B. 2-mev generator
C. cobalt 60
D. linear accelerator
E. betatron
REF. Silverstone SM: Arch Otolaryng, 97:43, Jan '73

74. The method of choice in the therapy of glomus jugulare tumors is:
A. 5,500 roentgens, 200 kv in a period of 30 days
B. 1,200 to 3,000 rads with the betatron (supervoltage radiation)
C. 5,500 to 7,000 rads with 2-mev generator, cobalt 60 or linear accelerator
D. irradiation (3,000 rads) followed by surgery
E. surgery, when feasible
REF. Rosenwasser H: Arch Otolaryng, 97:49, Jan '73

75. Glomus jugulare tumors are frequently overlooked and must be considered in the differential diagnosis when treating which of the following conditions?
A. unresolved middle ear infections
B. subacute otitis media
C. serous otitis media
D. congenital cholesteatoma
E. aneurysm
F. meningioma
G. idiopathic hemotympanum
H. fibrous dysplasia
REF. Rosenwasser H: Arch Otolaryng, 97:49, Jan '73

76. A reddish, circumscribed lesion visible behind the tympanic membrane with tinnitus and a mild conductive hearing loss may be a glomus jugulare tumor most likely:
A. confined to the tympanic cavity as an isolated growth
B. confined to the middle ear but attached to the jugular bulb
C. involving the middle ear, mastoid and under surface of the temporal bone
D. C with endocranial extension
E. C with nasopharyngeal extension
REF. Rosenwasser H: Arch Otolaryng, 97:49, Jan '73

77. Facial paralysis in glomus jugulare tumors are:
A. common
B. not a significant finding
C. usually due to tumor growth

D. postoperative facial paralysis is not frequent
E. postoperative facial paralysis occurs too frequently
REF. Rosenwasser H: Arch Otolaryng, 97:49, Jan '73

78. Metastasis and multicentricity in glomus jugulare tumors are significant but the basic mechanisms have not been elucidated. The mortality rate in percent is almost:
A. 2.0
B. 5.0
C. 11.0
D. 17.0
E. 28.0
REF. Rosenwasser H: Arch Otolaryng, 97:49, Jan '73

79. Tinnitus is one, if not the major, presenting symptom in glomus jugulare tumors. Following removal of the tumor, if the tinnitus does not disappear (or returns later) indicates:
A. nothing
B. incomplete removal of the tumor
C. development of an adjacent multicentric tumor
D. recurrence of the tumor
E. sudden increase rate of growth of an overlooked tumor focus during the original exploration
REF. Rosenwasser H: Arch Otolaryng, 97:49, Jan '73

80. The mortality and morbidity of glomus jugulare tumors can only be improved by determining the extent of the tumor prior to selection of the most appropriate treatment and this can only be done by which of the following procedures?
A. early diagnosis by being familiar with symptoms and signs
B. polytomography
C. jugularography
D. neurological exam
E. arteriography with special attention to the venous phase
REF. Rosenwasser H: Arch Otolaryng, 97:49, Jan '73

81. Which of the following materials which become extruded have been discarded in tympanoplasty by many otologists?
A. patient's ossicles
B. homograft ossicles
C. cartilage
D. bone chips
E. wire
F. plastic materials which contact the drum
G. autoplastic or homoplastic denatured incus (bone)
REF. Farrior JB, Crabtree JA, Harrison WH, Plester D, Smyth GDL: Arch Otolaryng, 97:55, Jan '73

82. In tympanoplasty to bridge the gap between the head of the stapes and malleus (destroyed or shortened long crus of incus), the procedures of choice appear to be:
A. incus transposition (House, Sheehy, and others)
B. malleus transposition
C. removal long crus incus (or part not destroyed) and position base of long crus in contact with head of stapes
D. small piece bone or cartilage between stapes head and handle malleus (David Austin malleus-stapes assembly)
E. myringostapedioplexy (Arthur Juers)
REF. Farrior JB, Crabtree JA, Harrison WH, Plester D, Smyth GDL: Arch Otolaryng, 97:55, Jan '73

83. In tympanoplasty when the stapes arch is missing but the stapes foot-plate is movable, the procedure of choice appears to be:
   A. no. 40 wire (38-gauge in Europe) inserted into nasal septal cartilage preserved in 70% alcohol, washed in normal saline for one hour before use, and then shaped like a boomerang and placed between foot-plate and undersurface of the grafted drum (Jansen technique)
   B. incus repositioned graft (short or long process in oval window, incus must project above the facial canal)
   C. malleus reposition (handle of)
   D. no effective surgical procedure
   E. fenestration
   REF. Farrior JB, Crabtree JA, Harrison WH, Plester D, Smyth GDL: Arch Otolaryng 97:55, Jan '73

84. In tympanoplasty with stapes fixation, the procedure of choice appears to be:
   A. stapedectomy with removal of tympanosclerosis, vein or fascia over oval window, and then boomerang cartilage strut no. 40 wire inserted into nasal cartilage placed between graft in oval window and drum
   B. tympanoplasty as a primary procedure with removal of most tympanosclerosis as in A. above except stapedectomy with insertion of the strut as a secondary procedure
   C. fenestration as a primary procedure
   D. fenestration as a secondary procedure after a primary double-blue line technique and tympanoplasty
   E. no effective surgical procedure
   REF. Farrior JB, Crabtree JA, Harrison WH, Plester D, Smyth GDL: Arch Otolaryng 97:55, Jan '73

85. In tympanoplasty the repositioned ossicles are best held in position by:
   A. absorable gelatin sponge (Gelfoam)
   B. drilling the ossicles to make impressions to anchor them
   C. glues
   D. silicone rubber (silastic sheeting)
   E. hydrocortisone (Hydrocortone) ointment
   REF. Farrior JB, Crabtree HA, Harrison WH, Plester D, Smyth GDL: Arch Otolaryng 97:55, Jan '73

86. In tympanoplasties hydrocortisone (Hydrocortone) in the middle ear:
   A. discourages adhesions
   B. encourages adhesions
   C. has no effect
   D. prevents healing
   E. creates loculated areas of unabsorbable material which must be removed later
   REF. Farrior JB, Crabtree JA, Harrison WH, Plester D, Smyth GDL: Arch Otolaryng, 97:55, Jan '73

87. In tympanoplasties reaeration of the middle ear is probably helped by:
   A. lining middle ear space, epitympanum and even the mastoid cavity with silicone rubber (silastic) sheeting
   B. filling middle ear with absorbable gelatin sponge (Gelfoam)
   C. instilling hydrocortisone (Hydrocortone) ointment
   D. glues to hold together the repositioned ossicles
   E. interdigitation of the fascial tympanic membrane graft (Fred Guilford Technique) with the handle of the malleus and maintaining the anterior - inferior tympanomeatal angle by placing the fascia underneath the anterior border of the perforation
   REF. Farrior JB, Crabtree JA, Harrison WH, Plester D, Smyth GDL: Arch Otolaryng, 97:55, Jan '73

88. In tympanoplasties the effect of glues (methylmethacrylate and isobutylsan or acrylic) in the middle ears of experimental animals and as it would be used in humans in small and precise amounts seems to result in:
A. excellent fixation between the repositioned ossicles
B. no effect
C. foot-plate fistulas
D. promontory fistulas
E. labyrinthitis
REF. Farrior JB, Crabtree JA, Harrison WH, Plester D, Smyth GDL: Arch Otolaryng, 97:55, Jan '73

89. In tympanoplasties what is the chief contraindication to reconstruction of an ossicular chain?
A. absence of a stapes superstructure
B. chronically infected mucosa throughout the entire middle ear and/or mastoid
C. complete destruction of the tympanic membrane including most, if not all, of the malleus
D. cholesteatoma
E. poor eustachian tube function with probable impaction of the reconstructed tympanoplasty with decreased hearing level
REF. Farrior JB, Crabtree JA, Harrison WH, Plester D, Smyth GDL: Arch Otolaryng, 97:55, Jan '73

90. In tympanoplasties when a perfect incus except for a very small piece of adherent cholesteatoma is removed, which of the following procedures should be considered by the surgeon?
A. autoclave before using
B. use in the next patient after denaturation in a mercury compound like thimerosal (Merthiolate)
C. discard
D. debride the incus and use
REF. Farrior JB, Crabtree JA, Harrison WH, Plester D, Smyth GDL: Arch Otolaryng, 97:55, Jan '73

91. The most critical period in days after a tympanic transplant because perforation (early necrosis) can occur is:
A. 6
B. 14
C. 21
D. 28
E. after 42
REF. Marquet J, Schepens P, Kuijpers W: Arch Otolaryng, 97:58, Jan '73

92. Tympanic transplants may be classified as: (See Fig. 8)
A. partial implants - fibrous layer only, fibrous annulus only, segment fibrous annulus with part fibrous layer
B. total implants - fibrous layer only, fibrous layer with complete annulus, complete fibrous annulus and part of the meatal periosteum
C. tympanomalleus
D. tympanomalleus-incus
E. tympanomalleus-incus-stapes
REF. Marquet J, Schepens P, Kuijpers W: Arch Otolaryng, 97:58, Jan '73

93. What appears to be the best preservative solutions for tympanic transplants?
A. 70% alcohol
B. buffered formaldehyde solution
C. alcoholic preparation 1 to 5000 of an organic mercury compound 2-(ethylmercurithio)-5-benzoxazol-carboxylic (cialit) - very similar to thimerosal (Merthiolate)

D. same as C. except an aqueous solution
E. deep freezing
REF. Derlacki EL, Brandow Jr, EC, Glasscock III ME, Marquet J, Perkins R, Smyth GDL; Arch Otolaryng, 97:67, Jan '73

94. Which of the following solutions destroy the proteins in the nuclear portion of cells and destroy all immunologic qualities in tympanic transplants?
A. 70% alcohol
B. buffered formaldehyde solution
C. aqueous solution of cialit - very similar to thimerosal (Merthiolate)
D. deep freezing
E. alcoholic preparation of merthiolate
REF. Derlacki EL, Brandow Jr. EC, Glasscock III ME, Marquet J, Perkins R, Smyth GDL: Arch Otolaryng, 97:67, Jan '73

95. Why are fresh ear drums usually rejected (about 18 days) when used as tympanic transplants?
A. more supple than preserved grafts, especially formalin - preserved, and therefore do not remain in position
B. usually infected
C. become infected
D. immunological reaction with rejection
E. shrinkage of the graft
REF. Derlacki EL, Brandow Jr. EC, Glasscock III ME, Marquet J, Perkins R, Smyth GDL: Arch Otolaryng, 97:67 Jan '73

96. Which of the following types of patients are selected for homograft transplants?
A. large perforation with missing malleus, or no ossicles
B. in a congenital ear
C. total drum defect (in order to maintain conical shape of the tympanic membrane)
D. blunting of the anterior sulcus
E. small perforations
REF. Derlacki EL, Brandow Jr. EC, Glasscock III ME, Marquet J, Perkins R, Smyth GDL: Arch Otolaryng, 97:67, Jan '73

97. When is a homograft transplant used in an infected ear?
A. never-no type of graft
B. only when necessary when infection does not improve with treatment
C. two stage procedure - first remove the infection and/or cholesteatoma, temporize with fascia graft to protect the middle ear, and in the second stage put in the homograft transplant
D. never-fascia results are superior in rate-take and function
REF. Derlacki EL, Brandow Jr. EC, Glasscock III ME, Marquet J, Perkins R, Smyth GDL: Arch Otolaryng, 97:67 Jan '73

98. What are the problems and complications created by homograft transplants not experienced (usually) with fascia graft and autogenous or transposed ossicular tissue?
A. failure of technique with later removal of thick mass of tissue creating a situation more difficult than the initial problem
B. 10% of the homografts perforate usually during first 10 to 15 days after surgery
C. blunting
D. infection
E. technically difficult
REF. Derlacki EL, Brandow Jr. EC, Glasscock III ME, Marquet J, Perkins R, Smyth GDL: Arch Otolaryng, 97:67, Jan '73

99. When are antibiotics used in homograft transplants?
  A. no prophylactic systemic antibiotics but ears are packed with Gelfoam soaked in Pyocidin-HC Otic solution
  B. no systemic antibiotics but local absorbable gelatin sponge (Gelfoam) soaked in Cortisporin
  C. no systemic antibiotics but artificial plastic sponges on top of the graft soaked with penicillin drops
  D. chloramphenicol (Chloromycetin) solution on Gelfoam
  E. systemic antibiotics (Ampicillin)
  REF. Derlacki EL, Brandow Jr. EC, Glasscock III ME, Marquet J, Perkins R, Smyth GDL: Arch Otolaryng, 96:67, Jan '73

100. There is an increasing interest in allograft tympanic transplantation (en bloc tympanic membrane and malleus with or without incus and stapes). Early non-technical failures suggest immunologic rejection is important. All of the following events occur to notify the host's immunological reacting centers which then mobilize in an attempt to destroy the graft. The first immunological event following vascularization of foreign tissue in a host and usually (experimentally) within ten minutes is:
  A. circulating lymphocytes in the graft pick up antigenic information destined to trigger the rejection reaction (so-called Lymphoid Sensitization)
  B. shedding of antigen by the graft into the invading blood vessels
  C. changes occur in the paracortical area (area situated between the true cortex and medulla of the regional lymph nodes draining the organ graft) Two lymph lines are found in the paracortical area-thymus dependent (T-cells) and gut dependent (bursa equivalent or B-cells). Enlargement of the paracortical area is due to proliferation of the T-cells now called immunoblasts and are also pyroninophilic because of taking special histologic stains
  D. paracortical immunoblasts differentiate into two cell lines-plasma cells producing antibodies and long lived lymphocytes with immunological memory
  E. exact role of the macrophage in lymphoid tissue (although paramount) in allograft rejection has not been entirely defined
  REF. Bergan J: Arch Otolaryng, 97:70, Jan '73

101. While the precise role of the macrophage in lymphoid tissue is paramount but unknown, in allograft rejection it appears to have which of the following functions?
  A. macrophages in lymphoid tissue seem to be needed for lymphoblast transformation
  B. difficult to induce immunity in absence of macrophages
  C. macrophages do not synthesize antibody molecules but facilitate formation of antibody perhaps by adsorbing isoantibody from the circulation and act as sensitized cells which adhere to and destroy allograph cells by close cell contact
  D. all of the above
  E. none of the above
  REF. Bergan J: Arch Otolaryng, 97:70, Jan '73

102. Which of the following mechanisms is important in allograft destruction?
  A. cellular-sensitized lymphoid cells (immunoblasts) destroy target cells (allograft) rapidly with cell to cell contact (release of lysosomal enzymes?)
  B. cellular-actual destruction of the graft is performed by polymorphonuclear leukocytes and macrophages
  C. primitive immunoblasts differentiate into mature plasma cells which produce antibodies and antibodies may sensitize a reaction with graft destruction

D. all of the above
E. none of the above
REF. Bergan J: Arch Otolaryng, 97:70, Jan '73

103. Clinically graft rejection involves which of the following?
A. platelets
B. polymorphonuclear leukocytes
C. lymphocytes
D. histiocytes
E. plasma cells
F. antibody and complement (immunofluorescent studies)
REF. Bergan J: Arch Otolaryng, 97:70, Jan '73

104. Short-term rejected graft has a histologic appearance containing which of the following?
A. perivascular edema
B. disruption of vessel endothelium
C. intravascular thrombosis
D. cellular infiltration - polymorphonuclear leukocytes, lymphocytes, histocytes, plasma cells, platelets
E. antibody and complement
REF. Bergan J: Arch Otolaryng, 97:70, Jan '73

105. Long-term allograft rejection may occur in tympanic membranes due to surface antigenic detection and although nonvascular tissue is damaged, the effects are chiefly in blood vessels and are usually as follows:
A. clumps of polymorphonuclear leukocytes decrease the blood vessel lumen
B. same as A with platelets
C. fibrin deposits occur within the vessels
D. arteriolar endothelial proliferation (response to complement mediated cytolytic damage) with graft ischemia
E. clumps of plasma cells and lymphocytes surround blood vessels with IgG deposition
REF. Bergan J: Arch Otolaryng, 97:70, Jan '73

106. In tissue transplantation in myringoplasty and in reconstruction of postmastoidectomy ears, which of the following must be considered?
A. viable cartilage will undergo far less resorption than dead cartilage
B. cartilage is immunogenic but there is little, if any, rejection due to mucopolysaccharide buffering produced by actively metabolizing chondrocytes
C. dead cartilage will undergo far less resorption than viable cartilage
D. bone allows successful grafting in a viable state
E. bone allows successful grafting in a nonviable state
F. osteocytes in bone die but graft stimulates new bone formation of host origin
REF. Bergan J: Arch Otolaryng, 97:70, Jan '73

107. The objective of the mastoid surgeon is:
A. eradication of all disease
B. eradication of disease but compromising if it interferes with any probable resultant hearing loss
C. eradication of disease with tympanoplasty as a one stage procedure even though minimal disease may remain
D. eradication of all disease regardless of the hearing result
E. always operate on the worse ear first and if it can be converted into the better ear, then operate on the other ear, if needed
REF. Tabb HG, Austin DF, Jansen C, Perkins R, Portmann M, Smith MFW: Arch Otolaryng, 97:74, Jan '73

108. Why should the bony canal wall be reconstructed in a mastoidectized ear?
A. eliminate a large wet cavity full of debris
B. increased periodic deafness elimination

C. increased discharge with odor elimination
D. intermittent vertigo elimination
E. dependence on physician care elimination
REF. Tabb HG, Austin DF, Jansen C, Perkins R, Portmann M, Smith MFW: Arch Otolaryng, 97:74, Jan '73

109. What are the contraindications to reconstruction of the bony canal wall in a mastoidectized ear?
A. carcinoma
B. complete obstruction of the eustachian tube
C. tympanic cavity completely filled with scar tissue
D. chronic infection which does not improve after adequate mastoid surgery
E. older patient with a dry ear and satisfied with the hearing level
REF. Tabb HG, Austin DF, Jansen C, Perkins R, Portmann M, Smith MFW: Arch Otolaryng, 97:74, Jan '73

110. What technique may be used in reconstructing the posterior bony canal wall in a mastoidectized ear assuming the patient has both adequate cochlear and eustachian tube function?
A. remove posterior osseous external canal wall with attached fibrous layer of the tympanic membrane, with attached malleus and incus (if present), remove all active disease as in a radical mastoid cavity, and then replace the tympanic membrane with attached ossicles as an autograft
B. aerated posterior cavity behind repositioned or replaced posterior bony canal wall using cartilage
C. temporalis fascia covered with canal skin
D. planned two-stage procedure with a radical mastoidectomy followed later after all disease has subsided by a second stage with an entire homograft using the external auditory osseous canal with attached fibrous layer and ossicles as needed
E. autogenous and homograft tissues - tympanic homograft and ossicles (adults), dura (infant). Autogenous bone is collected using constant heavy suction irrigation on the bone as it is drilled.
REF. Tabb HG, Austin DF, Jansen C, Perkins R, Portmann M, Smith MFW: Arch Otolaryng, 97:74, Jan '73

111. Is the use of silicone rubber (Silastic) sheeting necessary in the middle ear when performing a tympanoplasty?
A. never
B. always
C. only when there is no mucosa present
REF. Tabb HG, Austin DF, Jansen C, Perkins R, Portmann M, Smith MFW: Arch Otolaryng, 97:74, Jan '73

112. What size (thickness) silicone rubber (Silastic) sheeting should be used on the medial tympanic wall of the middle ear when performing a tympanoplasty?
A. 0.001
B. 0.003
C. 0.005
D. 0.007
E. 0.01
REF. Tabb HG, Austin DF, Jansen C, Perkins R, Portmann M, Smith MFW: Arch Otolaryng, 97:74, Jan '73

113. What size (thickness) silicone rubber (Silastic) sheeting should be used in a dumbbell shape from the epitympanic area through the aditus ad antrum to the mastoid antrum when performing a tympanoplasty?
A. 0.001
B. 0.005
C. 0.01
D. 0.04
E. 0.10
REF. Tabb HG, Austin DF, Jansen C, Perkins R, Portmann M, Smith MFW: Arch Otolaryng, 97:74, Jan '73

114. What hearing improvement in percent results in reconstruction of the mastoidectized ear?
A. 50-55
B. 60-65
C. 70-75
D. 80-85
E. 90-95
REF. Tabb HG, Austin DF, Jansen C, Perkins R, Portmann M, Smith MFW: Arch Otolaryng, 97:74, Jan '73

115. How should the surgeon handle the chorda tympani nerve covered with squamous epithelium (possible recurrence of cholesteatoma) when operating on a chronically infected ear?
A. resect the nerve
B. do nothing in the hope that the squamous epithelium will change in character
C. strip off the squamous epithelium and leave the nerve
REF. Tabb HG, Austin DF, Jansen C, Perkins R, Portmann M, Smith MFW: Arch Otolaryng, 97:74, Jan '73

116. What affect on the patient does resection of the chorda tympani nerve have when operating upon a chronically infected ear?
A. none
B. dry mouth (temporary)
C. taste disturbance (temporary)
D. dry mouth (permanent)
E. taste disturbance (permanent)
REF. Tabb HG, Austin DF, Jansen C, Perkins R, Portmann M, Smith MFW: Arch Otolaryng, 97:74, Jan '73

117. Which of the following types of spontaneous nystagmus is provoked by disease of the peripheral labyrinth or eighth nerve?
A. vertical
B. diagonal
C. rotatory
D. purely horizontal
E. combined horizontal-rotatory (horizontal-frontal)
REF. Jongkees LBW: Arch Otolaryng, 97:77, Jan '73

118. Which of the following types of spontaneous nystagmus is provoked by disease of the central nervous system (CNS)?
A. vertical
B. diagonal
C. rotatory
D. purely horizontal
E. combined horizontal-rotatory (horizontal-frontal)
REF. Jongkees LBW: Arch Otolaryng, 97:77, Jan '73

119. Which of the following are not indicative of peripheral disease of the vestibular system?
A. strong spontaneous nystagmus in a patient without vertigo
B. positional nystagmus showing a change in direction in different positions
C. disharmony between direction of the vestibulospinal reflexes and slow phases of a spontaneous nystagmus
D. vestibular tests provoke perverse reactions
E. spontaneous searching nystagmus without a quick or slow component (ocular)
REF. Jongkees LBW: Arch Otolaryng, 97:77, Jan '73

120. Electronystagmography is indispensable in:
A. recording of a cursory phenomenon which may not be observed visually - positional nystagmus
B. nystagmus at a certain time (not under treatment) with that at a later date (under treatment)
C. permanent record of patient which can be used on a scientific basis for later study

D. study of exact form of nystagmus beat
E. study, and perhaps significance, of nonnystagmic movements of the eyes
REF. Jongkees LBW: Arch Otolaryng, 97:77, Jan '73

121. In electronystagmography for many years authors have described nystagmus patterns called dysrhythmia, which were stated to be due to central lesions. It is now known that many of these various nystagmic variations are present without proving any disease. Which of the following patterns are now considered not significant?
A. arrhythmia
B. intermittent fast phase
C. dysmetria
D. petite écriture (small script)
E. salvos
F. different types group formation
G. secondary - phase nystagmus
H. square waves
I. jerks
J. sinusoidal movements
REF. Jongkees LBW: Arch Otolaryng, 97:77, Jan '73 (See Fig. 9)

122. In patients suffering from peripheral vestibular disease, nystagmus can be provoked, or changed, in a certain number of these patients by hyperventilation, valsalva maneuver or neck torsion. Which of the following statements are considered accurate?
A. hyperventilation should be performed for about 1 1/2 minutes
B. with A nystagmus change is greatest in patients with herpes zoster and acoustic neurinomas
C. valsalva maneuver is performed by forced expiration on the closed glottis for 15 seconds
D. with C nystagmus change is greatest in patients with tympanic or middle ear operations and greatest with fistula in the labyrinth
E. with either the hyperventilation of valsalva techniques, the nystagmus may be provoked, suppressed, or changed in direction
REF. Jongkees LBW: Arch Otolaryng, 97:77, Jan '73 (See Fig. 10)

123. It is important to stop all but life-support drugs for 48 hours to one week before electronystagmography. Which of the following can cause positional nystagmus of direction-changing type and gaze nystagmus?
A. phenobarbital
B. diphenylhydantoin sodium
C. diazepam
D. brain stem injury
REF. Pearson BW, Barber HO: Arch Otolaryng, 97:81, Jan '73

124. As an expert witness in whiplash injuries, the otologist should be cognizant of which of the following?
A. otovestibular damage or sequelae do occur as a result of whiplash: pure-tone, air and bone conduction hearing tests, speech discrimination tests and complete electronystagmograms (ENG) indicated
B. report only objective, positive findings and have at least two complete ENG recordings (and audiograms)
C. physician must be able to state that ENG and audio findings are consistent with head injury and whiplash
D. physician must be cognizant of impairment - or extent of patient's injury as it affects his personal activities of daily living
E. the legal profession must evaluate the social and economic effects of impairment
REF. Rubin W: Arch Otolaryng, 97:85, Jan '73

125. In head injuries the otoneurologist should be cautious in prognosis since the central nervous system (CNS) component of the injury may be more serious (prolonged or delayed) than a specific auditory or vestibular lesion. Which of the following disorders of higher nervous system function are common?
A. impairment of recent memory (amnesia)
B. loss of emotional control and insomnia
C. poor performance of psychometric tests

D. decreased ability to perform intellectual tests (subtracting from 100 by 7's)
E. overt psychiatric syndromes - depression and hysteria
REF. Pearson BW, Barber HO: Arch Otolaryng, 97:81, Jan '73

126. Otoneurologic sequelae of head injuries after a lateral blow are usually:
A. homolateral or bilateral cochlear loss at 4,000 and 8,000 Hz (8,000 Hz most frequent)
B. same as A but with cochlear loss in all frequencies
C. vestibular lesions that can be bilateral, homolateral, or contralateral
D. tinnitus is usually homolateral
E. tinnitus is usually bilateral
REF. Pearson BW, Barber HO: Arch Otolaryng, 97:81, Jan '73

127. Otoneurologic sequelae of head injuries after a lateral-oblique head blow are usually:
A. bilateral cochlear loss at 4,000 and 8,000 Hz (8,000 Hz most frequent) with contralateral loss greater than homolateral
B. same as A but in all frequencies
C. significant cochlear and vestibular losses occur regardless of severity of head injury
D. findings not related to presbycusis
E. normal hearing at 4,000 Hz may be present after severe head injury
REF. Pearson BW, Barber HO: Arch Otolaryng, 97:81, Jan '73

128. Otoneurologic sequelae of even minor head injuries may include traumatic perilymph fistula at the oval window requiring tympanotomy. Symptoms include:
A. episodic vertigo
B. postural spinning vertigo
C. conductive hearing loss
D. otalgia
E. fluctuating but progressive sensorineural hearing impairment
REF. Pearson BW, Barber HO: Arch Otolaryng, 97:81, Jan '73

129. In medicolegal consultation as an expert witness the otoneurologist must be cognizant of:
A. description of present hearing loss (at least two similar audiograms)
B. presentation of electronystagmograms (ENG)
C. in absence of hearing loss with a longitudinal fracture of the temporal bone, postural vertigo with positional nystagmus of benign paroxysmal type syndrome may occur
D. in C in absence of both hearing loss and vertigo, there may be severe or total destruction of vestibular function (ENG)
E. future risks - in longitudinal fracture of the temporal bone without any hearing loss or vestibular disturbance, there may develop meningitis or brain abscess years later or symptomatic presbycusis at a much earlier age
REF. Pearson BW, Barber HO: Arch Otolaryng, 97:81, Jan '73

130. In whiplash injuries with vestibular involvement which of the following facts are accurate?
A. vestibular suppressant drugs are of questionable value
B. patients with bilateral transverse petrous fractures will be permanently ataxic and disabled in the dark
C. dizziness caused by head injury gradually improves with time and improves especially with graduated physical activity

D. severely psychoneurotic patients may be permanently disabled
E. onset of vertigo is usually seven to ten days following the accident, occurs during head movement especially toward side of neck injured during the whiplash, seconds to minutes in duration without nausea or vomiting but may persist for months or years and spontaneous nystagmus beats in a direction opposite to the injured side

REF. Rubin W: Arch Otolaryng, 97:85, Jan '73

131. Ten aspects of auditory performance may be tested for diagnostic purposes. For this question, match each numbered item (typical test) with one lettered item (aspect of performance). Each choice may be used only once:

A. perception of loudness
B. recovery from excess adaptation
C. perception of pitch
D. adaptation to sustained tones
E. location of sound image
F. sensitivity for short tones
G. awareness of frequency change
H. binaural release from masking
I. distortion of tonal signals
J. Awareness of intensity change

1. critical off time
2. SISI
3. masking level difference
4. recruitment
5. directional audiometry
6. Békésy, tone decay
7. frequency DL
8. aural overload
9. brief tone audiometry
10. pitch matching

REF. Carhart R: Arch Otolaryng, 97:88, Jan '73

132. Which of the following auditory tests are now being generally used (though not perfect) and have demonstrated usefulness in the diagnosis of eighth cranial nerve and cerebellopontine angle tumors?

A. pure tone and speech
B. recruitment
C. Békésy audiometry
D. tone decay
E. SISI

REF. Carhart R: Arch Otolaryng, 97:88, Jan '73

133. Although there are no startling developments in special hearing tests for the diagnosis of acoustic neuromas or cerebellopontine angle tumors, which of the following tests are gaining increasing importance?

A. Békésy audiometry
B. impedance audiometry and tympanometry
C. tone decay
D. sensitized speech tests
E. measurement of cortical evoked response (electroencephalography)

REF. Carhart R: Arch Otolaryng, 97:88, Jan '73

134. Special hearing tests are concerned primarily with the differential diagnosis of cochlear or retrocochlear lesions. Which of the following would be considered such tests?

A. pure tone and speech audiometry
B. speech discrimination
C. loudness function
D. tone decay
E. impedance audiometry

REF. Johnson EW: Arch Otolaryng, 97:92, Jan '73

135. Hearing tests in Ménière's disease indicate:

A. poor discrimination (0 to 30%)
B. good discrimination (82% to 100%)
C. Békésy type I or type II
D. Békésy type III or type IV (excessive tone decay)
E. high SISI scores (75% to 100%)

REF. Johnson EW: Arch Otoloaryng, 97:92, Jan '73

136. Auditory test results in acoustic tumors indicate:
  A. high frequency loss
  B. low frequency loss
  C. poor or intermediate speech discrimination
  D. excellent speech discrimination
  E. Békésy III and IV patterns with poor SISI scores
  REF. Johnson EW: Arch Otolaryng, 97:92, Jan '73

137. Impedance audiometry was first reported by Metz 25 years ago and has been widely used in Europe. The value of impedance audiometry is of special importance in its clinical application to:
  A. confirms the presence of conductive impairment (especially in a child) when it is not possible to establish bone conduction thresholds
  B. acoustic reflex decay may occur when the hearing loss is relatively mild in the impaired ear in acoustic neuromas
  C. a higher than normal impedance is anticipated in otosclerosis with an absence of acoustic reflex (type A impedance curve)
  D. tympanometry curve type B in bilateral serous otitis media
  E. tympanometry type A curves in normal ears and in patients with cochlear involvement
  REF. Johnson EW: Arch Otolaryng, 97:92, Jan '73

138. Electric response audiometry (ERA) - also known as cortical evoked responses or averaged vertex response - has definite but limited diagnostic uses in clinical otology. The vertex response or ERA can be used with reasonable degree of accuracy to:
  A. determine objectively the thresholds of hearing in subjects who cannot be tested satisfactorily by conventional audiometric methods - infants, young children, mentally retarded individuals, patients with lesions of central nervous system
  B. differentiate conductive from sensorineural hearing loss - air and bone thresholds can be determined equally well and is therefore an objective test
  C. differentiate organic from functional hearing impairment
  D. distinguish between auditory and pseudoauditory air-bone gap in patients with severe hearing impairment since birth or early childhood - thus severely deaf children can be selected early who will benefit from amplification
  E. not been found to be of significant value in differentiating cochlear and retrocochlear lesions
  REF. Cody DTR: Arch Otolaryng, 97:96, Jan '73

139. In electronystagmography (ENG) - also known as electro-oculography and photoelectronystagmography - which of the following facts appear to be established that ENG has an advantage over visual observation of nystagmus?
  A. nystagmus is more prominent with the eyes closed (or dark room)
  B. permanent record for medical use - before and after treatment
  C. provides a record for legal use
  D. spontaneous nystagmus which cannot be detected even by microscopic lenses
  E. proves a patient really has vertigo
  F. calorically induced nystagmus results are useless unless the presence of a preexisting spontaneous nystagmus is known and taken in consideration in the calculations
  G. predominance of nystagmus in one direction or not can be determined in half a minute with the eyes closed in a rotatory chair
  H. tests for function of the otolith on the parallel swing
  REF. Barber HO, Jongkees LBW, Rubin W, MacMillan BB, Tonkin J: Arch Otolaryng, 97:104, Jan '73

140. What are the disadvantages of electronystagmography (ENG)?
A. electrical equipment stops working or does not perform properly
B. not available, or at least quick service from knowledgeable, electrical engineer
C. trained girls go elsewhere
D. single-channel apparatus suffices for office practice but many physicians tend to go over-board at first - and for protection against break-downs in apparatus in a remote area, exact ENG machine may be advisable
E. water-baths (warm and cool water) are advised and add to the expense
REF. Barber HO, Jongkees LBW, Rubin W, MacMillan BB, Tonkin J: Arch Otolaryng, 97:104, Jan '73

141. An electronystagmogram (ENG) tracing by itself gives the following:
A. specific diagnosis
B. pathological diagnosis
C. central or peripheral localization diagnosis
D. all of the above
E. none of the above
REF. Barber HO, Jongkees LBW, Rubin W, MacMillan BB, Tonkin J: Arch Otolaryng, 97:104 Jan '73

142. Which of the following drugs will increase the intensity of an ENG spontaneous nystagmus (which is difficult to demonstrate clinically)?
A. barbiturates
B. tranquilizers
C. alcohol
D. antivestibular drugs
E. amphetamines
REF. Barber HO, Jongkees LBW, Rubin W, MacMillan BB, Tonkin J: Arch Otolaryng, 97:104, Jan '73

143. Which of the following drugs may increase the intensity of a spontaneous nystagmus on an electronystagmogram (ENG)?
A. barbiturates
B. tranquilizers
C. alcohol
D. antivestibular drugs
E. amphetamines
REF. Barber HO, Jongkees LBW, Rubin W, MacMillan BB, Tonkin J: Arch Otolaryng, 97:104, Jan '73

144. Which of the following drugs may suppress the intensity of a spontaneous nystagmus on an electronystagmogram (ENG)?
A. barbiturates
B. tranquilizers
C. alcohol
D. antivestibular drugs
E. amphetamines
REF. Barber HO, Jongkees LBW, Rubin W, MacMillan BB, Tonkin J: Arch Otolaryng, 97:104, Jan '73

145. Which of the following drugs even when taken in a small amount can either suppress or increase the intensity of a spontaneous nystagmus on an electronystagmogram (ENG)?
A. barbiturates
B. tranquilizers
C. alcohol
D. antivestibular drugs
E. amphetamines
REF. Barber HO, Jongkees LBW, Rubin W, MacMillan BB, Tonkin J: Arch Otolaryng, 97:104, Jan '73

146. Prior to performing an electronystagmogram (ENG) the patient should be warned to stop all drugs, except life-saving, for at least two weeks and especially the following:
A. barbiturates
B. tranquilizers
C. antivestibular drugs
D. amphetamines
E. alcohol
F. narcotics (codeine in cough medicine, etc.)
G. marihuana
H. LSD
REF. Barber HO, Jongkees LBW, Rubin W, MacMillan BB, Tonkin J: Arch Otolaryng, 97:104, Jan '73

147. The Tack operation, modification of the Fick sacculotomy operation, is an endeavor used in endolymphatic hydrops for:
A. relief of fullness or pressure sensation in the ear
B. control of vertigo
C. disappearance of tinnitus
D. improvement in pure-tone and speech-reception thresholds
E. improvement in speech-discrimination scores
REF. Cody DTR: Arch Otolaryng, 97:109, Feb '73

148. Complications of the Tack operation appear to be:
A. further loss of hearing (also characteristic of endolymphatic hydrops)
B. perilymph fistula
C. worsening of the tinnitus
D. tympanomeatal flap cholesteatoma
E. further loss of speech discrimination
REF. Cody DTR: Arch Otolaryng, 97:109, Feb '73

149. Perilymph fistula is a definite complication in the Tack operation when the head of the tack is thicker in mm than:
A. 0.1
B. 0.2
C. 0.3
D. 0.4
E. 0.5
REF. Cody DTR: Arch Otolaryng, 97:109, Feb '73 (See Fig. 11)

150. Patients complaining of spatial disorientation (vertigo) of undetermined etiology before having a vestibular nerve section (translabyrinthine, middle fossa approach, suboccipital craniotomy approach) should have in addition to a thorough general medical examination:
A. neurological evaluation
B. complete audiological studies
C. vestibular function tests (electronystagmogram)
D. x-rays of skull and temporal bone including polytomes of internal auditory canals
E. posterior fossa myelogram (when in doubt to rule out an acoustic tumor or other life-endangering lesion)
REF. Glasscock III ME: Arch Otolaryng, 97:112, Feb '73

151. Which of the following are indications for vestibular nerve section by the middle fossa approach?
A. early cases of Ménière's disease
B. late cases of Ménière's disease with severe hearing loss
C. persistent vertigo after stapes or fenestration surgery after eliminating a perilymph fistula
D. head injury with fracture through a semicircular canal with vertigo but with normal hearing, or vertigo following a modified or radical mastoidectomy with a non-healing fistula of semicircular canal
E. postural vertigo with normal hearing (but be certain of involved ear-electronystagmogram)
F. sudden hearing loss syndrome with persistent vertigo
REF. Glasscock III ME: Arch Otolaryng, 97:112, Feb '73

152. Which of the following are indications for translabyrinthine vestibular nerve section?
A. late cases of Ménière's disease with severe hearing loss and vertigo
B. sudden hearing loss syndrome with permanent deafness and persistent vertigo
C. traumatic labyrinthitis due to head injury with deafness with fracture semicircular canal with incapacitating vertigo
D. early Ménière's disease
E. uncontrolled vertigo, no residual hearing, and in whom an acoustic tumor cannot be ruled out by other means
REF. Glasscock III ME: Arch Otolaryng, 97:112, Feb '73

153. In middle fossa vestibular nerve section, the postoperative morbidity and mortality consist of:
A. headache, usually mild
B. edema of scalp extending to the eye on the operated side
C. meningitis (responds to antibiotic therapy)
D. persistent cerebrospinal leaks
E. operative and postoperative hemorrhage with death
REF. Glasscock III ME: Arch Otolaryng, 97:112, Feb '73

154. In patients with late Ménière's disease with deafness and incapacitating vertigo, the operation of choice appears to be:
A. simple labyrinthectomy through the external auditory canal (transcanal labyrinthectomy such as the Cawthorne procedure)
B. transmastoid labyrinthectomy in which all three semicircular canals are removed
C. translabyrinthine vestibular nerve section
D. middle fossa vestibular nerve section
E. vestibular nerve section after suboccipital craniotomy
REF. Glasscock III ME: Arch Otolaryng, 97:112, Feb '73

155. In non-Ménière's patients with deafness and persistent vertigo, the operation of choice is:
A. transcanal labyrinthectomy
B. transmastoid labyrinthectomy
C. translabyrinthine vestibular nerve section
D. middle fossa vestibular nerve section
E. vestibular nerve section after suboccipital craniotomy
REF. Glasscock III ME: Arch Otolaryng, 97:112, Feb '73

156. In non-Ménière's patients without deafness but with vertigo, the operation of choice is:
A. transcanal labyrinthectomy
B. transmastoid labyrinthectomy
C. translabyrinthine vestibular nerve section
D. middle fossa vestibular nerve section
E. vestibular nerve section after suboccipital craniotomy
REF. Glasscock III ME: Arch Otolaryng, 97:112, Feb'73

157. Which of the following anatomical structures must be destroyed in order to assure that patients with non-Ménière's problems will not have some residual labyrinthine function (vertigo)?
A. superior vestibular nerve
B. inferior vestibular nerve (supplies saccule and posterior ampulla)
C. Scarpa's ganglion (nerves degenerate to the brain stem nuclei)
D. three semicircular canals
E. the saccule and utricle
REF. Glasscock III ME: Arch Otolaryng, 97:112, Feb '73

158. Medical treatment of Ménière's disease is effective in the following percent of patients and surgery does not have to be considered:
A. 15 - 18
B. 21 - 32
C. 47 - 54
D. 66 - 85
E. 91 - 97
REF. Bryan V, Bucy PC: Arch Otolaryng, 97:115, Feb '73

159. Objections to selective vestibular nerve section by the middle cranial fossa approach appear to be:
A. prolonged morbidity period
B. permanent hemiparesis
C. facial palsy, transient
D. limited to only a few trained otolaryngologists in comparison to neurosurgeons who are more experienced in brain surgery
E. not as reliable as the suboccipital craniotomy method in the relief of vertigo
REF. Bryan V, Bucy PC: Arch Otolaryng, 97:115, Feb '73

160. Fluctuant hearing loss disorder (Ménière's disease) has all of the following symptoms. Which one is usually the earliest and most constant complaint?
A. vertigo
B. fluctuation in hearing
C. tinnitus
D. fullness
REF. Shea JJ, Kitabchi AE: Arch Otolaryng, 97:118, Feb '73

161. Ménière's disease has all of the following symptoms. The last symptom to appear is usually:
A. vertigo
B. fluctuation in hearing
C. tinnitus
D. fullness
REF. Shea JJ, Kitabchi AE: Arch Otolaryng, 97:118, Feb '73

162. Tinnitus in Ménière's disease is usually:
A. roar
B. whistle, intermittent
C. ring
D. banging noise, intermittent
E. pulse
REF. Shea JJ, Kitabchi AE: Arch Otolaryng, 97:118, Feb '73

163. Electronystagmographic measurements in most patients with Ménière's disease show:
A. normal ENG
B. abnormal ENG
C. spontaneous nystagmus
D. postural nystagmus
E. abnormal caloric measurements
REF. Shea JJ, Kitabchi AE: Arch Otolaryng, 97:118, Feb '73

164. Excessive smoking has a suppressing effect on cochlear function by:
A. hypoglycemia
B. interference with oxidative enzymes
C. 20% of hemoglobin bound as inactive carboxyhemoglobin
D. breakdown of cyclic 3'- and 5'-adenosine monophosphate
E. fluid retention
REF. Shea JJ, Kitabchi AE: Arch Otolaryng, 97:118, Feb '73 (See Fig. 12)

165. Diagnosis of etiology of fluctuant hearing loss must consist of which of the following tests?
A. no drugs with high (3,000) caloric diet with at least 300 gm carbohydrates three days prior to glucose tolerance test
B. one hundred grams glucose given by mouth, and blood and urine samples collected every 30 minutes for four hours
C. thyroid function

D. liver function
E. kidney function
REF. Shea JJ, Kitabchi AE: Arch Otolaryng, 97:118, Feb '73

166. Which of the following oto-audiological tests should be performed on patients with fluctuating hearing loss ?
A. air and bone audiograms
B. positional and caloric electronystagmography
C. Békésy audiometry
D. short increment sensitivity index (SISI) and alternate binaural loudness balance
E. x-rays including polytomes of petrous pyramids to show internal auditory canals and cochlear aqueducts
REF. Shea JJ, Kitabchi AE: Arch Otolaryng, 97:118, Feb '73

167. Which of the following are features of fluctuant hearing loss (Ménière's disease)?
A. hearing loss usually one ear first and second ear much later
B. cochlear-type loss, ascending at first, flattens out later and eventually descending
C. discrimination usually good at first (unless sudden hearing loss and then there is a concomitant loss of discrimination)
D. usually Békésy type I (no discrimination loss) or type II (with some discrimination loss) but with sudden severe hearing loss (Békésy type IV). With successful treatment Békésy usually reverts back to type I.
E. high SISI scores (for the affected frequencies) and definite recruitment with great distortions in the quality of the sound heard in the affected ear with unusual sensitivity to sound
REF. Shea JJ, Kitabchi AE: Arch Otolaryng, 97:118, Feb '73

168. Specific hospital treatment for fluctuant hearing loss (Ménière's disease) should consist of?
A. complete bed rest, heavy sedation with a strong tranquilizer (diazepam) (Valium), 5 to 10 mg four times a day and glucose tolerance, thyroid, liver and kidney function tests
B. no smoking or tobacco in any form
C. low-salt, low-caloric, low-carbohydrate, and low-fat diet and one potassium-sparing diuretic (Dyazide) each morning and weigh patients daily
D. stop all drugs, especially birth-control and diet pills, both of these pills are suspected of causing fluctuant hearing loss (life-saving drugs-cardiac-may be necessary)
E. intravenous infusions of 250 ml of lactated Ringer's solution with 2.75 mg. histamine phosphate given slowly but to create a flush twice daily simultaneously with inhalations of a mixture 5% CO_2 and 95% O_2 for 30 minutes four times daily to increase the blood supply to the inner ear and dura surrounding the endolymphatic sac
REF. Shea JJ, Kitabchi AE: Arch Otolaryng, 97:118, Feb '73

169. Specific office treatment for fluctuant hearing loss (Ménière's) while patient is being hospitalized should consist of?
A. daily audiometric tests including discrimination scores
B. daily positional electronystagmography
C. complete allergy investigation including skin tests, nasal smears (Hansel), complete blood counts with differential for eosinophiles, provocative tests and leukocyte cytotoxic reaction test (Bryan and Bryan)
D. removal of all known allergens
E. cyproheptadine (Periactin) hydrochloride 4 mg two to three times a day to control the allergic component
REF. Shea JJ, Kitabchi AE: Arch Otolaryng, 97:118, Feb '73

170. In the etiology of fluctuant hearing loss (Ménière's disease) which of the following should be considered?
   A. obstruction endolymphatic duct and sac (polytome x-rays of cochlear aqueducts)
   B. abnormal glucose tolerance (high insulin and abnormally high (inactive) proinsulin levels - active, even hyperactive, insulin response from the pancreas but an inability of the inner ear to recognize and utilize this insulin)
   C. hyperlipemia
   D. excessive smoking
   E. fluid retention
   F. allergy
   G. anxiety
   REF. Shea JJ, Kitabchi AE: Arch Otolaryng, 97:118, Feb '73

171. Final results of either medical or surgical treatment of Ménière's disease is usually:
   A. good for control of vertigo
   B. less good for restoration of hearing
   C. good for fullness or pressure-sensation in the ear
   D. improvement in tinnitus
   E. cure of all symptoms if treatment is started early in the disease
   REF. Shea JJ, Kitabchi AE: Arch Otolaryng, 97:118, Feb '73

172. The operation of decompression and drainage of the endolymphatic sac is based on the longitudinal theory of endolymph flow (operative procedure of Georges Portmann, modified by House, modified by Yamacava and Naito). Longitudinal theory supposes the secretion of endolymphatic fluid by the stria vascularis of the anterior part of the labyrinth and reabsorption by the endolymphatic sac beyond the posterior part of the labyrinth. Which of the following facts confirm this theory?
   A. in 1926 Georges Portmann obliterated the sacs of certain fish by microcoagulation and produced endolymphatic hydrops
   B. in 1927 Guild, using injected India ink, proved the existence of longitudinal circulation
   C. Ormerod (1960), using radioactive methods, confirmed this theory
   D. Lindquist et al (1963) injected colloidal silver into scala media of guinea pigs and 24 hours later found all the particles within the endolymphatic sacs
   E. from standpoint of histology (electron microscope) stria vascularis contains structures suitable for secretion while endolymphatic sac has structures more consistent with the function of absorption
   REF. Portmann M: Arch Otolaryng, 97:125, Feb '73

173. Despite evidence in favor of the longitudinal theory of endolymphatic flow, several other investigations do not support this belief including:
   A. Lindsay et al blocked off the endolymphatic sac which did not result in histologic evidence of dilatation of the labyrinth
   B. Watzke and Bast in an anatomical study demonstrated in some specimens complete absence of the endolymphatic duct
   C. Schuknecht and Seiti showed that rupture of the cochlea at a certain point did not alter the electrophysiological properties of other areas of the cochlea
   D. Naftalin and Harrison formulated a radial theory of secretion and absorption which takes place on the spot at each segment of the cochlear duct or of the posterior part of the labyrinth
   E. Lawrence agrees with D.
   REF. Portmann M: Arch Otolaryng, 97:125, Feb '73

174. Difficulties in diagnosing Ménière's disease exist because the same symptoms appear in which of these various conditions?
A. primary Ménière's disease (or pure Ménière's disease)
B. retrolabyrinthine lesion - acoustic neuroma
C. retrolabyrinthine lesion - other cerebellopontine angle tumors
D. retrolabyrinthine lesion - neuronitis of the eighth nerve
E. retrolabyrinthine lesion - abnormal vascular lesions
REF. Portmann M: Arch Otolaryng, 97:125, Feb '73

175. For this question, match each lettered item with one numbered item. Each choice may be used more than once.
Operation:
A. decompression and drainage endolymphatic sac
B. neurectomy (scarpectomy) of vestibular division eighth nerve (sparing cochlear division) through middle cranial fossa route
C. destruction of labyrinth (transmeatal or transcochlear route)

Condition:
1. peripheral vertigo of uncertain origin (normal audiometry with atypical electronystagmography)
2. classical Ménière's disease with total deafness with demonstration of no endolymphatic duct (Valvassori)
3. typical primary Ménière's disease with not over 40 to 50 db hearing loss with demonstration of endolymphatic duct by Valvassori polytomography
4. same as 3 except with severe hearing loss over 50 to 70 db
REF. Portmann M: Arch Otolaryng, 97:125, Feb '73

176. A simple consistently effective method relieving vertigo while preserving hearing has not been achieved in Ménière's disease. Which of the following procedures appear to be somewhat effective?
A. selective ablation of the vestibular sense organ by ultrasound and cyro-surgery
B. section vestibular nerve by middle and posterior fossa approaches
C. prevention overaccumulation of endolymph by endolymphatic sac operation and tack operation
D. control vascular system inner ear and alter fluid physiology by ablation of the sympathetic nerve supply
E. labyrinthectomy with complete destruction of the labyrinth
REF. Schuknecht HF, Bucy PC, Fisch U, House WF, Portmann M: Arch Otolaryng, 97:129, Feb '73

177. Which one of the following is an unusual condition causing typical Ménière's-type symptoms?
A. acoustic neuroma
B. angioma between the facial and vestibular nerves
C. neuronitis of the eighth nerve
D. cerebellopontine angle tumors other than acoustic neuromas
E. endolymphatic hydrops
REF. Schuknecht HF, Bucy PC, Fisch U, House WF, Portmann M: Arch Otolaryng, 97:129, Feb '73

178. There are three categories of patients with Ménière's disease: (1) typical Ménière's disease, (2) those with sudden symptoms and (3) those with progressive hearing loss. In all cases of Ménière's disease when the internal meatus is filled with iophendylate (Valvassori), what percent of patients have a space-occupying lesion confined to one-half of the internal auditory meatus due to swelling of Scarpa's ganglion?
A. 0
B. 7
C. 11
D. 38
E. 53
REF. Schuknecht HF, Bucy PC, Fisch U, House WF, Portmann M: Arch Otolaryng, 97:129, Feb '73

179. Macroscopic and histologic examination by electron microscopy of Scarpa's ganglia or of vestibular ganglia resected for Ménière's disease disclose:
A. swelling (by the surgeon)
B. degeneration of nerve fibers
C. increase in vacuolization of cytoplasm in the ganglion cells
D. all of the above
E. none of the above
REF. Schuknecht HF, Bucy PC, Fisch U, House WF, Portmann M: Arch Otolaryng, 97:129, Feb '73

180. Acoustic neurinoma is a misnomer and better terminology is:
A. vestibular schwannoma
B. meningioma
C. glomus jugulare tumor
D. epidermal glioma
E. arachnoid cyst
REF. Schuknecht HF, Bucy PC, Fisch U, House WF, Portmann M: Arch Otolaryng, 97:129, Feb '73

181. Filling of the internal auditory meatus with iophendylate (Valvassori) is an accepted procedure in the diagnosis of acoustic neurinoma (vestibular schwannoma). Probability of this tumor can be indicated by fluid study obtained by a vestibular tap procedure which can be performed on patients (Schuknecht) with:
A. peripheral vertigo of uncertain origin with normal audiogram with an atypical electronystagmogram
B. peripheral vertigo of uncertain origin with hearing level around 30 decibels with an atypical electronystagmogram
C. peripheral vertigo with severe deafness with an atypical electronystagmogram
D. all of the above
E. none of the above
REF. Schuknecht HF, Bucy PC, Fisch U, House WF, Portmann M: Arch Otolaryng, 97:129, Feb '73

182. When performing a translabyrinthine neurectomy, why should Scarpa's ganglion be excised?
A. regeneration of nerve fibers cut distal to the ganglion
B. during revision surgery nerve fibers filling the posterior canal can be traced back to the singular nerve in the internal auditory canal
C. in experimental animal surgery the vestibular nerve does not regenerate
D. all of the above appears correct
E. none of the above is correct
REF. Schuknecht HF, Bucy PC, Fisch U, House WF, Portmann M: Arch Otolaryng, 97:129 Feb '73

183. Tinnitus can more often be relieved by:
A. vestibular neurectomy
B. labyrinthectomy
C. vestibular - cochlear neurectomy
D. no operative procedure can with certainty relieve tinnitus
E. section of the cochlear nerve
REF. Schuknecht HF, Bucy PC, Fisch U, House WF, Portmann M: Arch Otolaryng, 97:129 Feb '73

184. The cerebrospinal fluid pressure compared with the endolymphatic fluid pressure is:
A. higher
B. essentially the same
C. less
D. varies
E. debatable
REF. Schuknecht HF, Bucy PC, Fisch U, House WF, Portmann M: Arch Otolaryng, 97:129, Feb '73

185. The fluid pressures of the endolymphatic and perilymphatic systems are:
    A. higher perilymphatic
    B. lower perilymphatic
    C. higher endolymphatic
    D. lower endolymphatic
    E. equal pressures in the endolymphatic and perilymphatic systems in order for the basilar membrane to vibrate (Von Békésy)

    REF. Schuknecht HF, Bucy PC, Fisch U, House WF, Portmann M: Arch Otolaryng, 97:129, Feb '73

186. Decompression and drainage of the endolymphatic sac in the Portmann operation for Ménière's disease six months after the operation indicate relief from vertigo in the following percent of patients:
    A. 50
    B. 65
    C. 70
    D. 85
    E. 90

    REF. Schuknecht HF, Bucy PC, Fisch U, House WF, Portmann M: Arch Otolaryng, 97:129, Feb '73

187. The Portmann operation for Ménière's disease four years after the operation indicates relief from vertigo in the following percent of patients:
    A. 50
    B. 65
    C. 70
    D. 85
    E. 90

    REF. Schuknecht HF, Bucy PC, Fisch U, House WF, Portmann M: Arch Otolaryng, 97:129, Feb '73

188. Two methods can be used for ultrasound application in Ménière's disease: lateral canal versus round window approach. The percentage of failure in the lateral canal approach is:
    A. 5
    B. 10
    C. 20
    D. 40
    E. 60

    REF. Basek M: Arch Otolaryng, 97:133, Feb '73

189. The percentage of failure in the round window approach for ultrasound application in Ménière's disease is:
    A. 5
    B. 10
    C. 20
    D. 40
    E. 60

    REF. Basek M: Arch Otolaryng, 97:133, Feb '73 (See Fig. 13)

190. Complications of ultrasound application for Ménière's disease are:
    A. facial nerve paralysis
    B. tympanic membrane perforation
    C. complete hearing loss due to perforation round window membrane due to small probe (only 1 mm in diameter used)
    D. injury to the jugular bulb
    E. inefficiency or inconsistency in the energy output of the equipment

    REF. Basek M: Arch Otolaryng, 97:133, Feb '73

191. Since insufficient evidence is available concerning the basic pathophysiology of the major clinical entities of which vertigo is a primary symptom, treatment of vertigo is obviously difficult. Which of the following drug categories are used for treating vertigo?
    A. sedatives - tranquilizers
    B. antihistamines
    C. antiemetics and anticholinergics
    D. vasodilators including histamine
    E. anticoagulants
    F. diuretics

    REF. Rubin W: Arch Otolaryng, 97:135, Feb '73

192. Sedative - tranquilizers for controlling vertigo is based on the concept of a change in threshold response of vestibular receptors or of the synaptic connections in the vestibular pathways. Which of this group of drugs appear most effective?
A. barbiturates
B. phenothiazine - also causes possible extrapyramidal side-effects
C. droperidol (a respiratory depressant)
D. innovar (droperidol - fentanyl combination)
E. thiethylperazine accumulates in vestibular nuclear areas and vermis of the cerebellum
REF. Rubin W: Arch Otolaryng, 97:135, Feb '73

193. Antihistamines have been used extensively as vestibular drugs but their efficacy as a group has been rather poor for vestibular suppression. Dolowitz, however, states there is a central action which lowers the thresholds or interferes with the mediation of symptoms of dizziness. Which of the following appear to be effective?
A. diphenidol - occasional hallucinogenic side effects
B. cinnarazine (not available in U.S.)
C. phenergan
D. benadryl
E. pyribenzamine
REF. Rubin W: Arch Otolaryng, 97:135, Feb '73

194. The three objectives in surgery of chronic otitis media with or without mastoid involvement is:
A. lifesaving
B. elimination of infection
C. opening ear spaces for drainage
D. preservation of normal anatomic contours
E. restoration of function
REF. Sheehy JL: "Surgery of Chronic Otitis Media", in Otolaryngology, Hagerstown, MD.: W. F. Prior Co., Inc., 1972, Vol 1, Chap. 10

195. For this question, match each lettered item with one numbered item. Each choice may be used only once.
A. mastoid antrum, tympanum, and external auditory canal are converted into a common cavity exteriorized through the external meatus without retention of the tympanic membrane or ossicular remnants to preserve hearing
B. same as A with retention of the tympanic membrane and ossicular remnants to preserve hearing
C. repair of a tympanic membrane perforation
D. eradication of infection wherever present and obliteration of either a mastoid or fenestration cavity
E. eradication of disease only in the middle ear and reconstruction of the hearing mechanism with or without tympanic membrane grafting
F. same as E but with eradication of disease in both the middle ear and mastoid

1. mastoid obliteration
2. radical mastoidectomy
3. tympanoplasty with mastoidectomy
4. myringoplasty
5. modified radical mastoidectomy
6. tympanoplasty without mastoidectomy
REF. Sheehy JL: "Surgery of Chronic Otitis Media," in Otolaryngology, Hagerstown, Md: W. F. Prior Co., Inc., 1972, Vol.1, Chap. 10

196. Early symptoms of chronic otitis media are:
A. pain
B. discharge
C. vertigo
D. hearing impairment
E. facial nerve paralysis
REF. Sheehy JL: "Surgery of Chronic Otitis Media," in Otolaryngology, Hagerstown, Md. W.F. Prior Co., Inc., 1972, Vol. 1, Chap. 10

197. Advanced symptoms of chronic otitis media are:
A. pain
B. discharge
C. vertigo
D. hearing loss
E. facial nerve paralysis
REF. Sheehy JL: "Surgery of Chronic Otitis Media", in Otolaryngology, Hagerstown, Md: W. F. Prior Co., Inc., 1972, Vol. 1, Chap. 10

198. In the absence of cholesteatoma in chronic otitis media, which of the following conductive hearing loss levels usually indicates that the ossicular chain is intact?
A. 20 db or less
B. 30 db
C. 40 db
D. 50 db
E. 60 db
REF. Sheehy JL: "Surgery of Chronic Otitis Media", in Otolaryngology, Hagerstown, Md.: W. F. Prior Co., Inc., 1972, Vol. 1, Chap. 10

199. A progressive conductive hearing loss in the absence of active disease in chronic otitis media usually suggests (and may require a two stage operation):
A. tympanosclerosis
B. mastoid disease
C. unrecognized middle ear infection
D. round window bony overgrowth
E. otosclerosis
REF. Sheehy JL: "Surgery of Chronic Otitis Media", in Otolaryngology, Hagerstown, Md.: W. F. Prior Co., Inc., 1972, Vol. 1, Chap. 10

200. It is not unusual to find in an ear with an attic perforation and large cholesteatoma a hearing loss of:
A. no loss (normal hearing)
B. 10 - 19 db
C. 20 - 39 db
D. 40 - 59 db
E. greater than 60 db
REF. Sheehy JL: "Surgery of Chronic Otitis Media," in Otolaryngology, Hagerstown, Md.: W. F. Prior Co., Inc., 1972, Vol. 1, Chap. 10

201. The treatment for auricular hematoma in order to prevent the development of a "cauliflower ear" is:
A. oral enzymes
B. ice packs
C. aspiration of the hematoma (or an incision may be necessary) and application of a compressive dressing
D. excision of the overlying skin and perichondrium and split-thickness skin graft applied
E. steroids and antibiotics orally
REF. Grabb WC, Smith JW: Plastic Surgery: A Concise Guide to Clinical Practice, Boston, Little, Brown & Co., p. 254, 1973

202. Which of the following conditions causes eustachian tube blockage?
A. neoplasm of the nasopharynx
B. polyp in the nasopharynx
C. allergic reaction to specific allergens in coffee
D. intolerance or idiosyncrasy to caffeine in coffee
E. psychosomatic reaction
REF. Browning RW, Marlowe FI, McGovern JP: Consultant 15:15, Sept '75

203. Therapy considered in Herpes Zoster consists of:
A. topical anesthetic such as dimethisoquin lotion
B. systemic steroids
C. intralesional injections of corticosteroids along the course of each eruption (0.75 ml of a mixture of 1 ml or 25 mg of hydrocortisone acetate in 2 ml of procaine)
D. adenine arabinoside
E. gamma globulin or convalescent serum
F. antibiotics
G. deep x-ray therapy to the involved ganglia
H. vitamin B_1
I. vitamin B_{12}
J. repeated smallpox vaccinations
REF. Noojin RO: Consultant 15:59, Sept '75

204. Some of the complications of Herpes Zoster are:
A. involvement (vesicles) of the cornea and sometimes tip of the nose (supraorbital form)
B. vesicles on the pinna and in the external auditory canal (geniculate ganglion)
C. facial paralysis (geniculate ganglion)
D. vesicles on the soft palate (glossopharyngeal ganglion)
E. disturbances of the cerebrospinal nervous system with motor paralysis
REF. Noojin RO: Consultant 15:59, Sept '75

205. Patients who have ingested large amounts of ethchlorvynol (placidyl) usually have, when present, positional coarse nystagmus characterized by being:
A. horizontal
B. predominant in one direction
C. vertical
D. ocular in type without quick and slow components
E. nystagmus only with eyes open
REF. Ropper AH: JAMA 232:907, June '75

206. In positional nystagmus, a pattern of gaze nystagmus predominantly in opposite directions with differing body positions usually indicates a lesion in the:
A. semicircular canals
B. utricle
C. vestibular nerve
D. cerebellopontine angle
E. central nervous system
REF. Ropper AH: JAMA 232:907, June '75

207. The second most common single organism isolated from middle ear disease is:
A. hemophilus influenzae (H. influenzae)
B. streptococcus pneumoniae (pneumococcus)
C. staphylococcus aureus
D. escherichia coli
E. proteus vulgaris
REF. Howie VM: Ann Otol Rhinol Laryngol 84 (Supp. 19):67, Mar '75

208. IgM antibody production in patients treated with either ampicillin, erythromycin or sulfonamide for otitis media showed the greatest primary or IgM response to treatment with:
A. ampicillin
B. erythromycin
C. sulfonamide
D. B + C combination therapy
E. any of these
REF. Howie VM: Ann Otol Rhinol Laryngol 84 (Supp. 19):67, Mar '75

209. The immunology of otitis media is far from being determined but which of the following appear to be true?
A. evidence indicates that local specific antibody is associated with rapid clearing of middle ear fluid
B. IgG, IgM and IgA antibodies are found in middle ear aspirate
C. IgG, IgM and IgA antibodies are found in the serum of patients with otitis media
D. patients responding immunologically to pneumococcal otitis media increase with age
E. potential for immunization procedures in otitis media appears encouraging
REF. Howie VM: Ann Otol Rhinol Laryngol 84 (Supp. 19):67, Mar '75

210. The common denominator predisposing to an otitis media prone condition of six or more episodes requiring tubomyringotomy in a patient one to two years of age is an initial infection with:
A. hemophilus influenzae (H. influenzae)
B. streptococcus pneumoniae (pneumococcus)
C. staphylococcus aureus
D. escherichia coli
E. proteus vulgaris
REF. Howie VM: Ann Otol Rhinol Laryngol 84 (supp. 19):67, Mar '75

211. The major pathogen in acute otitis media is:
A. hemophilus influenzae (H. influenzae)
B. streptococcus pneumoniae (pneumococcus)
C. staphylococcus aureus
D. escherichia coli
E. proteus vulgaris
REF. Howie VM: Ann Otol Rhinol Laryngol 84 (Supp. 19):67, Mar '75

212. Of more than 80 types of streptococcus pneumoniae (pneumococcus), which of the following types are associated but less frequently with otitis media?
A. 1
B. 3
C. 5
D. 9
E. 18
REF. Howie VM: Ann Otol Rhinol Laryngol 84 (Supp. 19):67, Mar '75

213. Of more than 80 types of streptococcus pneumoniae (pneumococcus), which of the following types are associated with the vast majority (50%) of otitis media episodes?
A. 2
B. 6
C. 14
D. 19
E. 23
REF. Howie VM: Ann Otol Rhinol Laryngol 84 (Supp. 19):67, Mar. '75

214. Ventilatory (tubomyringotomy) tubes are usually indicated at the time of which acute episode of otitis media occurring within a year?
A. 1
B. 2
C. 3
D. 4
E. 6
REF. Howie VM: Ann Otol Rhinol Laryngol 84 (Supp. 19):67, Mar '75

215. With medical treatment and without serious complications, ventilatory (tubomyringotomy) tubes are usually indicated if middle ear fluid persists (following an acute episode) more than:
A. one week
B. two weeks
C. one month
D. six weeks
E. two months
REF. Howie VM: Ann Otol Rhinol Laryngol 84 (Supp. 19):67, Mar '75

216. Hearing defects may result from which of the following conditions?
A. congenital disorders of the immunologic system such as agammaglobulinemia
B. inborn errors of metabolism such as cystic fibrosis
C. hypobaric pressure in the middle ear (pathological secretion of mucosal glands in and around the eustachian tube)
D. craniofacial dysostosis of Apert and Crouzon
E. enlarged adenoids
REF. Pruzansky S: Ann Otol Rhinol Laryngol 84 (Supp. 19):55, Mar '75

217. A relatively new member of the tetracycline family of bacteriostatic agents, minocycline (minocin-Lederle) is more toxic to women than men and has which of the following distressing side effects:
A. dysphagia
B. urticaria and angioneurotic edema
C. photosensitivity
D. vertigo
E. discoloration of tooth enamel
REF. Wolber PGH, King SJ: Notes and tips, Harper & Row Pub., Inc. 5:131, Mar '75

218. The highly recommended so-called narcotic analgesic pentazocine (Talwin) has serious side effects which are:
A. vertigo
B. headache
C. hallucinations and toxic psychosis
D. respiratory depression
E. fatal hypotension
REF. Wolber PGH, King SJ: Notes and Tips, Harper & Row Pub., Inc., 5:131, Mar '75

219. The eustachian tube:
A. is closed normally and opens only momentarily during swallowing
B. causes a feeling of fullness in the middle ear during swallowing when the mouth and nose are closed (Toynbee Procedure)
C. results in air entering the middle ear under pressure during the Toynbee Procedure
D. results in a negative pressure in the middle ear during the Toynbee Procedure
E. opens by means of the tensor veli palatini muscle and closes partly by the elasticity of the eustachian tube cartilage
REF. Shapiro SL: EENT Monthly 54:105, Mar '75

220. The most common malfunction of the eustachian tube is:
A. failure of the tube to open
B. inability of the tube to close
REF. Shapiro SL: EENT Monthly 54:105, Mar '75

221. Patients with acute alcoholic hallucinosis have:
A. visual hallucinations
B. tactile hallucinations
C. disorientation for time and place
D. auditory hallucinations
REF. Lieb J, Slaby AE: Modern Med 85, Mar '75

222. Orthostatic hypotension (with vertigo) may occur as a side effect of treatment of psychoses or depression with:
A. tricyclic antidepressants
B. aliphatic phenothiazines
C. monoamine oxidase inhibitors
D. butyrophenones
REF. Lieb J, Slaby AE: Modern Med 81, Mar '75

223. By any route, the most effective glucocorticoid for dermatologic disorders such as eczematoid otitis externa is:
A. triamcinolone
B. methylprednisolone
C. dexamethasone
D. prednisolone
E. paramethasone
REF. Test: Drug therapy 5:154, Nov '75

224. Allergic contact dermatitis due to pierced ear lobes is most likely due to:
A. nickel
B. chrome
C. paraphenylinediamine
D. ethylenediamine in topical medications
E. rubber on pierced ear inserts
REF. Provost TT: Allergy News Bull 4:3, (Month=0) Issue 9, '75

225. The causes of cholesteatomas of the epitympanic areas are:
A. epithelial migration from Shrapnell's membrane as proliferation of the deeper layers of the epidermis
B. retraction of Shrapnell's membrane
C. epithelial rests from the first ectodermal branchial pouch
D. metaplasia of the cuboidal epithelium of the middle ear into a squamous stratified epithelium
E. debatable but probably all of the above
REF. Peron DL, Schuknecht HF: Arch Otolaryngol 101:498, Aug ' 75

226. Congenital cholesteatoma of the external auditory canal is usually associated with:
A. atresia due to a bony plate
B. an atretic cartilaginous canal
C. being medial to the area of atresia of the external auditory canal
D. erosion of bone of the external auditory canal
E. invasion and destruction of the middle ear structures
REF. Peron DL, Schuknecht HF: Arch Otolaryngol 101:498, Aug '75

227. Diagnosis of congential cholesteatoma of the middle ear indicates:
A. it usually arises in the hypotympanum
B. it usually arises in the epitympanum
C. erosion (x-ray) of the inferior margin of the lateral epitympanic wall
D. erosion of the superior wall with the inferior margin intact
E. extensive erosion of the ossicles
REF. Peron DL, Schuknecht HF: Arch Otolaryngol 101:498, Aug '75

228. Symptoms and signs of congenital cholesteatoma of the middle ear are:
A. otoscopy reveals the classical "whitish mass" (sometimes pink) behind an intact tympanic membrane
B. average age 11 years
C. hearing loss
D. otorrhea, otalgia and loss of taste
E. facial paralysis (dehiscence of fallopian canal)
REF. Peron DL, Schuknecht HF: Arch Otolaryngol 101:498, Aug '75

229. Symptoms and/or signs of congenital cholesteatoma of the mastoid are:
A. conductive hearing loss with associated infection, ossicular destruction, or perforation of the tympanic membrane
B. swelling of the posterior wall of the external auditory canal and of the postauricular area
C. postauricular pain
D. facial paralysis
E. vertigo with fistulae of the lateral semicircular canals
REF. Peron DL, Schuknecht HF: Arch Otolaryngol 101:498, Aug '75

230. A study of the incidence of tumor growths in the cerebellopontine angle indicates that the most common tumor is:
A. cholesteatoma
B. glioma
C. meningioma
D. vestibular schwannoma
REF. Peron DL, Schuknecht HF: Arch Otolaryngol 101:498, Aug '75

231. Total protein values in cerebrospinal fluid are elevated in which of the following tumors?
A. cholesteatoma of the petrous apex
B. glomus jugularis
C. salivary choristoma of the middle ear
D. meningioma
E. large vestibular schwannoma
REF. Peron DL, Schuknecht HF: Arch Otolaryngol 101:498, Aug '75

232. Diagnosis of congenital cholesteatoma of the petrous apex is indicated with:
A. radiological finding of a radiolucent defect in the petrous apex
B. posterior fossa myelography showing large lesions with a distinctive scalloped surface contour with occasional extension into the middle and posterior cranial fossae
C. with posterior cranial fossa extension only
D. normal total protein values in the cerebrospinal fluid
E. abnormal total protein values in the cerebrospinal fluid
REF. Peron DL, Schuknecht HF: Arch Otolaryngol 101:498, Aug '75

233. Signs of congenital cholesteatoma of the petrous apex are:
A. facial nerve paralysis
B. fifth cranial nerve involvement
C. sixth cranial nerve paralysis
D. ninth cranial nerve paralysis
E. cerebellar dysfunction
F. meningitis
G. decreased or absent vestibular response
H. sensorineural hearing loss with poor speech discrimination
I. sensory hearing loss with good speech discrimination
REF. Peron DL, Schuknecht HF: Arch Otolaryngol 101:498, Aug '75

234. Symptoms of congenital cholesteatoma of the petrous apex are:
A. first symptom is unilateral hearing loss
B. conductive deafness with good speech discrimination
C. progressive sensorineural hearing loss with poor speech discrimination
D. hemifacial spasm or facial weakness
E. vertigo with decreased or absent vestibular response
F. head pain
REF. Peron DL, Schuknecht HF: Arch Otolaryngol 101:498, Aug '75

235. Mononeuritis in infectious mononucleosis is relatively uncommon but occurs as:
A. anosmia, optic neuritis
B. oculomotor, trochlear and abducens palsy
C. dysfunction of cranial nerves five and eight to eleven
D. hypoglossal nerve involvement, isolated, and as a polyneuritic variant involving cranial nerves 9, 10, 11
E. facial nerve dysfunction, both unilaterally and bilaterally
REF. Michel RG, Pope TH, Jr., Patterson CN: Arch Otolaryngol 101:486, Aug '75

236. To prescribe two powerful hearing aids instead of one for severely deaf children can result in:
A. serious, permanent damage to residual hearing
B. interesting implications in dichotic listening skills of deaf children with a dominant ear and suppression of sounds in the other ear rather than integration as in normal listeners and choice of ear if only one aid is being purchased
C. deprivation of the user of subtle pinna and ear canal factors available to the normal listener
D. substantial temporary threshold shift (TTS) after as little as three and one-half hours of exposure and probably permanent threshold diminution as a result of protracted use of powerful instruments
E. even though language development is based on early auditory experience, there is no justification for fitting two hearing aids for simultaneous use but rather to alternate a single aid from ear to ear
REF. Jerger, JF: Arch Otolaryngol 101:480, Aug '75

237. Chronic otitis externa may result from:
A. traumatic injury to the external auditory canal
B. otitis media
C. parotid infection extending through the fissures of Santorini
D. cerumen (hard)
E. traumatic perforation of a foreign body from the oral cavity penetrating the deep tissues of the neck
REF. Stewart C, Passy V: Arch Otolaryngol 101:478, Aug '75

238. The radiographic view superior for evaluating the foot-plate and superstructure of the stapes is:
A. Guillen with the tympanic cavity viewed through the orbit and with the head tilted 15° to the side under investigation
B. lateral
C. straight anteroposterior (AP)
D. basal
E. projection 20° off straight anteroposterior toward the investigated side
REF. Babin RW, Hannafee WN, Ward PH: Arch Otolaryngol 101:474, Aug '75

239. Results of long-term treatment with transmyringeal aeration (tubomyringotomy) in children with chronic serous otitis media were not satisfactory in 20.9 percent of the ears because of:
A. hearing losses varying from 25 to 60 db
B. development of chronic otitis media
C. development of cholesteatoma
D. development of adhesive otitis media
E. perforations requiring myringoplasty
REF. Gundersen T, Tonning FM: Arch Otolaryngol 102:198, Apr '76

240. Air embolism in a scuba diver is a massive intra-arterial infusion of air caused by over-pressurization of the intrapulmonic space when a diver breathing compressed air becomes panicky and holds his breath until he swims to the surface. Which of the following symptoms may then occur?
A. unconsciousness
B. blindness
C. paralysis
D. dysarthria
E. convulsions
F. coma
G. death
H. pneumothorax
I. mediastinal and subcutaneous emphysema
J. choking, dyspnea, substernal pain, nonproductive cough
K. cyanosis
REF. Goodman HF: Emergency Med 7:187, June '75

241. Any aircraft flight within 24 hours of scuba diving can lead to decompression sickness because most aircraft are pressurized in feet to only:
A. 2000
B. 4000
C. 8000
D. 10,000
E. 12,000
REF. Goodman HF: Emergency Med 7:187, June '75

242. Air embolism due to a scuba diver breathing compressed air can occur after an ascent in feet of:
A. 66
B. 33
C. 22
D. 4 in a backyard swimming pool
E. all of these
REF. Goodman HF: Emergency Med 7:187, June '75

243. When a scuba diver stays at depths greather than 33 feet for too long and ascends too rapidly, which of the following gases dissolved in body fluids during hyperbaric pressure form bubbles as pressure is reduced on ascent and collects in plasma and tissues causing decompression sickness:
A. oxygen
B. carbon dioxide
C. nitrogen
D. A plus C
E. B plus C
REF. Goodman HF: Emergency Med 7:187, June '75

244. The purpose of audiometric screening in school is to:
A. screen as many children as possible but the screening test is not designed to identify slight hearing problems
B. identify hearing losses
C. identify the presence of an active ear disorder
D. refer abnormal cases to the physician
E. refer cases in need of rehabilitation to the proper authorities as soon as possible
REF. Lescouflair G: Arch Otolaryngol 101:469, Aug '75

245. Which of the following complications occur from ear lobe piercing for earrings?
A. hemorrhage
B. staphylococcus infection
C. metallic dermatitis
D. keloid formation
E. viral hepatitis
REF. Goff WF: EENT Monthly 54:41, Aug '75

246. The main cause of false-positive referrals from audiometric screening in schools is due to:
A. environment-ambient masking noise varying between 40 and 60 db of sound pressure level (SPL)
B. equipment-calibration of screening audiometers every four months, failure of
C. personnel-poorly trained
D. method-pure tone generated by an audiometer does not exist in normal life (no concrete reality for the child)
E. lack of attention and motivation in children during testing
REF. Lescouflair G: Arch Otolaryngol 101:469, Aug '75

247. A child with a bone-conduction (BC) hearing level of -5 db and an air conduction (AC) of 20 db will pass the usual school screening test although he actually has:
A. minimal hearing loss of no significance
B. hearing level within normal range
C. sensory deafness
D. neural deafness
E. conductive deafness requiring treatment
REF. Lescouflair G: Arch Otolaryngol 101:469, Aug '75

248. All of the following appear true but the endochondral layer of the otic capsule has been regarded as an arrested stage of development of bone in cartilage (metabolically inert in adult life) because of:
A. inability of fractured endochondral bone to form callus
B. changeover from acid to neutral mucopolysaccharides in the pericanalicular and perilacunar substance
C. inability to visualize osteocytes or osteocyte precursors in endochondral bone stained with hematoxylin-eosin
D. uptake of tetracycline labelled within the endochondral bone of the otic capsule
REF. Hawke M: Arch Otolaryngol 101:462, Aug '75

249. Which of the following disease states affects the otic capsule secondarily?
A. otosclerosis
B. ossifying panlabyrinthitis
C. Paget's disease
D. metabolic bone disease
REF. Hawke M: Arch Otolaryngol 101:462, Aug '75

250. Which of the following disease states affects the otic capsule primarily?
A. metabolic bone disease
B. ossifying panlabyrinthitis
C. Paget's disease
D. otosclerosis
REF. Hawke M: Arch Otolaryng 101:462, Aug '75

251. In the following question each lettered item is to be matched with one numbered item. Each choice may be used only once! The human otic capsule is unique histologically and physiologically and incorporates layers of bone that differ in morphology and staining characteristics:
A. endosteal (inner) layer
B. periosteal (outer) layer
C. outer regions
D. endochondral (middle) layer
1. not sharply defined and consists of coarse, fibrillar bone with lamellar elements
2. periosteal bone undergoing remodeling similar to skeletal bone
3. thin lamellar bone, poorly vascularized and considered to be of low metabolic activity
4. layer of an irregularly woven nonlamellar bone found only in the skeleton during fetal development and at fresh fracture sites and when fractured, cannot develop callus
REF. Hawke M: Arch Otolaryngol 101:462, Aug '75

252. The etiology of musical hallucinations in deafness appears to result from distortions in the normal processing of sensory information so that abnormal perceptions occur centrally. Distortions in the normal processing of sensory information result from damage to the:
A. inner and outer hair cells
B. entire organ of Corti
C. Deiter's and Hensen's cells
D. Claudius cells
E. unknown
REF. Ross ED, Jossman PB, Bell B, Sabin T, Geschwind N: JAMA 231:620, Feb '75

253. Other causes of formed auditory hallucinations can usually be excluded from musical hallucinations in deafness because in other causes there is present one or more of the following conditions:
A. a schizophrenic disorder
B. psychoses, such as delirium tremens and chronic alcoholic hallucinosis
C. voices, frequently offending but may be pleasant and even with a musical quality
D. not continuous but intermittent musical hallucinations, such as in some temporal lobe tumors
E. normal hearing
REF. Ross ED, Jossman PB, Bell B, Sabin T, Geschwind N: JAMA 231:620, Feb '75

254. The treatment of musical hallucinations in deafness is:
A. changing the tune by singing aloud
B. thinking about another melody
C. disappear with the use of a hearing aid
D. assuring the patient of the benign and non-psychiatric character of the disorder
E. patients seem to adjust to the musical hallucinations
REF. Ross ED, Jossman PB, Bell B, Sabin T, Geschwind N: JAMA 231:620, Feb '75

255. Which of the following characteristics occur in formed musical hallucinations in deafness?
A. generally preceded by a long history of progressive deafness with tinnitus and experienced predominantly in the ear with the most severe hearing loss
B. music is vivid and reflects past musical memories, such as singing, playing an instrument, band, or orchestra
C. repetition of same melody on awakening and continuous throughout the day
D. musical hallucinations may be disturbing or pleasing with the patient harmonizing
E. patients name the ear or head as the site of origin of the music
REF. Ross ED, Jossman PB, Bell B, Sabin T, Geschwind N: JAMA 231:620, Feb '75

256. Very few otologists and clinicians are aware of the existence of which one of the following causes of formed auditory hallucinations?
A. psychoses
B. schizophrenic disorders
C. temporal lobe epilepsy
D. temporal lobe tumors
E. acquired peripheral deafness
REF. Ross ED, Jossman PB, Bell B, Sabin T, Geschwind N: JAMA 231:620, Feb '75

257. Formed auditory hallucinations are generally considered to be manifestations of which of the following conditions?
A. schizophrenic disorders
B. psychoses, such as delirium tremens and chronic alcoholic hallucinosis
C. Ictal states, such as temporal lobe epilepsy
D. temporal lobe tumors
E. pure word deafness
REF. Ross ED, Jossman PB, Bell B, Sabin T, Geschwind N: JAMA 231:620, Feb '75

258. Which of the following auditory hallucinations are formed?
A. tinnitus
B. music
C. singing
D. sentences
E. spoken words
REF. Ross ED, Jossman PB, Bell B, Sabin T, Geschwind N: JAMA 231:620, Feb '75

259. Which of the following auditory hallucinations are unformed?
A. spoken words
B. sentences
C. singing
D. music
E. tinnitus
REF. Ross ED, Jossman PB, Bell B, Sabin T, Geschwind N: JAMA 231:620, Feb '75

260. In Calhoun versus Frazier, 125Sw2d, Tennessee, facial paralysis occurred two hours after a mastoidectomy. Judgment for the defendant was upheld on appeal because:
A. operation was necessary
B. surgeon was a Board-certified otolaryngologist
C. defendant's testimony that paralysis often results from infection or thrombosis as well as nerve damage
D. paralysis was not present immediately after surgery
E. theory of Res ipsa loquiter did not apply in the absence of positive evidence for the plaintiff
REF. Redden K, Frankel C: ORL Digest 37:31, Mar '75

261. A facial nerve paralysis followed a mastoidectomy. Judgment for the plaintiff (Marlow versus Patrick) was upheld on appeal because:
A. operation was not indicated
B. nerve, although not severed, was injured
C. surgeon, though as skilled as any other surgeon, produced no evidence of bone necrosis with unavoidable nerve injury
D. surgeon was not skilled
E. infection was not present
REF. Redden K, Frankel C: ORL Digest 37:31, Mar '75

262. Ibuprofen (motrin) is a nonsteroid drug with analgesic, antipyretic, and anti-inflammatory properties recently introduced for use in antiarthritis therapy. Which of the following otolaryngological complaints occur during therapy?
A. vertigo
B. headache
C. deafness
D. tinnitus
E. urticaria
REF. Lewis JR: JAMA 233:364, July '75; Blechman WJ, Schmid FR, April PA, Wilson CH, Brooks CD: JAMA 233:366, July '75

263. Which of the following neurologic symptoms and/or signs arise from the venous reflux through clot formation in otogenic sigmoid sinus thrombosis?
A. inflammatory alterations in the subdural area
B. increase in cerebrospinal fluid (CSF) pressure
C. cerebral edema
D. abducens paralysis
E. oculomotor paralysis
F. choked disc
G. labyrinthine spontaneous nystagmus
H. central spontaneous nystagmus
REF. Majer EH: ORL Digest 37:11, July '75

264. The frequently profuse neurologic symptomatology in otogenic complications is caused by the close topographic relationship between the temporal bone and the peripheral and central nervous sytem. Even today in this era of antibiotic therapy there have been increasing numbers of reports of atypical, masked mastoiditis in which complications make a sudden appearance after a latent period of several weeks. Otogenic meningitis remains a life-threatening complication even though with modern day treatment the mortality has been reduced from 75 percent to:
A. 1-3
B. 4-5
C. 7-13
D. 14-30
E. 31-47
REF. Majer EH: ORL Digest 37:11, July '75

265. Which of the following symptoms or signs appear in otogenic sigmoid sinus thrombosis with or without cholesteatoma?
A. usually septic temperature
B. chills
C. severe headache with vomiting
D. drowsiness or even unconsciousness
E. aphasia
REF. Majer EH: ORL Digest 37:11, July '75

266. Which of the following symptoms and/or signs occurs especially in otogenic basal meningitis?
A. loss of consciousness (sometimes apopleptic in nature)
B. headache
C. floccillation
D. positive Kernig sign
E. paralysis of cerebral nerves
REF. Majer EH: ORL Digest 37:11, July '75

267. Which of the following symptoms and/or signs occur in otogenic meningitis?
A. severe headache with sensitivity to light
B. confusion or loss of consciousness
C. floccillation
D. stiffness of the neck
E. positive Kernig symptom
REF. Majer EH: ORL Digest 37:11, July '75

268. Plaintiff (patient) had an ear drainage of long duration and x-ray revealed extensive disease in the left mastoid area and the possibility of cholesteatoma. During operation without using a surgical microscope, the facial nerve was partially severed causing a left side facial paralysis. The defendant physician was held liable for severing the cranial nerve by the Appeals Court based on expert ENT testimony that standard treatment applicable to this problem is that:
A. surgery was not necessary
B. surgical microscope is absolutely necessary
C. cholesteatoma wall should be left in the area of the facial nerve and the end state of the surgery is the same whether or not the skin (cholesteatomous wall) is removed
D. C same with granulation tissue
E. opening of the ear to release the pressure is sufficient
REF. Redden K, Frankel C: ORL Digest 37:29, July '75 (Livingood VS Howard, 295 N.E. 2d 736, 1973)

269. Round window rupture may occur:
A. after exertion or severe sneezing or coughing
B. after barometric pressure changes in the middle ear (scuba diving, forceful autoinflation)
C. spontaneously without A or B
D. in congenital inner ear abnormalities with patent cochlear aqueduct or patent modiolus with increased perilymphatic fluid pressure
E. tubal occlusion with negative middle ear hydrostatic pressure
REF. Healy GB, Strong MS, Sampogna D: Arch Otolaryngol 100:130, Aug '74

270. The diagnosis of an inner ear window rupture must be considered when there is no apparent reason for which of the following symptoms or signs?
A. vertigo
B. positional nystagmus
C. sensorineural hearing loss
D. positive Romberg sign
E. positive fistula test
REF. Healy GB, Strong MS, Sampogna D: Arch Otolaryngol 100:130, Aug '74

271. The most common area of the oval window to rupture is:
A. anterior
B. inferior
C. superior
D. posterior
E. central
REF. Healy GB, Strong MS, Sampogna D: Arch Otolaryngol 100:130, Aug '74

272. Inner ear window ruptures can be repaired by:
A. perichondrium
B. lobular fat
C. vein graft
D. silastic sheeting
E. canal skin
REF. Healy GB, Strong MS, Sampogna D: Arch Otolaryngol 100:130, Aug '74

273. High-tone, and occasionally low tone, sensorineural hearing losses occurring after chronic ear surgery regardless of the type of procedure are most likely due to:
A. late disarticulation of the incus before cleaning the attic
B. excessive stimulation of the ossicular chain during surgery
C. B with extensive stapes movements after removal of the incus
D. dissection of the malleus but not as one should in the direction of its handle
E. sensorineural loss being common in chronic otitis media
REF. Palva T, Kärjä J, Palva A: Arch Otolaryngol 98:176, Sept '73

274. Preoperative evaluation of eustachian tubal function to determine patency:
A. is essential for successful tympanoplastic surgery in most instances
B. does not always assure improved postoperative hearing results
C. assures improved postoperative hearing results
D. shows that excellent postoperative hearing results may occur in the presence of tubal obstruction
E. indicates that the electroacoustic impedance bridge is a practical method to determine eustachian tubal function
REF. Parisier SC: Mt Sinai J Med NY 41:687, Oct '74

275. Mycobacterium tuberculosis infection of the middle ear:
A. usually results when tubercle bacilli enter the eustachian tube from the nasopharynx
B. usually reaches the middle ear via the hematogenous route
C. may be the first sign of tuberculosis
D. perforates usually the lower half of the tympanic membrane
E. destroys the labyrinth with only rare labyrinthine symptoms
REF. Sahn SA, Davidson PT: Chest 66:104, July '74

276. Mycobacterium tuberculosis infects the mastoid cells by extension from the tympanic cavity or occasionally via the hematogenous route and is best treated by:
A. immediate surgery
B. surgery after chemotherapy for one month
C. B after therapy for 2-6 months or even longer
D. chemotherapy with multiple anti-ototoxic drugs, when possible, for at least two years
E. ototoxic drugs must be avoided
REF. Sahn SA, Davidson PT: Chest 66:104, July '74

277. Before considering surgery on the congenital ear, it is important to determine sensorineural function and perform anteroposterior polytomography in 2-mm and 1-mm sections. Polytomography indicates that:
A. patients with inner ear abnormality have external ear abnormality
B. cardiac malformations are common
C. renal malformations are common
D. the most common lesion is a large round cavity with a superior semicircular canal
E. lesions of the sixth and seventh cranial nerves are common
REF. Phelps PD: Arch Otolaryngol 100:11, July '74

278. High doses of irradiation to the middle ear for neoplasms in the head and neck area cause a high incidence of serous otitis media due to:
A. hyperemia and edema of the eustachian tube
B. A plus changes due to any surgical impairment of the tensor veli palatini muscle
C. damage to the lymphatics of the eustachian tube
D. probably all of the above
E. none of the above
REF. Brill AH, Martin MM, Fitz-Hugh GS, Constable WC: Arch Otolaryngol 99:406, June '74

279. A small semicircular canal labyrinthine fistula membrane can be removed by using a small-gauge aspirator and a sharp elevator. The area of the fistula should be:
A. left uncovered
B. covered with gelfoam
C. covered with a fascial graft
D. covered with a bone chip
E. D but held in place with fascia
REF. Gacek RR: Ann Otol Rhinol Laryngol (Suppl. 10):83, Jan '74

280. Especially when the ENG findings before the accident are unknown, electronystagmography (ENG) is only a useful and not a completely diagnostic procedure in evaluating audiovestibular findings following cervical spine trauma. Which of the following ENG findings occur following cervical spine trauma?
A. spontaneous nystagmus
B. directional preponderance
C. unilateral weakness
D. positional nystagmus
E. dead labyrinth
REF. Kosoy J, Glassman AL: Tex Med 70:66, Oct '74

281. The management of cholesteatomatous membrane over bony labyrinthine and cochlear fistulas is controversial but which of the following facts appear true?
A. dehiscence should always be expected whether the fistula test is positive or negative
B. membrane should not be removed when the cochlear wall is involved
C. B may be removed
D. membranes may be removed over small canal fistulas, facial nerves or dural surfaces
E. membranes should be left undisturbed over large canal fistulas
REF. Gacek RR: Ann Otol Rhinol Laryngol (Supp. 10):83, Jan '74

282. Ossicular bone destruction in middle ear disease is:
A. not necessarily linked with cholesteatoma
B. always associated with the presence of cholesteatoma
C. due to a "lytic" process by cholesteatoma
D. found in simple, noncholesteatomatous chronic otitis media
E. bone destruction limited topographically to the region immediately above the notch of Rivinus
REF. Sadé J, Halevy A: J Laryngol Otol 88:139, Feb '74

283. Tissue adhesive in reconstructive middle ear surgery would be very useful but to date such glues have been found either inadequate or dangerous. One report indicates that in experimental dogs 2-cyano-butyl-acrylate (histoacryl):
A. unites fascia to tympanum
B. A cartilage to foot-plate
C. A bone to foot-plate
D. A incus interposition between malleus and stapes
E. causes no tissue reaction except in the area of glue application
REF. Siedentop KH: Laryngoscope 84:1397, Aug '74

284. Petrositis has a high mortality rate and still occurs in spite of antibiotic therapy and:
A. can develop by direct extension from the middle ear without mastoid involvement
B. mastoiditis is always present
C. any facial or retrobulbar pain during or after otitis media is suspicious
D. Lempert approach is preferable when inflammation is confined to the petrous apex
E. D middle cranial fossa approach
REF. Hendershot EL, Wood JW: Arch Otolaryngol 98:426, Dec '73

285. Tobramycin ototoxicity, like all the aminoglycoside antibiotics, may cause inner ear toxicity and:
A. exact mechanism is known
B. A is unknown
C. related to the concentration and slow clearance of the drug from the endolymph
D. the drug has stronger and probably primary effects in the organ of Corti
E. concomitant renal toxicity may occur
REF. Logan TB, Prazma J, Thomas WG, Fischer ND: Arch Otolaryngol 99: 190, Mar '74

286. An adequate external auditory meatus following tympanoplasty, mastoidectomy, acquired atresia, stenosis and congenital atresia is necessary:
A. for the passage of sound to the tympanum
B. to prevent accumulation of debris (self-cleansing)
C. for good postoperative care with removal of debris
D. for aeration of the mastoid cavity
E. to allow proper drainage so infection does not develop
REF. Anthony WP: Laryngoscope 84:1118, July '74

287. Causes of failure in tympanomastoidectomy are due to:
A. closed technic for cholesteatoma
B. early surgery of acute traumatic perforations
C. ossicular reconstruction without interlocking or fascia tie techniques
D. incomplete mastoid surgery
E. posteroanterior types of tympanomastoidectomy in poorly developed infected mastoids
REF. Farrior JB: Trans Am Acad Ophthalmol Otolaryngol 78:378 (ORL), Sept '74

288. Intracranial complications of otogenic origin have declined markedly but morbidity remains high due to:
A. epilepsy
B. hemiplegia
C. ataxia
D. coma
E. neck rigidity and fever
REF. Wright JLW, Grimaldi PMGB: J Laryngol Otol 87:1085, Nov '73

289. The most useful radiologic study in intracranial complications of otogenic origin is:
A. skull x-rays
B. A plus mastoid x-rays
C. unidirectional tomography
D. polytomography (cycloidal)
E. cerebral angiography
REF. Wright JLW, Grimaldi PMGB: J Laryngol Otol 87:1085, Nov '73

290. The earliest symptom in a patient with an intracranial complication due to a discharging ear is usually:
A. headache
B. vertigo
C. tinnitus
D. deafness
E. ataxia
REF. Wright JLW, Grimaldi PMGB: J Laryngol Otol 88:1085, Nov '73

291. One of the postoperative complications of stapedectomy is granuloma in the oval window and in the vestibule with cochlear damage and severe sensorineural deafness. The etiology of granuloma may be due to:
A. infection since inflammatory cells are present
B. noninfectious cause since the granulomas contain chronic lymphocytes
C. B with the presence of plasma cells
D. toxicity or hypersensitivity to the oval window grafting material (autoimmune reaction)
REF. Gromer R, Kietzer G, Oda M, Paparella M: Arch Otolaryngol 100:168, Sept '74

292. The etiology of poststapedectomy granulomas is unknown but some findings suggest a foreign body contaminant. Symptoms and/or signs of a granuloma are:
A. sensorineural hearing loss
B. vertigo
C. severe loss in speech discrimination
D. edematous tympanomeatal flap
E. granulomatous mass in the oval window or middle ear
REF. Burtner D, Goodman ML: Arch Otolaryngol 100:171, Sept '74

293. Sudden unilateral sensorineural hearing loss may occur with:
A. vascular conditions
B. viral lesions
C. otosclerosis
D. streptomycin therapy
E. neuroma
REF. Clemis JD: Laryngoscope 83:1959, Dec '73

294. Findings suggestive of acoustic tumor include all of the following but the most definitive finding is based on:
A. reduced caloric response, unilateral
B. asymmetrical sensorineural loss
C. retrocochlear audiometric signs, including greatly reduced discrimination score
D. tomography of the internal auditory canal
E. posterior fossa myelogram
F. increased protein in the cerebrospinal fluid
G. other ipsilateral cranial nerve involvement
REF. Clemis JD: Laryngoscope 83:1959, Dec '73

295. What percent of patients with neuroma give a history of sudden hearing loss?
A. none
B. 10
C. 20
D. 30
E. over 50
REF. Clemis JD: Laryngoscope 83:1959, Dec '73

296. Although all of the following occur, which one of the following conditions must be given first consideration when a patient displays symptoms of endolymphatic hydrops after stapedectomy?
A. perilymph fistula
B. neuroma
C. viral lesions
D. dual disease (A plus B)
E. occlusion of the cochleovestibular branch of the internal auditory artery
REF. Clemis JD: Laryngoscope 83:1959, Dec '73

297. Facial paralyses of lower motor neuron origin are caused by malignant involvement in what percent of patients?
A. less than 1
B. 3
C. 5
D. 9
E. around 14
REF. Neely JG, Alford BR: Arch Otolaryngol 100:298, Oct '74

298. The surgical procedure of choice in chronic recurrent parotiditis appears to be:
A. parotidectomy, superficial lobe
B. parotidectomy, total
C. parotid duct ligation
D. tympanic neurectomy
E. C plus D
REF. Morgan WR: Arch Otolaryngol 98:179, Sept '73

299. The advantages of hypoglossofacial anastomosis for facial palsy are:
A. complete or almost complete facial symmetry at rest
B. applicable to patients with facial palsy due to interruption of the nerve on the cranial side of the parotid
C. improvement in facial tone usually complete within one year of operation
D. operation may be performed 10-14 months after onset of paralysis
E. operation must be performed within six months after onset of paralysis
REF. Evans DM: Br J Plast Surg 27:251, July '74

300. Tympanic neurectomy in the "crocodile tears" syndrome appears successful; this syndrome is recognized by:
A. following peripheral facial paralysis
B. being always unilateral
C. most often following "chilling paralysis"
D. responsible lesion being situated at the level of the geniculate ganglion or higher
E. tearing always appearing late after facial paralysis
REF. Rosen G, Konak S: Ann Otolaryngol Chir Cervicofac 90:723, Dec '73

301. The treatment of choice in long-standing facial paralysis (as long as 33 years) is:
A. none-nerve paralysis is irreversible
B. facial nerve graft
C. spinal accessory-facial nerve anastomosis
D. masticatory muscle transposition
E. hypoglossal cross-over
F. neuromuscular rehabilitation augmented by B, D, E, whichever is indicated
REF. Conley J: Trans Am Acad Ophthalmol Otolaryngol 78:386 (ORL), Sept '74

302. The differential diagnosis of a red mass involving the tympanic membrane and/or external auditory canal include:
A. pyogenic granuloma
B. hemangioma
C. cholesteatoma
D. embryonal rhabdomyosarcoma
E. glomus tympanicum (as early as 22 months)
REF. Busby DR, Hepp VE: Arch Otolaryngol 99:377, May '74

303. The treatment of choice in glomus jugulare tumors is:
A. irradiation as primary therapy
B. en bloc dissection for large tumors
C. surgery alone for small tumors
D. high-dose preoperative radiotherapy plus en bloc dissection for large tumors
E. radiotherapy for unresectable lesions
REF. Spector GJ, Maisel RH, Ogura JH: Ann Otol Rhinol Laryngol 83:26, Jan '74

304. Effect of fistulae of the horizontal canal, superior canal, common crus and utricle on experimentally induced endolymphatic hydrops indicated:
A. significant improvement when made immediately before obliteration of the endolymphatic duct
B. A no effect
C. A when made several months after obliteration of the endolymphatic duct or when a polyethylene strut is introduced into the membranous labyrinth
D. C no effect
E. that procedures designed to surgically fistulize the membranous labyrinth are of questionable value in the treatment of Ménière's disease and may have an adverse effect on the sensorineural elements
REF. Kimura RS, Schuknecht HF: Ann Otol Rhinol Laryngol 84:271, May '75

305. The mammalian tectorial membrane of the organ of Corti is:
A. thin and ribbon-like
B. thick, massive-appearing structure permeated by cavities (probably facilitating the diffusion of endolymph) as in chickens
C. in contact with the tips of the sensory hairs and attached to the supporting cells by fine fibrils
D. not in contact with the tunnel rods and Deiters Cells
E. believed to move across the hair cells so that a shearing type force is exerted on the hairs
REF. Tanaka K, Smith CA: Ann Otol Rhinol Laryngol 84:287, May '75

306. Electrocochleography (E CochG) employs electrodes placed on or near the cochlea and computer averaging to record low voltage electrical potentials from the human inner ear. These potentials and their variations with changes in acoustic stimuli are used in assessment of hearing impairment. Extra-tympanic electrodes include:
A. earlobe clips
B. mastoid-vertex skin
C. needle in external auditory canal
D. ball in external auditory canal
E. wick in external auditory canal
REF. Crowley DE, Davis H, Beagley HA: Ann Otol Rhinol Laryngol 84:297, May '75

307. The electrode method of choice in electrocochleography (E CochG) appears to be:
A. earlobe clips
B. placement through existing perforated tympanic membrane
C. mastoid-vertex skin
D. ball in external auditory canal
E. needle electrodes placed on the cochlear promontory through the tympanic membrane
REF. Crowley DE, Davis H, Beagley HA: Ann Otol Rhinol Laryngol 84:297, May '75

308. Electrocochleography (ECochG) appears to be extremely beneficial in testing the hearing level in young children and neonates with which of the following conditions?
A. neurologic or psychiatric disorders, such as retardation
B. autism
C. hyperactivity or brain damage
D. congenital malformations or general development delay
E. nonverbal and nonresponsive child to other tests
REF. Crowley DE, Davis H, Beagley HA: Ann Otol Rhinol Laryngol 84:297, May '75

309. Electrocochleography (ECochG) appears to be most useful in testing the hearing level in adults with which of the following conditions?
A. nonorganic hearing loss associated with psychiatric or neurological disturbances
B. nonorganic hearing loss due to simulation or malingering in legal situations
C. otosclerosis
D. otitis media
E. preoperative cochlear evaluation with masking problems
REF. Crowley DE, Davis H, Beagley HA: Ann Otol Rhinol Laryngol 84:297, May '75

310. Electrocochleography (ECochG) requires local anesthesia for adults and a general anesthetic for children when the electrodes are placed on the cochlear promontory through the intact tympanic membrane or in the skin of the external auditory canal. The local anesthetics of choice appear to be:
A. ear canal injection with one percent lidocaine
B. A with one percent lidocaine with 1/100,000 dil. epinephrine
C. A with one percent lidocaine with 1/200,000 dil. epinephrine
D. A with 0.5 percent lidocaine with 1/200,000 dil. epinephrine
E. two percent piperocaine hydrochloride with and without epinephrine
F. 10 percent topical spray lidocaine
G. 14 percent benzocaine topical spray
REF. Crowley DE, Davis H, Beagley HA: Ann Otol Rhinol Laryngol 84:297, May '75

311. The implant of choice to prevent adhesions and maintain a middle ear space following a one-stage mastoidectomy-tympanoplasty where the mucosa has been removed from the promontory is:
A. gelfilm
B. teflon
C. polyethylene
D. paraffin
E. silastic
REF. Falbe-Hansen J, Jr., Tos M: Ann Otol Rhinol Laryngol 84:315, May '75

312. Unilateral lesions of which of the following cerebellar structures result in a complete loss or a significant reduction in visual suppression of vestibular nystagmus?
A. vermis
B. uvula
C. paraflocculus
D. cerebellar cortex
E. fastigial nuclei
F. interpositus nuclei
G. flocculus
H. nodulus
I. dentate nucleus
REF. Takemori S: Ann Otol Rhinol Laryngol 84:318, May '75

313. The intermediators in the cerebellar area through which the visual system can alter visual reflexes in visual suppression of vestibular nystagmus appear to be:
A. flocculus
B. vermis
C. cerebellar cortex
D. fastigial or interpositus nuclei
E. nodulus
REF. Takemori S: Ann Otol Rhinol Laryngol 84:318, May '75

314. Vestibular nystagmus has which of the following features?
A. spontaneous nystagmus is more prominent with eyes open (fixation)
B. A with eyes closed or in a dark room
C. nystagmus provoked by caloric stimulation is more prominent in darkness
D. C in light
E. nystagmus initiated by rotation is more prominent in darkness
REF. Takemori S: Ann Otol Rhinol Laryngol 84:318, May '75

315. The eustachian tubes of patients with unrepaired palatal clefts:
 A. appear more pliant
 B. appear less pliant
 C. have wider bihamular measurements
 D. have a wider nasopharynx than normal
 E. show decreased action potentials by electromyography in the levator and tensor veli palatini muscles
 F. demonstrate hypoplasia of the tensor veli palatini muscle at autopsy in newborns
 REF. Bluestone CD, Berry QC, Cantekin EI, Paradise JL: Ann Otol Rhinol Laryngol 84:333, May '75

316. All of the following growths occur as cerebellopontine angle lesions but the most common is:
 A. cholesteatoma
 B. meningioma
 C. arachnoid cyst
 D. acoustic neuroma
 E. brain stem lesions
 F. cerebellar lesions such as medulloblastoma
 REF. Britton BH: Ann Otol Rhinol Laryngol 84:364, May '75

317. All of the following growths occur as cerebellopontine angle lesions but the least common is:
 A. acoustic neuroma
 B. arachnoid cyst
 C. meningioma
 D. cholesteatoma
 E. cerebellar lesions
 F. brain stem lesions
 REF. Britton BH: Ann Otol Rhinol Laryngol 84:364, May '75

318. Which one of the following large growths usually shows enlargement of the internal auditory canal?
 A. cerebellar
 B. acoustic neuroma
 C. brain stem
 D. cholesteatoma
 E. meningioma
 F. arachnoid cyst
 REF. Britton BH: Ann Otol Rhinol Laryngol 84:362, May '75

319. Cerebellar medulloblastoma is:
 A. an uncommon lesion in the adult
 B. a common lesion in the adult
 C. a malignant growth originating from the granular layer of the cerebellar parenchyma
 D. usually a mid-line lesion in children
 E. usually a lateral lesion in adults
 F. frequently associated with positional nystagmus as an early sign
 REF. Britton BH: Ann Otol Rhinol Laryngol 84:364, May '75

320. In the differential diagnosis of large acoustic neuromas versus medulloblastomas, match the following letters with the correct numbers. Each choice may be used more than once:
 A. difficulty with coordinated movements
 B. cerebellar signs
 C. sensorineural hearing loss
 D. vertigo
 E. x-ray (routine) normal internal auditory canal (IAC)
 F. x-ray (routine) abnormal internal auditory canal (IAC)
 G. pantopaque - abnormal without filling internal auditory canal
 H. pantopaque - angle mass with possible filling of internal auditory canal

 1. large acoustic neuroma
 2. medulloblastoma
 REF. Britton BH: Ann Otol Rhinol Laryngol 84:364, May '75

321. Clinical electronystagmography (ENG) has proven useful in the evaluation of patients with vertiginous and/or audiologic symptoms. Recently employed independent eye movement measuring techniques suggest that:
A. eyes do not move conjugately in ENG
B. A do as has been assumed
C. disconjugate eye movements can occur only when pathology involves the medial longitudinal fasciculus (MLF)
D. C without involvement of MLF
E. disconjugate eye movements can occur with no detectable pathology involving cranial nerves III, IV, or VI
REF. Kimm J, MacLean JB: Ann Otol Rhinol Laryngol 84:368, May '75

322. The most common electronystagmographic (ENG) abnormality in central nervous system disease is:
A. calibration overshoot
B. gaze nystagmus
C. failure of fixation suppression
D. abnormal optokinetic nystagmus
E. abnormal pendulum tracking
REF. Spector M: Ann Otol Rhinol Laryngol 84:374, May '75

323. Useful central signs with eyes open in electronystagmographic (ENG) findings are:
A. calibration overshoot
B. gaze nystagmus
C. abnormal pendulum tracking
D. failure of fixation suppression
E. abnormal optokinetic nystagmus
REF. Spector M: Ann Otol Rhinol Laryngol 84:374, May '75

324. The most common cause of failure of fixation suppression in electronystagmographic (ENG) findings appears to be:
A. acoustic neuroma
B. multiple sclerosis
C. brain stem lesion
D. cerebellar pathology
E. drugs such as alcohol and valium
REF. Spector M: Ann Otol Rhinol Laryngol 84:374, May '75

325. The lesion most likely present when the predominant optokinetic nystagmus is toward the side of the lesion and the defective optokinetic toward the contralateral side in electronystagmographic findings (ENG) is in the:
A. brain stem
B. parietal lobe
C. internal auditory canal
D. cerebellum
E. medial longitudinal fasciculus (MLF)
REF. Spector M: Ann Otol Rhinol Laryngol 84:374, May '75

326. Which of the following methods have been tried in attempts to relieve symptoms of Ménière's disease by creating fistulae in the walls of the involved membranous labyrinths?
A. fistulization of the horizontal membranous semicircular canal
B. puncture of the saccule
C. insertion of a tack through the footplate of the stapes into the vestibule
D. implantation of a plastic tube to create an endolymph to perilymph shunt
E. all of the above
F. none of the above
REF. Kimura RS, Schuknecht HF: Ann Otol Rhinol Laryngol 84:271, May '75

327. Optokinetic nystagmus in electronystagmographic (ENG) findings is deranged in:
A. severe basilar arterial insufficiency involving the brain stem
B. far-advanced neurologic disease
C. Ménière's disease
D. vestibular neuronitis
E. parietal lobe
REF. Spector M: Ann Otol Rhinol Laryngol 84:374, May '75

328. Bilateral caloric weakness with normal optokinetic reaction in electronystagmographic (ENG) tests indicate:
A. a peripheral lesion
B. brain stem lesion
C. general vascular disease
D. cerebellar disease
E. multiple sclerosis
REF. Spector M: Ann Otol Rhinol Laryngol 84:374, May '75

329. Hypoactive or absent caloric responses in electronystagmography (ENG) may occur in:
A. acoustic neuroma
B. Ménière's disease
C. schizophrenia
D. streptomycin toxicity
E. cerebellopontine angle meningioma
REF. Spector M: Ann Otol Rhinol Laryngol 84:374, May '75

330. Electronystagmography (ENG) may be abnormal when the pendulum tracking test with eyes open is performed in patients with:
A. brain stem lesions (complete ataxia)
B. general vascular disease
C. cerebellar disease (fast movements)
D. posterior fossa lesions
E. disease of the tegmentum of the pons and midbrain
F. schizophrenia and related mental disorders
REF. Spector M: Ann Otol Rhinol Laryngol 84:374, May '75

331. A large acoustic schwannoma (neurinoma) in the cerebellopontine angle is suggested by involvement of which of the following cranial nerves?
A. V
B. VI
C. VII
D. VIII
E. IX
REF. Applebaum EL, Ferguson RJL: Ann Otol Rhinol Laryngol 84:379, May '75

332. A pontine vascular lesion (latero-medial inferior pontine syndrome) is suggested by involvement of which of the following cranial nerves?
A. V
B. VI
C. VII
D. VIII
E. IX
REF. Applebaum EL, Ferguson RJL: Ann Otol Rhinol Laryngol, 84:379, May '75

333. Signs consistent with a pontine vascular lesion with a lateral-inferior pontine syndrome would include some combination of:
A. ipsilateral facial palsy
B. loss of taste from the anterior two-thirds of the tongue
C. ipsilateral hearing loss
D. ipsilateral analgesia of the face
E. ipsilateral Horner's syndrome
F. contralateral loss of pain and temperature sensation from the trunk and extremities
G. paralysis of lateral conjugate gaze movements
REF. Applebaum, EL, Ferguson RJL: Ann Otol Rhinol Laryngol 84:379, May '75

334. Signs consistent with a pontine vascular lesion with a medial inferior pontine syndrome would include:
A. ipsilateral facial weakness
B. ipsilateral hearing loss
C. loss of taste from the anterior two-thirds of the tongue
D. ipsilateral lateral rectus palsy
E. contralateral hemiplegia
REF. Applebaum, EL, Ferguson RJL: Ann Otol Rhinol Laryngol 84:379, May '75

335. Elevation of the pure tone thresholds throughout the whole frequency range is often caused by which of the following conditions?
A. Ménière's disease
B. multiple sclerosis
C. tumor invasion of the auditory nuclei of the brain stem
D. severe cerebral edema
E. widespread, diffuse pathology in the cerebrum and brain stem in aged patients
REF. Makishima K, Ogata J: Ann Otol Rhinol Laryngol 84:391, May '75

336. Elevation of the threshold at 8 kHz has been observed in:
A. otosclerosis
B. drug ototoxicity
C. diabetes
D. small lesion VIII nerve
E. large lesion VIII nerve
REF. Makishima K, Ogata J: Ann Otol Rhinol Laryngol 84:391, May '75

337. Sensorineural hearing loss is often bilateral in patients with:
A. acoustic neuroma
B. sudden hearing loss syndrome
C. cortical dysacusis when lesion is localized in a single hemisphere
D. early Ménière's disease
E. brain stem lesions
REF. Makishima K, Ogata J: Ann Otol Rhinol Laryngol 84:391, May '75

338. Hearing loss in a patient with an acoustic neurinoma is typically:
A. profound, unilateral with tinnitus
B. mild, unilateral with tinnitus
C. profound, unilateral without tinnitus
D. mild, unilateral without tinnitus
E. late-developing with low frequency loss extending into the high frequencies and without tinnitus
REF. Makishima K, Ogata J: Ann Otol Rhinol Laryngol 84:391, May '75

339. A patient with spontaneous nystagmus, persistent (and of immediate onset) direction-changing positional nystagmus with normal and symmetrical responses to bithermal caloric stimulation has a lesion highly indicative of:
A. small acoustic neurinoma
B. small internal auditory canal syndrome
C. Ménière's disease
D. otosclerosis (late)
E. central pathology
REF. Makishima K, Ogata J: Ann Otol Rhinol Laryngol 84:391, May '75

340. A patient with spontaneous nystagmus, direction-changing positional nystagmus, normal and symmetrical responses to bithermal caloric stimulation, disturbances of gait and balance may have a brain stem tumor with impingement on the:
A. vestibular nuclei
B. reticular formation
C. medial longitudinal fasciculus and long tracts
D. A plus C
E. A, B, C
REF. Makishima K, Ogata J: Ann Otol Rhinol Laryngol 84:391, May '75

341. Risk of complications by opening the internal auditory canal whether through the translabyrinthine or transvestibular route include:
A. increased risk of CSF leak
B. meningitis
C. facial nerve injury
D. intracranial hemorrhage
E. injury to the anterior-inferior cerebellar artery which is vital to the brain stem
REF. Glasscock, III ME: Ann Otol Rhinol Laryngol 84:403, May '75

342. All of the following members of the aminoglycoside group of antibiotics produce cochlear damage. Which one drug, although primarily vestibulotoxic, produces cochlear damage, even from topical application to thermal burns when the patients appeared to be within the range of safety by serum level monitoring of the drug?
A. gentamicin
B. dihydrostreptomycin
C. kanamycin
D. streptomycin
REF. Dayal VS, Whitehead GL, Smith EL: Can J Otolaryngol 4 (No. 2):348, No month '75

343. Strong solutions of which one of the following aminoglycoside group of antibiotics show vestibular and cochlear hair cell damage when instilled in the middle ears of cats?
A. streptomycin
B. dihydrostreptomycin
C. kanamycin
D. gentamicin
REF. Dayal VS, Whitehead GL, Smith EL: Can J Otolaryngol 4 (No. 2):348, No month '75

344. Serial facial nerve excitability tests (N.E.T.) in Bell's palsy have which of the following advantages?
A. easy to perform
B. objective and reliable
C. assists accurate prognosis
D. capable of differentiating between a physiological block of conduction, partial denervation, and complete destruction
E. detection of denervation more rapidly (72 hours) than an electromyogram (10-12 days)
REF. Leclaire R, Tremblay L, Dupuis M: Can J Otolaryngol 4 (No. 2):352, No month '75

345. The most common sympton in patients with medium-sized and large acoustic neuromas is:
A. tinnitus
B. vertigo
C. reduced facial sensitivity
D. reduced corneal sensitivity
E. hearing loss
REF. Thomsen J, Zilstorff K: Acta Otolaryngol 80:276, Sept '75

346. The most common symptoms in order of frequency in patients with medium-sized and large acoustic neuromas are:
A. tinnitus
B. vertigo
C. facial nerve paralysis
D. reduced corneal sensitivity
E. hearing loss
REF. Thomsen J, Zilstorff K: Acta Otolaryngol 80:276, Sept '75

347. Apart from VIII cranial nerve symptoms, the most significant evidence of medium-sized acoustic neuromas is in order of frequency:
A. defective nasolacrimal reflex
B. loss of corneal sensitivity
C. facial nerve motor dysfunction
D. reduced sensitivity of the posterior wall of the external auditory canal
E. loss of taste sensation of the anterior two-thirds of the tongue
REF. Thomsen J, Zilstorff K: Acta Otolaryngol 80:276, Sept '75

348. All of the following VIII cranial nerve symptoms occur in patients with large acoustic neuromas. Name the symptoms in order of frequency:
A. spontaneous nystagmus
B. abolished caloric reaction
C. decreased caloric reaction
D. anacusis
E. hearing loss
F. positional nystagmus
G. defective optokinetic nystagmus
REF. Thomsen J, Zilstorff K: Acta Otolaryngol 80:276, Sept '75

349. Most all of the following VIII cranial nerve symptoms occur in patients with medium-sized acoustic neuromas. Name the symptoms in order of frequency:
A. abolished caloric reaction
B. decreased caloric reaction
C. anacusis
D. hearing loss
E. spontaneous nystagmus
F. positional nystagmus
G. defective optokinetic nystagmus
REF. Thomsen J, Zilstorff K: Acta Otolaryngol 80:276, Sept '75

350. If the serial nerve excitability tests (N.E.T.) in Bell's palsy remain normal for 32 days after the onset of the paralysis, recovery should be complete within a period of:
A. two weeks
B. one month
C. two months
D. three months
E. six to nine months
REF. Leclaire R, Tremblay L, Dupuis M: Can J Otolaryngol 4 (No. 2):352, No month '75

351. Reversal of nystagmus direction during the same recording in the same position in electronystagmographic (ENG) findings indicates frequently:
A. acoustic neuroma
B. extensive vascular disease
C. multiple sclerosis
D. brain stem lesion
E. cerebellar pathology
REF. Spector M: Ann Otol Rhinol Laryngol 84:374, May '75

352. All of the following V and VII cranial nerve findings are diminished and occur in patients with large acoustic neuromas. Name the findings in order of frequency:
A. taste
B. corneal sensitivity
C. facial sensation
D. naso-lacrimal-reflex
REF. Thomsen J, Zilstorff K: Acta Otolaryngol 80:276, Sept '75

353. The pacinian corpsule is a pressure sensor (mechanoreceptor) commonly found in numerous parts of the body such as in the connective tissue near tendons and joints, external genitalia, etc. The middle ear corpuscles of von Troeltsch appear to be:
A. not true pacinian corpuscles
B. of unknown function
C. easily destroyed by inflammation and related to the absence of earache in chronic ear disease
D. related to the process of mesenchymal tissue resorption in the middle ear and mastoid because of their consistent absence in subjects less than six years of age
E. specialized nerve endings unique in the middle ear and mastoid and concerned with pressure sensation in these areas
REF. Lim D, Jackson D, Bennett J: Laryngoscope 85:1725, Oct '75

354. Histopathology of Ménière's disease (initially reported by Hallpike and Cairns) consists of:
A. endolymphatic hydrops
B. dilatation of the cochlear duct with displacement of Reissner's membrane into the scala vestibuli
C. dilatation of the saccula
D. frequent contact of the saccular membrane with the vestibular surface of the stapes footplate
E. dilatation involving the utricle mainly at its junction with the ampullae of the semicircular canals
REF. Wolfson RJ, Leiberman A: Laryngoscope 85:1762, Oct '75

355. Although there is some difference of opinion, profound unilateral sensorineural hearing loss as the initial symptom appears to be extremely rare in:
A. measles
B. mumps
C. viral infections
D. sudden hearing loss syndrome
E. Ménière's disease
REF. Wolfson RJ, Leiberman A: Laryngoscope 85:1762, Oct '75

356. Histopathologic changes in viral labyrinthitis are almost always confined to:
A. degeneration or destruction of the organ of Corti
B. A of the stria vascularis
C. A of the tectorial membrane
D. collapse of the cochlear duct
E. distension of the cochlear duct
REF. Wolfson RJ, Leiberman A: Laryngoscope 85:1762, Oct '75

357. All of the following V and VII cranial nerve findings are diminished and occur in patients with medium-sized neuromas. Name the findings in order of frequency:
A. taste loss
B. corneal sensitivity
C. facial sensation
D. naso-lacrinal-reflex
REF. Thomsen J, Zilstorff K: Acta Otolaryngol 80:276, Sept '75

358. The conchal setback operation is a simple and useful technique for correction of many prominent ear deformities. Disadvantages of this technique are:
A. meatal stenosis of the external auditory canal which cannot be prevented
B. A which can be prevented
C. external meatus is most significantly narrowed when the antihelix is most poorly developed
D. surgical correction of the meatal stenosis at the time of the setback operation is simply performed
E. D cannot be performed
REF. Small A: Laryngoscope 85:1782, Oct '75

359. Transtympanic cochleography is a powerful tool when all other tests fail in the detection of the presence or the absence of cochlear function in patients. The most pressing diagnostic problem and need for transtympanic cochleography is in a child below the age of two years with:
A. suspected but undiagnosed hearing loss
B. A plus rubella syndrome
C. A plus mental retardation
D. A plus aphasia
E. A plus autism
REF. Simmons FB: Laryngoscope 85:1564, Sept '75

360. Transtympanic cochleography with promontory recording of the N_1 response from normal and abnormal ears is superior to external auditory canal measurements of the N_1. Promontory recording is more hazardous than the use of ear canal electrodes because:
A. electrode can slip into the cochlea via the round window
B. A via the oval window
C. ossicles can be fractured
D. stapes can be dislodged into vestibule with sensorineural deafness
E. stapes can be dislodged against the facial nerve with paralysis
F. tympanic membrane perforations can develop
G. otitis media from infection
H. labyrinthitis from infection
REF. Simmons FB: Laryngoscope 85:1564, Sept '75

361. It has been suggested that rupture of the tympanic membrane during the positive phase of a blast might tend to lessen inner ear damage by reducing the efficiency of transmission through the middle ear. The human tympanic membrane ruptures at blast waves in db of:
A. 110
B. 130
C. 150
D. 170
E. 180
REF. Eames BL, Hamernik RP, Henderson D, Feldman A: Laryngoscope 85: 1582, Sept '75

362. Recurrent attacks of severe vertigo preceded by profound unilateral sensorineural deafness of undetermined etiology but most likely in most instances by viral labyrinthitis is best treated by:
A. valium
B. phenobarbital
C. dilantin sodium
D. dramamine
E. destructive labyrinthectomy
REF. Wolfson RJ, Leiberman A: Laryngoscope 85:1762, Oct '75

363. The reasons for uniformly deficient results following so-called successful repairs of traumatized facial nerve trunks regardless of the types of procedures and independent of the sites of the lesions are:
A. peripheral axons are arranged in a separate specific compartmental fashion
B. A are not
C. peripheral axons intermingle and are distributed among various bundles which together constitute the main trunk
D. C do not and are not
E. each bundle of peripheral axons represents one specific region of the face
F. E represents the whole face
REF. Sadé J: Ann Otol Rhinol Laryngol 84:695, Sept '75

364. What dose of streptomycin in g/day is indicated in a patient with severe bilateral Ménière's disease who is unable to work, realizing that some variation in dose might be needed depending upon the patient's response to therapy?
A. 0.5
B. 1.0
C. 2.0
D. 3.0
E. 4.0
REF. Fulk R, Schuknecht HF, Glasscock M: Ann Otol Rhinol Laryngol 84:704, Sept '75

365. Hearing improvement has been observed following treatment of Ménière's disease with:
A. endolymphatic sacotomy
B. section of the superior division of the vestibular nerve
C. fenestration of the lateral semicircular canal
D. streptomycin therapy
REF. Schuknecht HF: Ann Otol Rhinol Laryngol 84:704, Sept '75

366. The most effective functional results that can be expected of so-called successful surgical repairs of traumatized facial nerve trunks whether the procedures are end-to-end suture or grafting and independent of the sites of the lesions are:
A. excellent tonus at rest
B. ability to close the affected eye to a useful degree when the other eye is closed
C. some ability to close the affected eye in association with some mass action of the affected face
D. ability to produce a faint smile in a small proportion of patients
E. ability to move the corner of the mouth, to smile fully or to whistle
F. ability to move isolated groups of muscles as can a healthy person
REF. Sadé J: Ann Otol Rhinol Laryngol 84:695, Sept '75

367. Which one of the following methods of treatment is advisable in a patient with severe bilateral Ménière's disease who is unable to work?
A. bilateral endolymphatic sacotomies
B. bilateral vestibular nerve sections
C. bilateral endolymphatic shunt procedures
D. streptomycin therapy
E. vasodilators, steroids and anticoagulation therapy
REF. Fulk R, Schuknecht HF, Glasscock M: Ann Otol Rhinol Laryngol 84:704, Sept '75

368. The most likely diagnosis of a diffuse homogenous sclerotic process involving only the petrous and mastoid portions of the temporal bone is:
A. osteoma
B. meningioma
C. Paget's disease
D. monostotic fibrous dysplasia
E. osteopetrosis (marble bone disease)
REF. Fulk R, Weber A, Schuknecht HF: Ann Otol Rhinol Laryngol 84:704, Sept '75

369. Lesions that should be considered in the differential diagnosis of a diffuse, homogenous, sclerotic process involving the petrous and mastoid portions of the temporal bone are:
A. osteoma
B. meningioma
C. Paget's disease
D. osteopetrosis (marble bone disease)
E. Engleman's disease
F. Pyle's disease
G. monostotic fibrous dysplasia
H. polyostotic fibrous dysplasia
REF. Fulk R, Weber A, Schuknecht HF: Ann Otol Rhinol Laryngol 84:704, Sept '75

370. Meningioma usually:
A. involves the petrous temporal bone in a homogenous manner
B. A does not involve
C. is associated with osteolytic destruction
D. C is not
REF. Fulk R, Weber A, Schuknecht HF: Ann Otol Rhinol Laryngol 84:704, Sept '75

371. Paget's disease:
A. not uncommonly involves the petrous part of the temporal bone
B. is usually associated with diffuse involvement of the skull table
C. causes expansion of the involved bone

D. has poorly delineated and difficult to define anatomic structures such as the cochlea and internal auditory canal
E. D well delineated and easy to define
REF. Fulk R, Weber A, Schuknecht HF: Ann Otol Rhinol Laryngol 84:704, Sept '75

372. Which one of the following conditions sometimes causes recurrent facial palsy presumably because of narrowing of the facial canal?
A. osteoma
B. otosclerosis
C. meningioma
D. tympanosclerosis
E. osteopetrosis (marble bone disease)
REF. Fulk R, Weber A, Schuknecht HF: Ann Otol Rhinol Laryngol 84:704, Sept '75

373. Complications from paracentesis or the insertion of tympanostomy tubes have been:
A. persistent permanent perforations
B. suppurative otitis media
C. cholesteatoma
D. tympanosclerosis
E. attic retraction
F. necrosis long crus of the incus
G. displacement of the stapes from the incus
H. total deafness
I. incision of a high jugular bulb in a dehiscent bony floor of the middle ear with possible death
J. atelectasis of the tympanic membrane
K. mastoidectomy necessary
REF. Kokko E: Acta Otolaryngol (Suppl.) 327:13, No month '74

374. As a rule, tympanostomy tubes should be:
A. removed at three months
B. removed at six months
C. removed at nine months
D. removed after one year
E. allowed to be spontaneously extruded
REF. Kokko E: Acta Otolaryngol (Suppl.) 327:34, No month '74

375. Which of the following on the basis of protein and enzyme analyses of middle ear effusions shows levels equally high in the serum and middle ear?
A. alkaline phosphatase
B. lactate and malate dehydrogenase
C. acid phosphatase
D. asparate aminotransferase
E. alanine aminotransferase
F. nonspecific esterase
REF. Kokko E: Acta Otolaryngol (Suppl.) 327:11, No month '74

376. Following facial nerve injury, absence of lacrimation indicates nonfunction of which of the following nerves?
A. auditory
B. greater superficial petrosal
C. lesser superficial petrosal
D. Jacobson's
E. Arnold's
REF. Alford BR, Carder HM: Am Acad Ophthalmol Otolaryngol (Abs Acad Videotape) 1 (No. 7):1, No month '74

377. A facial nerve injury resulting in loss of taste in the anterior two-thirds of the tongue but not impairing the function of the stapedial reflex probably has its site of injury between:
A. internal auditory meatus and the Fallopian canal
B. internal auditory meatus and the stapedius branch
C. stapedius branch and the chorda tympani
D. stapedius branch and stylomastoid foramen
REF. Alford BR, Carder HM: Am Acad Ophthalmol Otolaryngol (Abs Acad Videotape) 1 (No. 7):2, No month '74

378. Herpes zoster oticus affects the facial nerve at the level of:
A. internal auditory meatus
B. geniculate ganglion
C. stapedius muscle
D. chorda tympani nerve
E. stylomastoid foramen
REF. Alford BR, Carder HM: Am Acad Ophthalmol Otolaryngol (Abs Acad Videotape) 1 (No. 7):2, No month '74

379. The distal portion of a completely severed facial nerve will retain its ability to conduct stimuli for:
A. 0 minutes (no conduction)
B. 15 minutes
C. one hour
D. three days
E. two weeks
REF. Alford BR, Carder HM: Am Acad Ophthalmol Otolaryngol (Abs Acad Videotape 1 (No. 7):2, No month '74

380. Which of the following factors may have an influence on the results of the Schirmer test?
A. failure to removed pooled tears prior to testing
B. failure to stimulate lacrimation with spirits of ammonia or similar substances
C. repeated blinking during the test period
D. use of atropine-like substances by the patient before testing
E. all of the above
REF. Alford BR, Carder HM: Am Acad Ophthalmol Otolaryngol (Abs Acad Videotape) 1 (No. 7):2, No month '74

381. In evaluating the electrogustometry test, electrical taste may be mediated in part by fibers of which one of the following cranial nerves?
A. Vth
B. IXth
C. Xth
D. XIth
E. XIIth
REF. Alford BR, Carder HM: Am Acad Ophthalmol Otolaryngol (Abs Acad Videotape) 1 (No. 7):2, No month '74

382. One of the major advantages of the submaxillary salivary gland secretion study is that it:
A. requires no special training to perform
B. may be performed quickly
C. causes no discomfort to the patient
D. may have some prognostic value in determining future nerve degeneration
E. has been shown as the most effective method of determining whether the nerve has undergone axonotmesis or neurotmesis
REF. Alford BR, Carder HM: Am Acad Ophthalmol Otolaryngol (Abs Acad Videotape) 1 (No. 7):8, No month '74

383. Surgical decompression of the facial nerve is indicated when facial nerve paralysis develops during:
A. acute otitis media
B. chronic otitis media when there is no immediate improvement with medical therapy
C. herpes zoster oticus

D. idiopathic Bell's palsy
E. scleroderma
REF. Alford BR, Carder HM: Am Acad Ophthalmol Otolaryngol (Abs Acad Videotape) 1 (No. 7):8, No month '74

384. Which portion of the facial nerve is injured when there is parlysis of the lower portion of the face but spares the forehead and eyebrow?
A. supranuclear
B. nuclear
C. cerebellopontine angle
D. internal auditory canal
E. horizontal (middle ear) portion above the oval window
REF. Alford BR, Carder HM: Am Acad Ophthalmol Otolaryngol (Abs Acad Videotape) 1 (No. 7):1, No month '74

385. Which of the following conditions can cause facial nerve paralysis?
A. diabetes mellitus
B. sarcoidosis
C. metastatic disease to the temporal bone
D. subclinical disseminated collagen disease
E. all of the above
REF. Alford BR, Carder HM: Am Acad Ophthalmol Otolaryngol (Abs Acad Videotape) 1 (No. 7):9, No month '74

386. One of the most common problems following stapedectomy is fluctuating hearing which may be caused by:
A. fistula of oval window
B. secondary endolymphatic hydrops
C. vestibular infection (labyrinthitis)
D. vestibular granuloma
E. loose prosthesis on crus of incus
REF. Schuknecht HF, Sheehy J, Fulk R, Kiang N, Silverstein H: Ann Otol Rhinol Laryngol 84:704, Sept '75

387. The etiology of secretory otitis media is unclear and neither the hydrops ex vacuo theory nor the infection theory explain adequately the pathogenesis of this condition. Synonyms used in secretory otitis media are:
A. serous otitis media
B. adhesive otitis media
C. otosalpingitis
D. tubotympanitis
E. hydrotympanum
F. glue ear
REF. Kokko E: Acta Otolaryngol (Suppl.) 327:11, No month '74

388. The effusion in chronic secretory otitis media may show bacteria or be sterile. Sterility may be attributed to:
A. viral etiology (RS viruses)
B. bactericidal and bacteriostatic effect of middle ear effusion (IgA secreted by the mucous glands)
C. B but IgE secreted
D. previous antibiotic therapy
E. proof that the pathogenesis of this condition may be partly due to the hydrops ex vacuo theory
REF. Kokko E: Acta Otolaryngol (Suppl.) 327:10, No month '74

389. Ménière's disease is characterized by:
A. vertigo, which is often accompanied by nausea and vomiting
B. vertigo without any nausea
C. tinnitus
D. fluctuating hearing loss
E. progressive hearing loss without fluctuation
F. pressure or fullness in the involved ear
G. usually occurring in patients of middle age (30 to 50 years)
REF. Wolfson RJ, Leiberman A: Laryngoscope 85:1762, Oct '75

390. Of patients with complete Bell's paralysis and no response to serial nerve excitability tests (N.E.T.), what percent show an unsatisfactory recovery?
A. 31
B. 48
C. 69
D. 73
E. 100
REF. Leclaire R, Tremblay L, Dupuis M: Can J Otolaryngol 4 (No. 2):352, No month '75

391. Numerous hypotheses concerning the pathogenesis of otosclerosis have been proposed but which of the following beliefs are generally accepted?
A. destruction of enchondral bone mediated by osteocytes and osteoclasts
B. formation of immature basophilic bone
C. repetition of the remodeling process of resorption and new bone formation which becomes highly mineralized and acidophilic having a mosaic-like appearance
D. otosclerosis develops in predilected areas of the temporal bone and stapes
E. implication of genetic factors
REF. Lim DJ, Saunders WH: Acta Otolaryngol 80:255, Sept '75

392. Otoconia in man and other mammals have which of the following characteristics?
A. consist of crystalline calcium carbonate in the form of calcite
B. consist of calcim phosphate as the complex salt carbonite-apatite
C. embedded in the otolithic membrane
D. C not embedded
E. form a separate crystalline layer loosely held together by an unidentified organic substance
F. there is a definite loss and renewal of the otoconia
REF. Preston RE, Johnsson L-G, Hill JH, Schacht J: Acta Otolaryngol 80: 269, Sept '75

393. "Cupulolithiasis" is a term suggested by Schuknecht to indicate a form of disequilibrium due to:
A. dislodgement of otoconia in the saccule
B. dislodgement of utricular otoconia into the posterior ampulla
C. inflammation of the otolithic membrane in the saccule
D. C in the utricle
E. C plus D
REF. Preston RE, Johnsson L-G, Hill JH, Schacht J: Acta Otolaryngol 80: 269, Sept '75

394. Any patient with unilateral sensorineural hearing loss of undetermined origin should have ruled out:
A. otitis media
B. otosclerosis
C. acoustic neurinoma
D. drug toxicity
E. Ménière's disease
REF. Thomsen J, Zilstorff K: Acta Otolaryngol 80:276, Sept '75

395. Which of the following conditions should be considered in a patient with an excellent result from a stapedectomy for 11 years but develops sudden hearing loss and decrease in discrimination with a scratchy vibrating sensation?
A. fistula oval window
B. fistula round window
C. partial incus necrosis
D. loose prosthesis with acoustic distortion and poor discrimination
E. loose prosthesis with sound waves causing the wire to make a noise against the incus
REF. Belal A, Wehrs R, Robinson M, Sheehy J, Fulk R, Kiang N, Silverstein H, Schuknecht HF: Ann Otol Rhinol Laryngol 84:704, Sept '75

396. Experimental cochlear hair cell damage with hearing loss results from:
A. excessive noise
B. large doses of ototoxic antibiotic drugs
C. kanamycin in toxic doses
D. noise and kanamycin combined when safe in doses by themselves
REF. Dayal VS, Barek WG: Laryngoscope 85 (Suppl. 1):8, Nov '75

397. Experiments show definite damaging effects of noise with kanamycin. Results indicate:
A. some vulnerability to such damage in the apical section of the cochlea
B. more damage toward the base starting about one-third of the way from the apex of the cochlea
C. maximum area of damage is in the area of greater noise intensity
D. apical lesions are difficult to explain but this region may represent a metabolically more vulnerable part of the cochlea
E. mechanism by which potentiation of noise and kanamycin develops has been determined
REF. Dayal VS, Barek WG: Laryngoscope 85 (Suppl. 1):11, Nov '75

398. Experimental and pathologic studies of hair cell changes as a result of aging indicate:
A. initial changes start in the outer hair cells at the apex and with increasing age extend further basally
B. A start in the inner hair cells
C. more basal changes have been reported in humans compared with animals
D. early audiometric changes in humans occur in the high tones and may be due to ambient environmental noise and not aging
E. hair cells are only one of several cochlear areas involved in aging
REF. Dayal VS, Barek WG: Laryngoscope 85 (Suppl. 1):17, Nov '75

399. Osteoma in the temporal bone is usually limited to:
A. external auditory canal
B. middle ear
C. mastoid
D. outer table
E. squamosal portion of temporal bone
REF. Fulk R, Weber A, Schuknecht HF: Ann Otol Rhinol Laryngol 84:704, Sept '75

400. Which of the following electronystagmographic (ENG) findings indicate central nervous system disease?
A. dysrhythmia with eyes closed
B. directional preponderance
C. reversal of nystagmus direction during same recording in the same position
D. hyperexcitability on a caloric test with eyes closed
E. consistent nystagmus in the presence of normal calorics
REF. Spector M: Ann Otol Rhinol Laryngol 84:374, May '75

401. Consistent nystagmus with normal calorics in electronystagmogrphic (ENG) findings may indicate:
A. central lesion
B. Ménière's disease
C. acoustic neuroma
D. vestibular neuronitis
E. multiple sclerosis
REF. Spector M: Ann Otol Rhinol Laryngol 84:374, May '75

402. Calibration overshoots in electronystagmographic (ENG) findings indicate:
A. intracranial arteriosclerosis
B. a central lesion
C. acoustic neuroma
D. multiple sclerosis
E. vestibular neuronitis
REF. Spector M: Ann Otol Rhinol Laryngol 84:374, May '75

403. A left beating nystagmus eyes open and a right beating nystagmus eyes closed by electronystagmographic (ENG) findings indicate:
A. acoustic neuroma
B. extensive vascular disease
C. multiple sclerosis
D. brain stem lesion
E. cerebellar pathology
REF. Spector M: Ann Otol Rhinol Laryngol 84:374, May '75

404. Rebound nystagmus accompanied by enhanced caloric responses and deranged optokinetic nystagmus in electronystagmogrphic (ENG) findings indicate:
A. acoustic neuroma
B. extensive vascular disease
C. multiple sclerosis
D. brain stem lesion
E. chronic cerebellar disease
REF. Spector M: Ann Otol Rhinol Laryngol 84:374, May '75

405. Assessment of eustachian tube function indicates:
A. open in its resting state
B. A closed
C. unequal air pressure on each side of the tympanic membrane causes a sensation of fullness or discomfort relieved by swallowing or yawning
D. Valsalva maneuver creates a positive middle ear pressure
E. D negative
F. Toynbee maneuver creates either a positive or negative middle ear pressure
G. F negative
REF. Williams PS: Ann Otol Rhinol Laryngol 84:339, May '75

406. Osteogenesis imperfecta congenita (Lobstein's disease, fragilitas ossium) is manifested by:
A. fragile, thin stapedial crura and long bones
B. blue sclerae
C. ears appearing to bend outward by a supraaural prominence due to numerous islands of membranous bone in the skull
D. infant being usually stillborn
E. D not usually stillborn
REF. Zajtchuk JT, Lindsay JR: Ann Otol Rhinol Laryngol 84:350, May '75

407. Osteogenesis imperfecta tarda (van der Hoeve's syndrome) is characterized by:
A. blue sclerae
B. fragile bones including stapedial crura
C. deafness characteristic of otosclerosis with footplate fixation with secondary labyrinthine changes in advanced cases
D. C hearing impairment not always progressive
E. onset of deafness may occur during the second and third decades of life
REF. Zajtchuk JT, Lindsay JR: Ann Otol Rhinol Laryngol 84:350, May '75

408. Pathology in the temporal bone in osteogenesis imperfecta congenita (Lobstein's disease, fragilitas ossium) shows:
A. occasional preservation of unusual large remnants of cartilage with many intact cartilage cells during ossification
B. generalized but variable delay in the deposition of the skein-like bone in the endochondrial layer and a paucity and delay in the periosteal bone formation with fragility of the stapedial crura
C. deficient deposition of bone with fragility and paucity of the septae in the air-cell system or marrow spaces
D. scarcity of osteoblasts with some irregularity in their size and shape in both the endochondral and periosteal layers
E. occasional concretions in the stria vascularis
F. E observed in several types of genetic disorders but most frequently in renal insufficiency
REF. Zajtchuk JT, Lindsay JR: Ann Otol Rhinol Laryngol 84:350, May '75

409. Experimentally induced hydrops by ablation of the endolymphatic sac in guinea pigs is histopathologically similar to human hydrops in Ménière's disease. Which of the following changes have appeared following blockage of endolymphatic ducts in guinea pigs?
A. increase in sodium concentration in the endolymph
B. normal sodium but increased potassium concentration in the endolymph
C. high protein concentration in the endolymphatic sac fluid compared to that in the cochlear and vestibular endolymph
D. it is certain that disturbances in endolymph osmolarity occur before distention of the endolymphatic wall
E. D secondary to distention of the endolymphatic wall
REF. Kimura RS, Schuknecht HF: Ann Otol Rhinol Laryngol 84:271, May '75

410. Endolymph biochemical studies in humans with Ménière's disease showed concentrations of:
A. increased sodium
B. decreased sodium
C. increased potassium
D. decreased potassium
E. normal sodium, potassium and total proteins
REF. Kimura RS, Schuknecht HF: Ann Otol Rhinol Laryngol 84:271, May '75

411. Intermixing of the cochlear fluids without blockage of the endolymphatic duct is known to:
A. abolish the microphonic response
B. A not abolish
C. produce localized atrophy of the sensory cells
D. C not produce atrophy
E. not affect the population of the cochlear sensory cells nor the position of Reissner's membrane when fistulae were created in the saccule (experimental in squirrel monkeys and cats)
REF. Kimura RS, Schuknecht HF: Ann Otol Rhinol Laryngol 84:271, May '75

412. Experimental hydrops in the utricle, semicircular canal and ampulla is generally moderate and hardly demonstrable but severe in the saccule and cochlear duct due probably to:
A. difference in the thickness of the epithelial cells of Reissner's membrane and of the semicircular canal, etc.
B. difference in thickness of the subepithelial connective tissue fibrils in utricle, semicircular canal and ampulla
C. B and also supported by a trabecular meshwork of fibrocytes and fibrils reaching the endosteal layer
D. utriculo-endolymphatic valve
E. difference in size in the utricular and saccular ducts
REF. Kimura RS, Schuknecht HF: Ann Otol Rhinol Laryngol 84:271, May '75

413. A red or white round soft-tissue mass which may or may not pulsate behind an intact tympanic membrane (microscopic otoscopy), confined throughout the middle ear with absence of the normal proximal carotid artery canal and with an anomalous artery entering the temporal bone between a dehiscent area on the floor of the posterior part of the middle ear between the jugular fossae and the vertical segment of the facial nerve (tomographically), and with a narrowing of the carotid at the base of the skull (arteriography), is most likely:
A. glomus jugulare
B. high jugular bulb
C. aberrant or ectopic carotid artery
D. cholesterol granuloma
E. glomus tympanicum
REF. Valvassori GE, Buckingham RA: Ann Otol Rhinol Laryngol 83:606, Sept '74

414. A red-purple soft-tissue mass behind an intact tympanic membrane (microscopic otoscopy) eroding the floor of the middle ear and extending into the mastoid cells (tomographically) and obstructing the jugulare vein (retrograde jugular venography) and delineating the feeding vessels (subtraction arteriography) is most likely:
A. glomus jugulare
B. high jugular bulb
C. aberrant or ectopic carotid artery
D. cholesterol granuloma
E. glomus tympanicum
REF. Valvassori GI, Buckingham RA: Ann Otol Rhinol Laryngol 83:606, Sept '74

415. A vascular mass in the middle ear behind an intact tympanic membrane is usually:
A. glomus jugulare
B. high jugular bulb
C. aberrant or ectopic carotid artery
D. cholesterol granuloma
E. glomus tympanicum
REF. Valvassori GI, Buckingham RA: Ann Otol Rhinol Laryngol 83:606, Sept '74

416. The percent of failures of medical treatment in Ménière's disease is approximately:
A. 7
B. 11
C. 25
D. 33
E. 57
REF. Gardner G: South Med J 68:611, May '75

417. "Otitis prone" patient has been described as a child who has six or more episodes of otitis media before the age of six years. Which of the following two factors appear to favor otitis proneness?
A. onset of the first attack of otitis media during the first year of life
B. A after the first year of life
C. infection with staphylococcus (coagulase-positive)
D. C with alpha streptococcus
E. C with pneumococcus
REF. Hussey HH: JAMA 233:274, July '75

418. Acupuncture studies indicate:
A. no value in the treatment of sensorineural hearing loss
B. acupuncture "anesthesia" is not anesthesia
C. acupuncture "anesthesia" is not analgesia
D. acupuncture "anesthesia" is hypalgesia
E. acupuncture "anesthesia" is "natural surgery"
REF. Madell JR: ORL Digest 37:22, July '75; Traub A: Med World News 16: 41, July '75

419. Which of the following must usually be biopsied through an exploratory tympanotomy in order to establish a diagnosis?
A. glomus jugulare
B. high jugulare bulb
C. aberrant or ectopic carotid artery
D. cholesterol granuloma
E. glomus tympanicum
REF. Valvassori GE, Buckingham RA: Ann Otol Rhinol Laryngol 83:606, Sept '74

420. A red-purple, soft-tissue mass behind an intact tympanic membrane (microscopic otoscopy) and confined to the middle ear without erosion of the middle ear floor and without mastoid changes of chronic infection (tomographically) is most likely:
A. glomus jugulare
B. high jugular bulb
C. aberrant or ectopic carotid artery
D. cholesterol granuloma
E. glomus tympanicum
REF. Valvassori GE, Buckingham RA: Ann Otol Rhinol Laryngol 83:606, Sept '74

421. A red-purple, soft-tissue mass behind an intact tympanic membrane (microscopic otoscopy) confined to the middle ear without erosion of the middle ear floor but with evidence of chronic mastoid disease (tomographically) is most likely:
A. glomus jugulare
B. high jugular bulb
C. aberrant or ectopic carotid artery
D. cholesterol granuloma
E. glomus tympanicum
REF. Valvassori GF, Buckingham RA: Ann Otol Rhinol Laryngol 83:606, Sept '74

422. Which of the following findings by Palva, et al. indicate that middle ear effusion cannot be a transudate but must result from active secretion since middle ear effusion shows considerable higher levels of:
A. alkaline phosphatase levels
B. lactate and malate dehydrogenase
C. acid phosphatase
D. asparate aminotransferase
E. alanine aminotransferase
F. nonspecific esterase
REF. Kokko E: Acta Otolaryngol (Suppl.) 327:11, No month '74

423. The most common bacteria in chronic secretory otitis media in order of frequency are:
A. pseudomonas aeruginosa
B. hemophilus influenzae
C. staphylococcus aureus
D. Neisseria catarrhalis
E. staphylococcus albus
REF. Kokko E: Acta Otolaryngol (Suppl.) 327:18, No month '74

424. Which of the following, on the basis of protein and enzyme analyses of middle ear effusions, show levels in the serum higher than in the middle ear effusion?
A. alkaline phosphatase
B. lactate and malate dehydrogenase
C. acid phosphatase
D. asparate aminotransferase
E. alanine aminotransferase
F. nonspecific esterase
REF. Kokko E: Acta Otolaryngol (Suppl.) 327:11, No month '74

425. Facial nerve neuromas may appear with:
A. vague pain without facial paralysis
B. A with facial paralysis
C. parotid mass
D. symptoms and signs of acoustic tumors
E. Bell's palsy (sudden onset)
F. electric excitability for years
G. electromyographic recovery from degeneration
H. clinical recovery from degeneration
REF. Neely JG, Alford BR: Arch Otolaryngol 100:298, Oct '74

426. Roentgenographic study of temporal bones by the Stenvers approach in otosclerosis can show otosclerotic changes in the region of the:
A. oval window
B. cochlear capsule
C. semicircular canals
D. internal auditory meatus
E. none of these
REF. Gukovich VA, Rosenfeld LG: Arch Otolaryngol 99:281, Apr '74

427. A study of the incidence of diagnosed clinical otosclerosis showed:
A. higher incidence rate in females
B. A in males
C. incidence rates in both sexes peaked at ages 39-49 years
D. C at ages 29-48
E. C at ages 19-28
REF. Pearson RD, Kurland LT, Cody DTR: Arch Otolaryngol 99:288, Apr '74

428. Blue mantles in otosclerosis:
A. occur in the region of the semicircular canals in diffuse otosclerosis
B. A in the cochlear capsule
C. A in the outer periphery of otosclerotic foci
D. are a precursor of otosclerosis
E. are a sign of susceptibility of the deep layer of the otic capsule to the genetic disorder of which otosclerosis is a focal manifestation
REF. Lindsay JR: Ann Otol Rhinol Laryngol 83:33, Jan '74

429. Ultrastructure studies of the middle ear mucosa in tympanosclerosis show:
A. degenerative changes in the epithelium
B. degenerative changes in the subepithelial mucosa
C. that the pathogenesis remains partly obscure
D. mucous glands may be absent
E. lamina propria may be thickened with only a few cells and show an increase in collagen fibers and hyaline degeneration
REF. Tos M, Bak-Pedersen K: J Laryngol Otol 88:119, Feb '74

430. Experimental studies using cochlear microphonic (CM) voltage in guinea pigs indicate that employees exposed to noise (80-93 decibels):
A. can develop hearing loss
B. cannot develop hearing loss
C. can retain an adaptive capacity
D. have the greatest loss at 2,000 and 6,000 Hz
E. can with ototoxic drug intake, especially during exposure to noise, predispose ears to damage with industrial noise
REF. Krochmalska E: Acta Otolaryngol 77:44, Jan '74

431. Acoustic reflex using the elctroacoustic impedance bridge in eighth nerve disorders indicates that:
A. it may fail to diagnose tumors in the retrocochlear area
B. the success ratio is relatively high
C. the success ratio is so low that it is a useless procedure
D. it is a valuable weapon in the clinician's armamentarium
E. only acoustic neuromas can be diagnosed
REF. Jerger J, Harford E, Clemis J, Alford B: Arch Otolaryngol 99:409, June '74

432. Central hearing disorders due to injuries in the central hearing pathways and auditory cortex:
A. can be demonstrated by ordinary tone audiometry
B. A cannot
C. cannot be demonstrated by ordinary speech audiometry

D. may be revealed in the early stages of disease by distorted speech audiometry
E. cannot be diagnosed by distorted speech audiometry as a valid specific diagnostic test
REF. Korsan-Bengtsen M: Acta Otolaryngol (Suppl.):310, '73

433. Transmeatal suction clearance has long been used for chronic ear disease followed by topical application of medication such as 13 percent aluminum acetate, nystatin powder for fungus infection or tri-adcortyl ointment for infected, fissured or crusted canals and otosporin or gentian drops for moist canals or mastoid cavities. Transmeatal suction followed by medication is most successful in patients with:
A. attic cholesteatoma
B. postero-superior quadrant cholesteatoma
C. mixed A and B
D. central perforations
E. keratosis obturans
REF. Cronin J, Dogra TS, Khan IA: J Laryngol Otol 88:113, Feb '74

434. Destructive labyrinthectomy is an operation of last recourse and is usually contraindicated:
A. in a deaf ear with persistent vertigo
B. in a deaf ear with persistent tinnitus
C. in a deaf ear with pressure sensation
D. in a deaf ear with distortion of sound
E. when the opposite ear is devoid of caloric vestibular function
REF. Pulec JL: Laryngoscope 84:1552, Sept '74

435. Which one of the following operative procedures appears to give the most complete relief from vertigo, tinnitus, pressure or distortion of sound in a deaf ear?
A. transcanal labyrinthectomy with destruction of the utricle
B. post-auricular labyrinthectomy
C. translabyrinthine section of the eighth nerve
D. decompression of the endolymphatic sac
E. transcanal labyrinthectomy with destruction of the utricle (and saccule) and contents of the semicircular canals with a right-angled hook
REF. Pulec JL: Laryngoscope 84:1552, Sept '74

436. Deafness due to ototoxic drug concentration in patients with renal failure and due to hemodialysis and kidney transplantation may be due to:
A. immunologic factors (possible immunological relationship between the stria vascularis and the glomerular tubule of the kidney)
B. electrolyte imbalance due to hemodialysis with changes in the biochemical nature of inner ear fluids
C. vascular injury
D. ototoxic drug effects
E. osmotic changes due to recurrent hemodialysis
REF. Oda M, Preciado MC, Quick CA, Paparella MM: Laryngoscope 84:1489, Sept '74

437. Screening tests for deafness during the neonatal period (0-2 months) are:
A. dependent upon monitoring facial and eye muscle activity due to intense sound stimulation ("Moro's reflex", "quasi-Moro's reflex", "auropalpebral reflex", "arousal reflex", "cessation reflex")
B. tests delivered to each ear separately
C. tests delivered (sound field) to both ears at the same time
D. responses elicited in sound pressure levels ranging from 50 to 115 db with an average response of around 77 db SPL
E. mass neonatal screening recommended and it is not necessary to formulate a special high-risk category of patients with genetic syndromes
REF. Adams DM III, Istre CO, JR.: South Med J 68:605, May '75

438. Which of the following conditions can mimic Ménière's disease?
A. acoustic neurinoma
B. otosclerosis
C. otitis media, transudative or secretory
D. Lues
E. food allergy
REF. Gardner G: South Med J 68:611, May '75

439. Serial tympanometry shows systematic changes during progression in serous otitis media from types:
A. A to A to A
B. A to C to B
C. B to A to A
D. A to C to A
E. C to A to A
REF. Lewis N, Dugdale A, Canty A, Jerger J: Arch Otolaryngol 101:722, Dec '75

440. Serial tympanometry shows systematic changes during remission in serous otitis media from types:
A. A to C to B
B. B to B to B
C. C to C to C
D. B to C to A
E. C to B to B
REF. Lewis N, Dugdale A, Canty A, Jerger J: Arch Otolaryngol 101:722, Dec '75

441. Ménière's disease is a disorder of the membranous inner ear with endolymphatic hydrops due to fluid-producing dilatation of the endolymphatic system. Clinically, it is characterized by:
A. recurrent attacks of vertigo
B. sensorineural (nerve type) hearing loss, progressive without fluctuation
C. B but with fluctuation
D. tinnitus (always)
E. tinnitus (usually)
REF. Gardner G: South Med J 68:611, May '75

442. Patients with Ménière's disease appear to have:
A. frequent high hematocrits
B. high cholesterol levels at times
C. low mortality rates
D. potential latent chemical diabetes
E. improvement with a safe, long-acting vasodilating drug or drugs-papaverine, concentrated liquid nicotinic acid, histamine
REF. Turner JS, Jr., Saunders AZ, Per-lee JH: Laryngoscope 83:1816, Nov '73

443. Which one of the following disturbed structures by itself does not appear to cause nystagmus?
A. anterior semicircular canal
B. posterior semicircular canal
C. horizontal semicircular canal
D. utricle
REF. Fluur E, Siegborn J: Acta Otolaryngol 76:438, Dec '73

444. The relatively high incidence of cochlear otosclerosis as a cause of progressive, hereditary sensorineural hearing loss has been substantiated by strontium-85 studies and histological evaluation of footplates removed before and after treatment with:
A. tetracycline
B. irradiation
C. corticosteroids
D. sodium fluoride
E. hormones
REF. House HP, Linthicum FH, Jr.: Arch Otolaryngol 100:427, Dec '74

445. Tests for deafness in the young child (2 to 5 years) are:
A. tests for identification
B. tests to determine the extent of the loss
C. conditional play audiometry (pegboard, various toys)
D. speech reception threshold testing (picture spondees)
E. use of amplification with a hearing aid on a rental-purchase arrangement even when auditory input is questionable to determine any improvement in language and speech development
REF. Adams DN III, Istre CO, Jr.: South Med J 68:605, May '75

446. Tests for deafness during the infantile period (4 to 24 months) are:
A. tests based more upon localization and distractability
B. uncalibrated noise makers such as cowbells, snappers, and toy telephones often used in office evaluation
C. noise makers which produce frequencies below and above the prominent audible frequency
D. C but frequencies which are within the usual speech range
E. based on conditioned orientation reflex (Cor) with pure tone signals presented in a sound field for the speech frequencies and helpful in children with delayed language development
F. averaged evoked audiometry which is very accurate as an objective test
G. impedance audiometry which is probably most objective of all procedures
REF. Adams DM III, Istre CO, Jr.: South Med J 68:605, May '75

447. An adult patient had a facial paralysis immediately following surgery. The lower court declared the surgeon liable but the appellate court's decision was "no" because:
A. surgeon stated the paralysis was due to anesthesia and would recover
B. second operation by another surgeon revealed a severed nerve
C. clear evidence of considerable necrosis of bone and an unavoidable accident
D. first surgeon was negligent in not referring patient for second operation immediately after the paralysis
E. testimony indicated good surgical practice required waiting period to allow complete healing of the original infection before second operation should be performed
REF. Redden K, Frankel C: ORL Digest 37:31, Mar '75

448. Which of the following triad of symptoms are most significant in otogenic cerebellar abscess?
A. vomiting
B. apathy
C. restlessness
D. vertigo with central nystagmus
E. headache in the posterior cranial fossa on the diseased side
REF. Majer EH: ORL Digest 37:11, July '75

449. The otogenic extradural (epidural) or perisinuous abscess rarely causes symptoms but suspicious symptoms and signs include:
A. nightly hemialgia
B. seriously ill appearance
C. paralysis
D. cramps
E. cerebral irritation
REF. Majer EH: ORL Digest 37:11, July '75

450. Whenever there is suspicion of otogenic brain abscess, which of the following investigations are indicated?
A. E.E.G.
B. scintigraphy
C. angiography
D. ventriculography
REF. Majer EH: ORL Digest 37:11, July '75

451. In the treatment of vertigo, one must remember that phenobarbital can:
A. increase dizziness
B. increase drowsiness
C. increase unsteadiness
D. decrease level of arousal
E. decrease awareness of surroundings and orientation in space
REF. Eviator L, Eviator A: Emergency Med 7:167, June '75

452. The vestibular pathways are coordinated in the:
A. anterior superior portion of the temporal lobe
B. reticular formation
C. frontal lobe
D. parietal lobe
E. occipital lobe
REF. Eviator L, Eviator A: Emergency Med 7:167, June '75

453. Post-traumatic vertigo has:
A. normal responses to torsion swing stimulation
B. normal responses to bithermal labyrinthine stimulation
C. abnormal positional nystagmus on electronystagmography (ENG)
D. abnormal electroencephalogram tracings
E. excellent response to phenobarbital
REF. Eviator L, Eviator A: Emergency Med 7:167, June '75

454. The treatment for post-traumatic vertigo is:
A. phenobarbital
B. methylphenidate (ritalin)
C. meclizine (antivert)
D. primidone (mysoline) starting with 50 mg three times daily increasing to 250 mg
E. dimenhydrinate (dramamine) in a daily dose of 5 mg/kg
REF. Eviator L, Eviator A: Emergency Med 7:167, June '75

455. The cortical representation for the vestibular system is in the temporal lobe in the:
A. anterior superior portion
B. anterior inferior portion
C. mid portion
D. posterior superior portion
E. posterior inferior portion
REF. Eviator L, Eviator A: Emergency Med 7:167, June '75

456. Vestibular neuronitis is distinguished by:
A. acute onset of vertigo with nausea and is a self-limiting condition
B. loss of postural control without loss of consciousness
C. labyrinthine preponderance on bithermal caloric stimulation tests with normal electronystagmogram (ENG)
D. exacerbation of vertigo with phenobarbital
E. control of vertigo with dimenhydrinate
REF. Eviator L, Eviator A: Emergency Med 7:167, June '75

457. The treatment for vestibular neuronitis is:
A. phenobarbital
B. methylphenidate (ritalin)
C. meclizine (antivert)
D. primidone (mysoline) starting with 50 mg three times daily increasing to 250 mg
E. dimenhydrinate (dramamine) in a daily dose of 5 mg/kg
REF. Eviator L, Eviator A: Emergency Med 7:167, June '75

458. Congenital cholesteatomata take origin from displaced epithelial rests present at birth and occur in the temporal bone in the following sites:
A. petrous apex
B. mastoid
C. middle ear
D. both middle ear and mastoid
E. external auditory canal
REF. Peron DL, Schuknecht HF: Arch Otolaryngol 101:498, Aug '75

459. Which of the following conditions or substances have a profound effect on both the inner ear and kidney?
A. Alport disease
B. diabetes mellitus
C. aminoglycoside antibiotics
D. ethacrinic acid
E. furosemide
F. potassium bromate
G. concomitant developmental anomalies of the ears and kidneys
REF. Quick CA, Chole RA, Mauer M: Arch Otolaryngol 101:494, Aug '75

460. Potassium bromate ($KBrO_3$) is used as a neutralizer for permanent waving solutions in hair styling and as a preservative in making bread; toxic doses can cause deafness most likely due to vacuolization of the:
A. inner hair cells
B. outer hair cells
C. Henson's cells
D. Deiter's cells
E. stria vascularis
REF. Quick CA, Chole RA, Mauer M: Arch Otolaryngol 101:494, Aug '75

461. Although all of the following have been reported, dehiscence of the bony otic capsule between the perilymphatic space and middle ear-mastoid complex with resulting fistulae occurs most commonly as a sequel of:
A. temporal bone fracture
B. otologic trauma other than A
C. syphilitic osteitis of the bony capsule
D. tuberculous otitis media
E. chronic otitis media
F. neoplastic process
G. congenital fistulae of the stapedial footplate
H. cholesteatoma
I. partial labyrinthine agenesis with fistula
J. poststapedectomy fistula
REF. Smith RR, Lowe JT, Farmer JC: Arch Otolaryngol 101:490, Aug '75

462. Which of the following side-effects occur in the use of hydroxychloroquine in the treatment of rheumatoid arthritis?
A. vertigo (positional)
B. minor neuropsychiatric disturbances
C. ototoxicity
D. headache
E. nausea
REF. Prince DS, Hardin JG: JAMA 233:984, Sept '75

463. Experimental recordings from chorda tympani nerves indicate which of the following animals do not have any taste for water?
A. rabbit
B. cat
C. dog
D. rhesus monkey
E. man
F. rat
REF. Diamant H: Trans Am Acad Ophthalmol Otolaryngol 80:ORL-362, July '75

464. Nondivided, even though stretched, chorda tympani nerves following stapes surgery regain their functions in the following percent of patients:
A. none
B. 10-20
C. 30-40
D. 70-80
E. 100
REF. Diamant H: Trans Am Acad Ophthalmol Otolaryngol 80:ORL-362, July '75

465. Primary cholesteatomas of the petrous apex require a choice of the following surgical procedures:
A. exteriorization via a mastoid approach
B. exteriorization via a translabyrinthine approach
C. transsphenoid approach
D. tympanomastoidectomy
E. canal plasty with mastoidectomy
REF. Peron DL, Schuknecht HF: Arch Otolaryngol 101:498, Aug '75

466. A four-year-old boy hospitalized with pneumonia and otitis media for at least the fifth occasion has an electropherogram showing absence of gamma globulin and a history indicating a congenital sex-linked agammaglobulinemia. Which of the following statements relating to his condition are true?
A. infections usually start within the first nine months of life
B. infections are usually caused by gram-negative organisms
C. infections caused by pyogenic organisms are frequent
D. does not tolerate viral infections well
E. usually has negative skin tests to antigens such as candida, trichophytin, PPD, streptokinase, and mumps
F. rheumatoid arthritis - like syndrome observed (in 50 percent of these patients usually disappears with replacement therapy)
REF. Graf MW: Modern Med 43:134, Mar '75, Samter M (Editor): Immunologic diseases, 2nd Ed., Little, Brown & Co., Boston, pp. 499-503, 1971

467. Which of the following are major causes of otitis media and sinus infection but are uncommon as pathogens associated with simple pharyngotonsillitis?
A. haemophilus influenzae
B. diplococcus pneumoniae
C. streptococcus pyogenes
D. staphylococcus aureus
E. adenovirus
REF. Klein JO: Ann Otol Rhinol Laryngol 84 (Suppl. 19):30, Mar '75

468. The elimination of bacterial pathogens (streptococcus pyogenes) from the oropharynx in the treatment of tonsillitis and/or otitis media by an adenotonsillectomy is:
A. temporary
B. consistent for up to five years
C. evident in rheumatic fever patients
D. of probable value in viral-bacterial and bacterial-bacterial synergistic infections
E. the proven method by substantive data to reduce the incidence or severity of recurrent infections of the oropharynx or ears of children
REF. Sprinkle PM: Ann Otol Rhinol Laryngol 84 (Suppl. 19):25, Mar '75

469. Electrocochleography appears to be emerging as the best and most accurate objective measurement of cochlear function and:
A. ear canal electrodes is the easiest and most accurate method of placing recording electrodes
B. transtympanic technic is better than A above
C. typical canal recording has a threshold 40 db higher than typical promontory recording
D. canal and promontory recordings are the same
E. cochleography is performed in a highly select group of children when behavior audiometry and evoked response audiometry are equivocal
REF. Simmons FB: Ann Otol Rhinol Laryngol 83:312, May '74

470. Which of the following should be considered in the treatment of otitis externa?
A. insufflation of sulfonamide powder may be iatrogenic
B. patch tests (contact dermatitis)
C. biopsy always indicated
D. rule out psoriasis
E. bacteriologic study of the ears, nares and perianal region
REF. Peterkin GAG: J Laryngol Otol 88:15, Jan '74

471. Ear piercing by lay people, jewelers, nurses and even physicians may be an important means of transmission of serum infectious hepatitis. Hepatitis virus can only be killed when instruments are sterilized by:
A. 100 percent alcohol
B. 70 percent alcohol
C. zephiran solution
D. autoclaving
E. boiling for 20 minutes
REF. Johnson CJ, Anderson H, Spearman J, Madson J: JAMA 227:1165, Mar '74

472. Abnormally patulous eustachian tube syndrome include symptoms of tympanophonia and autophony relieved by lying down or bending forward and diagnosed partly by motion of the tympanic membrane synchronous with quiet respiration. At the present time the most practical treatment is:
A. tubomyringotomy
B. weight loss
C. surgical destruction of the nasopharyngeal orifice of the eustachian tube
D. tubal catheterization and insufflation with 1:4 salicylic acid and boric acid
E. tensor veli palatini transposition
REF. Misurya VK: J Laryngol Otol 88:877, Sept '74

473. Idiopathic thrombocytopenic purpura (ITP) can be preceded by which of the following conditions?
A. infection
B. postviral
C. drugs
D. infectious mononucleosis
E. cytomegalovirus
REF. McClure PD: Emergency Med 7:84, June '75

474. The treatment for benign paroxysmal vertigo is:
A. phenobarbital
B. methylphenidate (ritalin)
C. meclizine (antivert)
D. primidone (mysoline) starting with 50 mg three times daily increasing to 250 mg
E. dimenhydrinate (dramamine) in a daily dose of 5 mg/kg
REF, Eviator L, Eviator A: Emergency Med 7:167, June '75

475. Benign paroxysmal vertigo is characterized by:
A. self-limited disorder with vestibular dysfunction
B. unsteadiness
C. vertigo and loss of postural control
D. loss of consciousness
E. abnormal responses to ice-cold stimulation with normal electroencephalogram (EEG)
REF. Eviator L, Eviator A: Emergency Med 7:167, June '75

476. Bellucci suggests a classification of tympanoplasty into four groups which predicts before surgery the potential for obtaining dry, stabilized ears. Any type of tympanoplasty cannot survive in the presence of active middle ear infection. Patients with retained nasopharyngeal malformations have a strong tendency toward chronic middle ear infection. In the following question each lettered item is to be matched with one numbered item. Each choice may be used only once:
A. Group I with good prognosis
B. Group II with fair prognosis
C. Group III with poor prognosis
D. Group IV with very poor prognosis

1. with a stable middle ear except during upper respiratory tract infection
2. with continuous ear infection and obvious nasopharyngeal abnormalities
3. free from infection in the middle ear for extended time despite upper respiratory infection
4. with a continuous ear infection
REF. Bellucci RJ: Laryngoscope 83:1754, Nov '74

477. Pure-tone audiometric findings and acoustic impedance measurements in Type I tympanoplasty indicate that:
A. periosteum appears to be stiffer than temporalis fascia
B. best results occur with temporalis fascia and gelfoam in the underlay position
C. B with periosteum onlay
D. B with temporalis fascia onlay
E. B with temporalis fascia plus gelfoam onlay
F. "dead ears" occur as a result of Type I tympanoplasty
REF. Booth JB: J Laryngol Otol 87:1039, Nov '73

478. When cryptococcosis caused by cryptococcus neoformans infects the brain and meninges from the temporal bone, it is characterized by:
A. a disease closely simulating tuberculous meningitis
B. A brain abscess
C. A brain tumor
D. best treated by amphotericin B which is ototoxic
E. D which is not ototoxic
REF. Igarashi M, Weber SC, Alford BR, Coats AC, Jerger J; Arch Otolaryngol 101:577, Sept '75

479. The crura of normal human stapes when studied with the scanning electron microscope show:
A. two layers of mucosa and bone
B. three layers of mucosa, periosteum and bone
C. the covering mucosa to be squamous epithelium
D. C to be respiratory type epithelium
E. periosteal fibroblasts are never present where the mucosa has been stripped off
REF. Graham MD, House HP: Arch Otolaryngol 101:548, Sept '75

480. The typical patient with idiopathic sensorineural hearing loss who suddenly becomes hard of hearing, more hard of hearing (if a previous unrelated loss is present) or deaf in one ear is associated frequently with:
A. tinnitus
B. quality distortion of sound
C. recruitment
D. loud sound intolerance
E. fullness in the ear
F. vertigo
REF. Haug O, Draper WL, Haug SA: Arch Otolaryngol 102:5, Jan '76

481. Excluding idiopathic sensorineural hearing loss, which of the following conditions are known to produce abrupt, usually unilateral sensorineural loss?
A. mumps
B. measles
C. meningitis
D. encephalitis
E. acoustic tumors
F. ear surgery
G. skull fracture
H. ototoxic drugs
I. perilymphatic fistula from exertion
J. I from barotrauma
K. otosclerosis
L. tympanosclerosis
M. otitis media acute without fluid
REF. Haug O, Draper WL, Haug SA: Arch Otolaryngol 102:5, Jan '76

482. The etiology of sudden idiopathic sensorineural hearing loss is thought to be:
A. vascular resulting in hemorrhage into the cochlea
B. viral resulting in hemorrhage into the cochlea
C. due to bacterial infection
D. vascular resulting in reduced blood supply to the cochlea
E. viral resulting in reduced blood supply to the cochlea
REF. Haug O, Draper WL, Haug SA: Arch Otolaryngol 102:5, Jan '76

483. Idiopathic sensorineural hearing loss is being treated by which of the following methods?
A. none at all by one-third of otolaryngologists
B. vasodilators
C. anticoagulants
D. vitamins
E. adrenocorticotropic hormone
F. steroids
G. sedatives
H. tranquilizers
I. diuretics
J. smallpox vaccinations
K. stellate ganglion blocks
REF. Haug O, Draper WL, Haug SA: Arch Otolaryngol 102:5, Jan '76

484. Stellate ganglion block for idopathic sensorineural hearing loss is controlled by the onset of Horner's syndrome which is featured by:
A. enophthalmos
B. exophthalmos
C. anhydrosis
D. ptosis
E. miosis of the pupil
F. E mydriasis
G. drooping of the corner of the mouth
H. nasal congestion
I. nasal secretion
REF. Haug O, Draper WL, Haug SA: Arch Otolaryngol 102:5, Jan '76

485. Which of the following symptoms indicate signs of successful treatment in idiopathic sensorineural hearing loss?
A. high-frequency tinnitus
B. low-frequency tinnitus
C. absence of vertigo
D. absence of fullness in the ear
E. fullness in the ear
REF. Haug O, Draper WL, Haug SA: Arch Otolaryngol 102:5, Jan '76

486. Which of the following symptoms indicate a poor prognosis in the treatment of idiopathic sensorineural hearing loss?
A. vertigo
B. fullness in the ear
C. low-frequency tinnitus
D. high-frequency tinnitus
E. absence of vertigo
REF. Haug O, Draper WL, Haug SA: Arch Otolaryngol 102:5, Jan '76

487. Even many months following surgery, post stapedectomy otitis media, meningitis and labyrinthitis may be present when a patient complains of:
A. otalgia
B. otorrhea
C. loss of hearing
D. disturbance of balance
E. headache
REF. Newlands WJ: Arch Otolaryngol 102:51, Jan '76

488. The predominant infecting organism in post-stapedectomy meningitis is:
A. staphylococcus pyogenes
B. B-hemolytic streptococcus
C. pseudomonas
D. hemophilus influenzae
E. pneumococcus
REF. Newlands WJ: Arch Otolaryngol 102:51, Jan '76

489. The antibiotics in order of choice in post-stapedectomy otitis media and meningitis are:
A. erythromycin
B. penicillin
C. cephaloridine (Loridine)
D. chloramphenicol
REF. Newlands WJ: Arch Otolaryngol 102:51, Jan '76

490. What percent of patients suffer from bilateral Ménière's disease if only the combination of sensorineural hearing loss, recruitment and tinnitus is accepted as definite proof of the diagnosis?
A. 10
B. 15
C. 28
D. 59
E. 73
REF. Greven AJ, Oosterveld WJ: Arch Otolaryngol 101:608, Oct '75

491. All of the following pathologic conditions occur behind central perforations of tympanic membranes in which order of frequency?
A. exposure of the facial nerve
B. dural exposure
C. fistula in the horizontal semicircular canal with a negative fistula test preoperatively
D. erosion of the incus
E. stapes superstructure partly or totally absent
REF. Rice DH: Arch Otolaryngol 101:626, Oct '75

492. Which one of the following findings is rare in Ménière's disease but is common in acoustic nerve tumors?
A. sensorineural hearing loss
B. conductive hearing loss
C. decreased discrimination score
D. recruitment
E. total absence of caloric response
REF. Weymuller, Jr. EA: Arch Otolaryngol 101:630, Oct '75

493. A two year study of performance of hearing aids and wearer satisfaction showed that:
A. eyeglass aids are stronger and more durable than other types
B. A more fragile
C. most patients are satisfied with their aids
D. degree of satisfaction with aids correlates with aided discrimination score
E. D does not correlate
REF. Birt BD, Alberti PW: Can J Otolaryngol 4 (No. 3):529, No month '75

494. Which of the following living membranes may be used to seal the oval window during a stapedectomy?
A. mucosa from the promontory
B. perichondrium
C. fascia
D. subcutaneous tissue
E. fat
REF. Shea JJ: Tr Am Acad Ophthal Otolaryngol 82:ORL-21, Jan '76

495. The complications found in transcanal tympanoplasty for chronic suppurative otitis media and atelectatic otitis media (adhesive otitis media) are:
A. failure of ossicular reconstruction
B. sensorineural hearing loss
C. retraction or collapse of the reconstructed drumhead
D. persistent disease in the unexplored mastoid
E. persistent perforation with frequent extrusion of a polymeric silicone (silastic) film
REF. Austin DF: Tr Am Acad Ophthal Otolaryngol 82:ORL-30, Jan '76

496. Homograft tympanic membranes obtained from fresh unembalmed cadavers preserved in 70 percent ethyl alcohol and used in conjunction with canal skin or fascia have a graft-take in percent over:
A. 50
B. 60
C. 70
D. 80
E. 90
REF. Wehrs RE: Tr Am Acad Ophthal Otolaryngol 82:ORL-39, Jan '76

497. Which of the following causes have usually precipitated the perilymphatic fistulas of the oval or round windows?
A. trauma from sneezing, coughing, and the "valsalva maneuver"
B. head injuries such as falls, windshield trauma
C. explosive sound at close range
D. barotrauma due to swimming and diving
E. exertion
F. spontaneous
G. stapedectomy
H. temporal bone fractures
I. ossicular chain disruption
REF. Healy GB, Friedman JM, Strong MS: Tr Am Acad Ophthal Otolaryngol 82:ORL-44, Jan '76

498. The initial complaints in patients with perilymphatic fistulas of the oval or round windows in order of frequency are:
A. sudden hearing loss
B. hearing loss
C. tinnitus
D. fluctuating hearing
E. positional vertigo
F. episodic vertigo
G. gait disturbance
REF. Healy GB, Friedman JM, Strong MS: Tr Am Acad Ophthal Otolaryngol 82:ORL-44, Jan '76

499. Primary Epstein-Barr virus infections have heen associated with:
A. infectious mononucleosis
B. Guillain-Barré syndrome
C. Bell's palsy
D. meningoencephalitis
E. transverse myelitis
REF. Proctor B, Corgill DA, Proud G: Tr Am Acad Ophthal Otolaryngol 82:ORL-70, Jan '76

500. Pathology of Bell's palsy throughout the entire course of the facial nerve from the internal auditory meatus to the stylomastoid foramen shows:
A. phagocytosis of myelin by macrophages
B. beginning axonal swelling
C. increased cellularity due to lymphocytic infiltration
D. moderate proliferation of schwann cells
E. moderate proliferation of fibroblasts
F. absence of D and E
REF. Proctor B, Corgill DA, Proud G: Tr Am Acad Ophthal Otolaryngol 82: ORL-70, Jan '76

501. Pathology of Bell's palsy shows:
A. acute inflammatory changes in the nerve trunk in the fallopian canal
B. compression of the vascular channels in the fallopian canal
C. inflammatory changes in the chorda tympani nerve
D. positive Hilger's sign-markedly dilated blood vessels associated with the swollen chorda tympani nerve crossing the tympanum
E. evidence of vascular occlusion commonly considered as an etiologic factor as a consequence to chilling of the face
REF. Proctor B, Corgill DA, Proud G: Tr Am Acad Ophthal Otolaryngol 82: ORL-70, Jan '76

502. Which two of the following are associated with a significant number of complications in transcanal tympanoplasty for chronic suppurative otitis media and atelectatic otitis media (adhesive otitis media)?
A. polymeric silicone film
B. absorbable gelatin film
C. ossicular bone transplants
D. homograft nasal cartilage
REF. Austin DF: Tr Am Acad Ophthal Otolaryngol 82:ORL-30, Jan '76

503. Sudden sensorineural hearing impairment may be caused by:
A. oval window fistula
B. round window fistula
C. acoustic tumor (first symptom)
D. upper respiratory infection
E. unknown factors in most cases
REF. Shaia FT, Sheehy JL: Laryngoscope 86:389, Mar '76

504. Although all of the following appear to be effective in the medical treatment of sudden sensorineural hearing impairment, dramatic results at times occur with:
A. 2.75 mg histamine phosphate in 250 cc saline administered on three consecutive days at 50-60 drops per minute
B. 25 cc of one percent procaine in 250 cc saline (substituted for I.V. histamine in asthmatic patients and in those who arc hyper-reactors to histamine)
C. 50 mg nicotinic acid tablets 30 minutes before breakfast and the evening meal
D. large doses of vitamin C and the lemon bioflavanoid complex (Lipoflavanoid)
E. dramamine (Merazine or Bonine) every six hours
REF. Shaia FT, Sheehy JL: Laryngoscope 86:389, Mar '76

505. Unfavorable prognostic factors in sensorineural hearing impairment are:
A. absence of vertigo
B. early treatment (within one month)
C. severe vertigo
D. late treatment (after one month)
E. diabetes
REF. Shaia FT, Sheehy JL: Laryngoscope 86:389, Mar '76

FIGURES FOR SECTION I

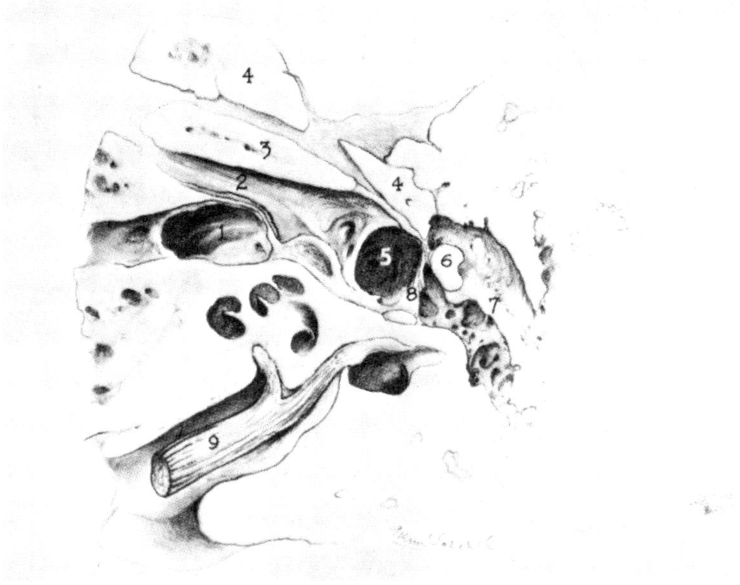

Fig. 1. Horizontal cut through a temporal bone at the level of the protympanum(2). Upper half of cut shows a supratubal recess (5), there being no anterior compartment to the attic. Carotid canal (1) with tiny bony carotid wall separating it from the protympanum. Intertympanosquamosal crest of the petrosa (3). Note how this edge of the petrosa is directed posterior in the line of the malleus head (6) to continue on as the petrosquamosal crest (7). Overriding of the squamosa here can be a cause of malleus fixation and conductive deafness. Squamosa (4). Processus cochleariformis (8); and auditory nerve (9). (Courtesy of Proctor, B.: Arch Otolaryng 97:2, Jan '73)

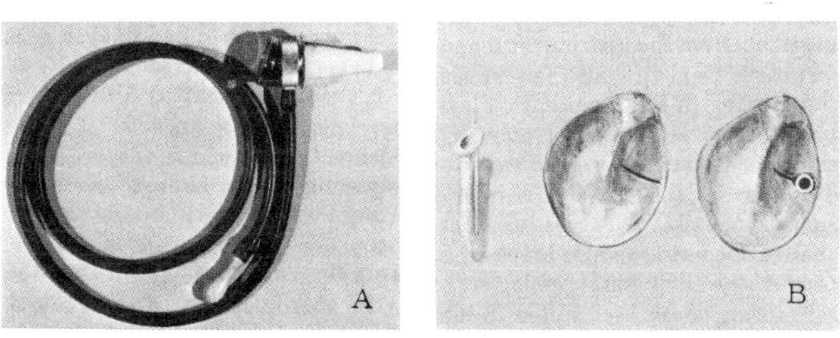

Fig. 2. (A) Pneumatic otoscope fitted with pliable polyvinyl chloride speculum and diagnostic tube. (B) Wide flanged beveled polytef (Teflon) tube; incision in anterosuperior quadrant; tube in place against annular fibers. (Courtesy of Armstrong, B. W.: Arch Otolaryng 97:13, Jan '73)

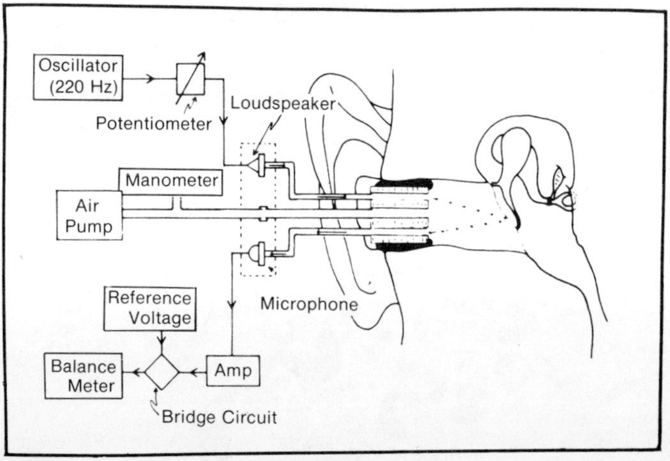

Fig. 3. Functional components of the Madsen electroacoustic bridge (model ZO 70). (Courtesy of Harford, ER: Arch Otolaryng 97:17, Jan '73)

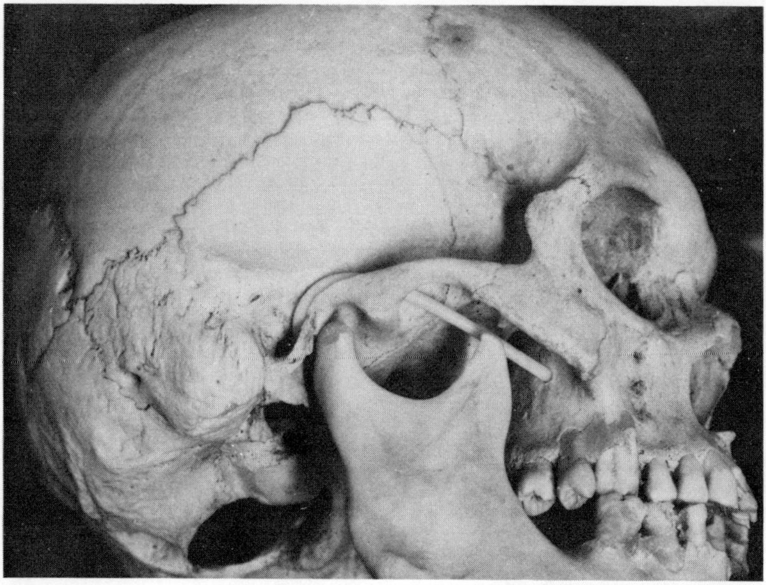

Fig. 4. Position of the tympanomaxillary shunt. Tympanomaxillary shunt is a method for obtaining permanent ventilation of the middle ear in cases with long-term obstruction of the Eustachian tube. The shunt establishes a permanent communication between the middle ear and the maxillary sinus by way of a silicone-rubber tube. It leaves the tympanic membrane and the auditory canal intact. It also permits positive pressure ventilation, e.g., by the Valsalva technique. The method has been used in five patients. The observation times are now between two months and four years. (Courtesy of Ekvall, L and Drettner, B: Arch Otolaryng 97:21, Jan '73)

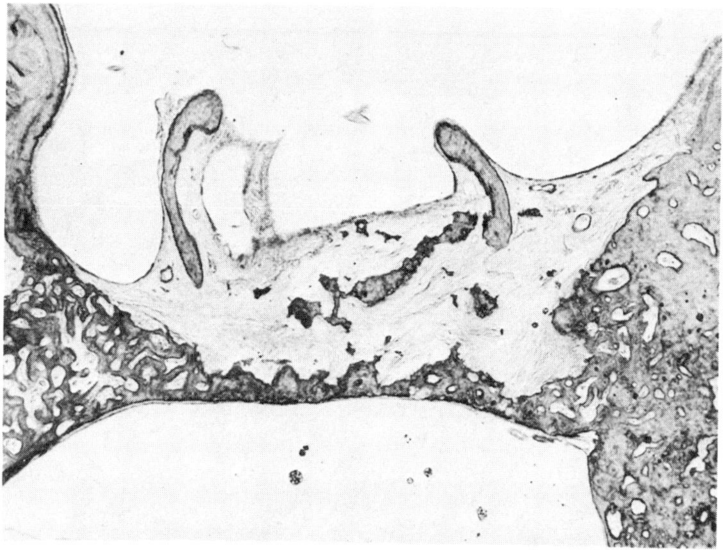

Fig. 5A. Otosclerosis forms lower border of oval window niche. Extensive fibrosis has formed in niche in which separate spicules of new bone are seen between crura of stapes (original magnification x31). (Courtesy of Lindsay, JR: Arch Otolaryng 97:24, Jan'73)

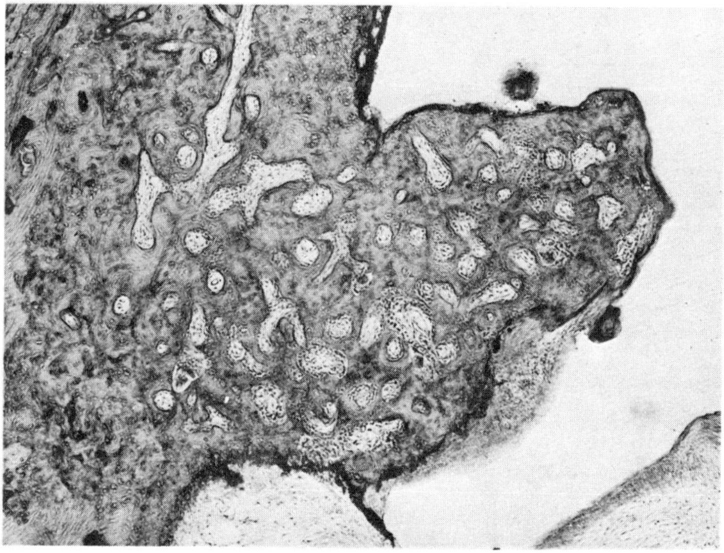

Fig. 5B. Woman of age 61. Bilaterally symmetrical hearing impairment for over five years. Averaging 52 dB for air conduction and bone conduction. Family history of hearing impairment. Single focus of otosclerosis at round window, bilateral (x75). (Courtesy of Lindsay, JR: Arch Otolaryng 97:24, Jan'73)

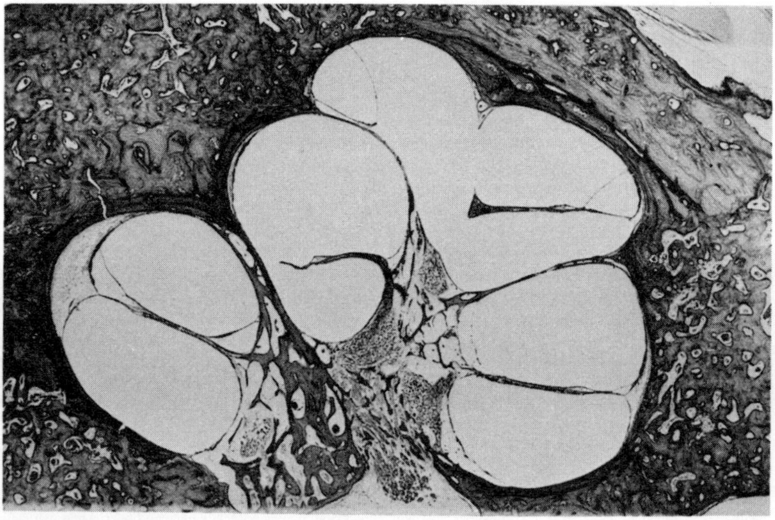

Fig. 6A. Multiple foci of otosclerosis in cochlear capsule of woman age 45. Bone-conduction level averaged 33 dB in speech frequencies (original magnification x20). (Courtesy of Lindsay, JR: Arch Otolaryng 97:24, Jan '73)

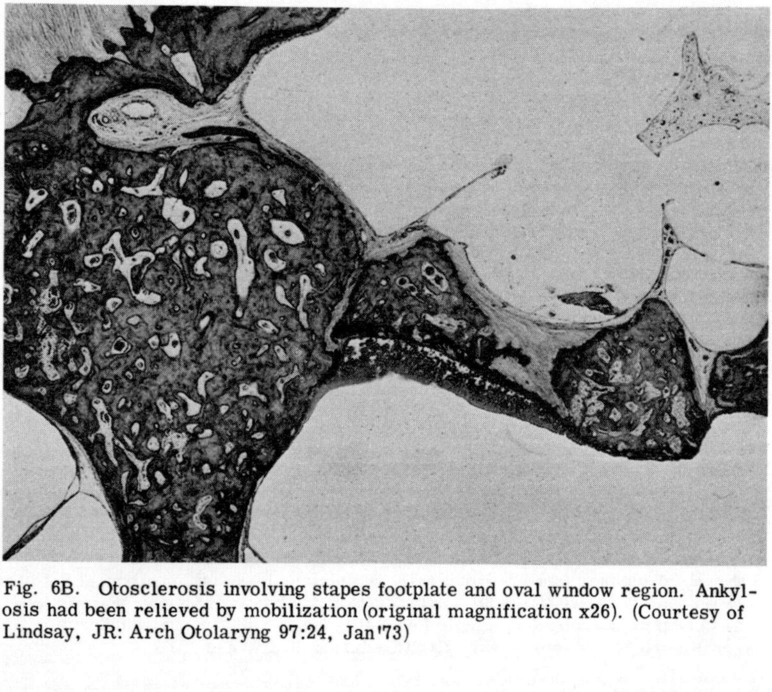

Fig. 6B. Otosclerosis involving stapes footplate and oval window region. Ankylosis had been relieved by mobilization (original magnification x26). (Courtesy of Lindsay, JR: Arch Otolaryng 97:24, Jan '73)

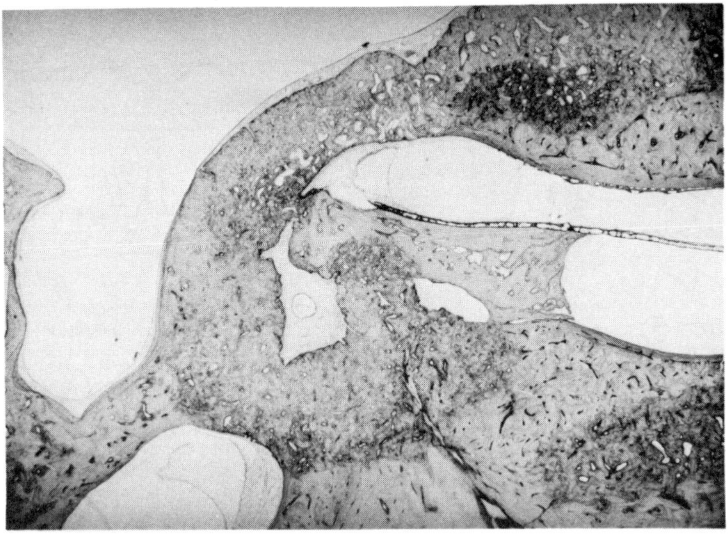

Fig. 7. Man of age 65. Profound deafness. Had used bone-conduction hearing aid for many years. Multiple extensive foci of otosclerosis. Both windows blocked. Labryinthitis ossificans in lower end of scala tympani with ingrowth of otosclerosis (original magnification x18). (Courtesy of Lindsay, JR: Arch Otolaryng 97:24, Jan'73)

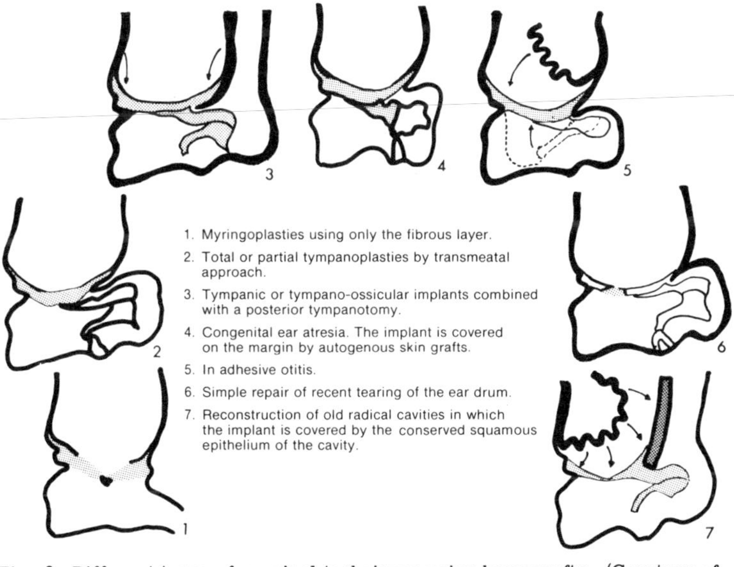

Fig. 8. Different types of surgical techniques using homografts. (Courtesy of Marquet, J, et al.: Arch Otolaryng 97:58, Jan'73)

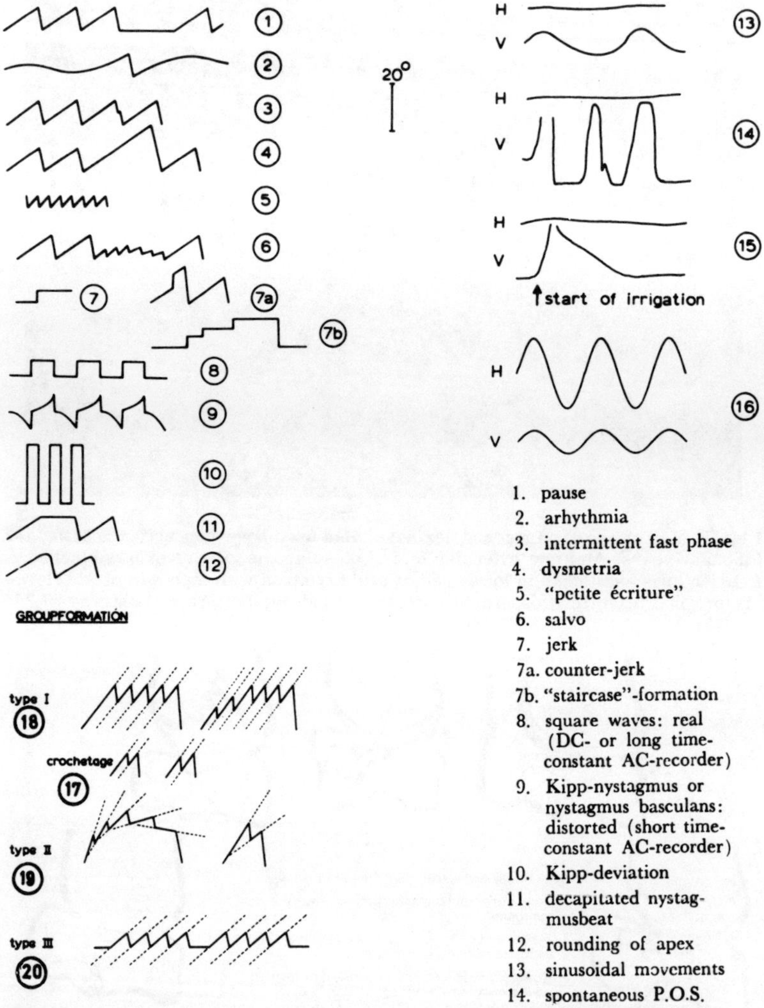

1. pause
2. arhythmia
3. intermittent fast phase
4. dysmetria
5. "petite écriture"
6. salvo
7. jerk

7a. counter-jerk

7b. "staircase"-formation

8. square waves: real (DC- or long time-constant AC-recorder)
9. Kipp-nystagmus or nystagmus basculans: distorted (short time-constant AC-recorder)
10. Kipp-deviation
11. decapitated nystagmusbeat
12. rounding of apex
13. sinusoidal movements
14. spontaneous P.O.S.
15. irrigation P.O.S.
16. pendular movements
17. "crochetage"
18. groupformation type I
19. groupformation type II
20. groupformation type III

Fig. 9. Variations of the nystagmus pattern as recorded by ENG (electronystagmography. (Courtesy of Jongkees, LBW: Arch Otolaryng 97:77, Jan'73)

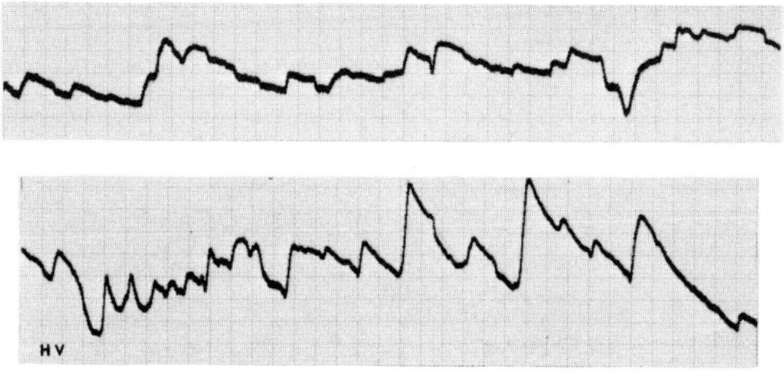

Fig. 10. Hyperventilation (HV) provokes a nystagmus not previously present. (Courtesy of Jongkees, LBW: Arch Otolaryng 97:77, Jan'73)

Table 1.—Postoperative Results of Vertigo Relief in 140 Patients

Result	Patients No.	Patients %
Satisfactory	115	82
Complete relief	88	63
Marked improvement (75 to 95%)	27	19
Failure	25	18
Improved (50 to 70%)	9	6
Improved with recurrence	12	9
No change	4	3
Worse	0	0

Table 2.—Satisfactory Postoperative Results of Vertigo Control in 42 Patients

Results	Follow-up, mo	Patients No.	Patients %
Initial report	6-21	38	90
Present status	52-67	35	83

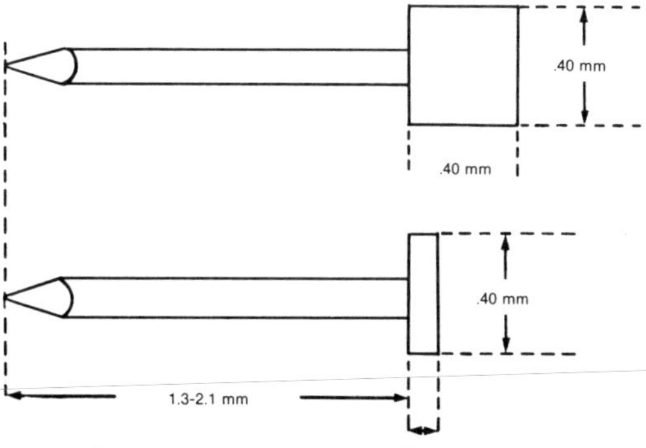

Diagram of two stainless steel tacks.

Table 3.—Satisfactory Postoperative Results of Vertigo Control in 140 Patients

	Group 1 (50 Patients)	Group 2 (90 Patients)
Tack, millimeter		
Head thickness	0.1	0.4
Mean length (range)	1.5 (1.0-1.9)	1.8 (1.5-1.9)
Follow-up, mo		
Mean (range)	57 (49-67)	37 (23-49)
With satisfactory results		
Patients	42	73
Percentage	84	81

Table 4.—Postoperative Results of Hearing in 140 Patients

Audiometric Test	Improved by 20 dB or 20% No.	Improved by 20 dB or 20% %	Worse by 20 dB or 20% No.	Worse by 20 dB or 20% %
Pure-tone and speech-reception thresholds	23	16	23	16
Speech-discrimination score	25	18	28	20
Pure-tone threshold, speech-reception threshold, speech-discrimination score	34	24	34	24

Table 5.—Postoperative Results of Tinnitus and Pressure or Ear Fullness in 140 Patients

Result	Patients No.	Patients %
Tinnitus (133 patients)		
Total improved	62	47
Complete relief	13	10
Worse	3	2
Fullness (101 patients)		
Total improved	92	91
Complete relief	58	57
Worse	0	0

Fig. 11. Tack operation. (Courtesy of Cody, DTR: Arch Otolaryng 97:109, Feb'73)

Ear	SRT	PB Max
R	23 dB	76 %
L	53 dB	54 %

Ear	SRT	PB Max
R	23 dB	86 %
L	43 dB	82 %

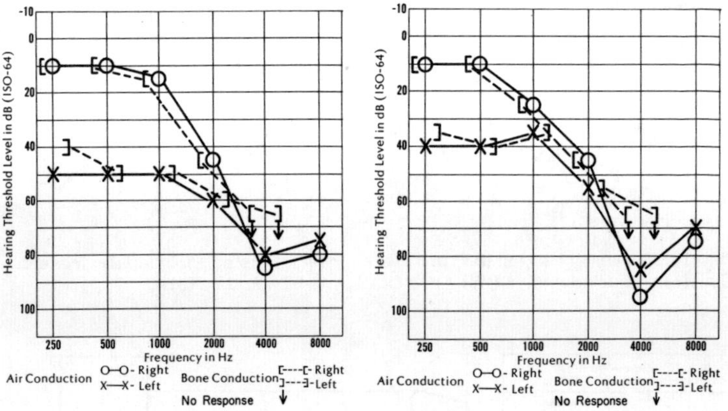

Fig. 12A. A 56-year-old clerk with sudden hearing loss in left ear and great distortion of sounds. Partial improvement on treatment for two months with sudden and complete recovery when patient stopped smoking two packs of cigarettes a day because of excision of cancer of lip.

Ear	SRT	PB Max
R	12 dB	96 %
L	52 dB	78 %

Ear	SRT	PB Max
R	12 dB	96 %
L	12 dB	96 %

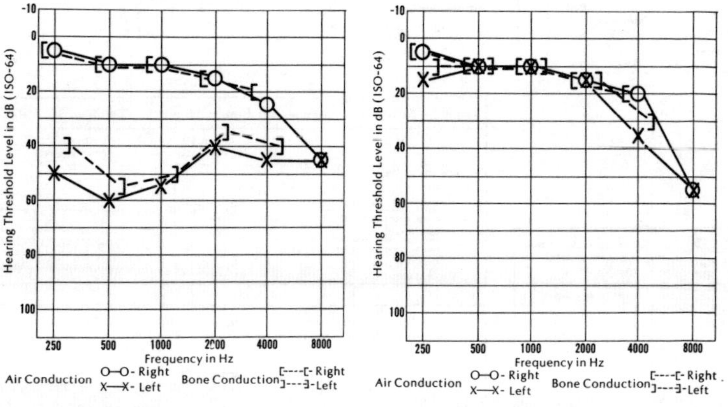

Fig. 12B. A 53-year-old tense cigarette smoking traveling salesman whose hearing went down suddenly in his left ear after eating a lot of salted peanuts. Complete recovery with diuresis of 12 pounds of fluid in 3 days. Patient's hearing went down again in his left ear when he ate more peanuts, and once again, he recovered on treatment. (Courtesy of Shea, JJ and Kitabchi, AE: Arch Otolaryng 97:118, Feb'73)

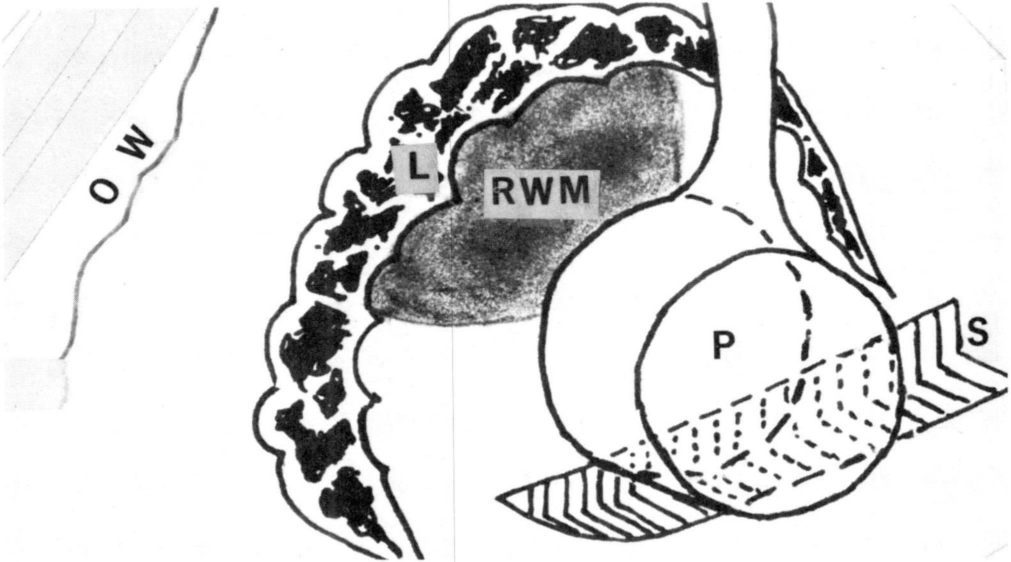

Fig. 13. Ultrasonic probe (P) resting against the step (S) drilled on the floor of the round window niche; OW indicates the oval window niche; L, the drilled away lip of the round window niche to properly expose the round window membrane (RWM). Two methods of ultrasound application for treatment of Ménière's disease are compared: lateral canal vs. round window approach. The experience of 14 years and 560 cases is evaluated. The percentage of failure for both methods is the same, 20%. The round window method is easier, faster, and more pleasant for the patient. Lateral canal approach, on the other hand, has the advantage of a long follow-up which proved its value. Ultrasound as such, however, has proven itself in treatment of Ménière's disease as a valuable contribution in controlling this bothersome illness. (Courtesy of Basek, M: Arch Otolaryng 97:133, Feb '73)

506. The most common mucocele encountered in the paranasal sinuses is located in the:
A. anterior ethmoid
B. posterior ethmoid
C. frontal
D. maxillary
E. sphenoid
REF. Zizmor J, Noyek AM, Chapnik JS: Canadian J Otolaryngol, supp. No. 1, 3: 1,'74

507. An infected mococele, the pyocele, is found occasionally in children with:
A. adenoiditis
B. tonsillitis
C. rhinosinusitis, allergic
D. choanal atresia
E. cystic fibrosis
REF. Zizmor J, Noyek AM, Chapnik JS: Canadian J Otolaryngol, supp. No. 1, 3:1,'74

508. Obstruction to a minor seromucinous gland in the submucosa of any given sinus will most likely produce:
A. mucocele
B. pyocele
C. osteoma
D. simple mucous retention cyst
E. polyps
REF. Zizmor J, Noyek AM, Chapnik JS: Canadian J Otolaryngol, supp. No. 1, 3:1,'74

509. Which one of the following sinus lesions is rarely, if ever, bone-destructive?
A. mucous retention cyst
B. pyocele
C. mucocele
D. osteoma
E. carcinoma
REF. Zizmor J, Noyek AM, Chapnik JS: Canadian J Otolaryngol, supp. No. 1, 3:1,'74

510. The most important of the extrinsic factors causing a mucocele of the frontal sinus is:
A. injury or surgery to the naso-frontal duct
B. deviated nasal septum
C. polyps
D. congenital obstruction or absence of the naso-frontal duct
E. obstruction of a minor seromucinous gland in the submucosa
REF. Zizmor J, Noyek AM, Chapnik JS: Canadian J Otolaryngol, supp. No. 1, 3:1,'74

511. Which of the following conditions have caused mucoceles of the frontal sinuses?
A. Paget's disease
B. osteoma
C. septal deviation
D. injury to the naso-frontal duct
E. surgery of the anterior ethmoid cells
REF. Zizmor J, Noyek AM, Chapnik JS: Canadian J Otolaryngol, supp. No. 1, 3:1,'74

512. Which of the following are the operative procedures of choice for a mucocele of the frontal sinus?
A. incision and drainage
B. submucous resection with anterior ethmoidectomy and enlargement of the naso-frontal duct
C. external osteotomy with catheter inserted into naso-frontal duct
D. osteoplastic external frontal
E. fronto-ethmoidal sinusectomy
REF. Zizmor J. Noyek AM, Chapnik JS: Canadian J Otolaryngol, supp. No. 1, 3:1,'74

513. Advanced neuroradiologic studies such as angiography and pneumoencephalography are rarely indicated in the diagnosis of sinus mucocele except for questionable disease in the:
A. frontal
B. anterior ethmoid
C. maxillary
D. sphenoid
E. sellar area
REF. Zizmor J, Noyek AM, Chapnik JS: Canadian J Otolaryngol, supp. No. 1, 3:1,'74

514. Mucoceles are most rare in which of the following sinuses?
A. frontal
B. anterior ethmoid
C. posterior ethmoid
D. maxillary
E. sphenoid
REF. Zizmor J, Noyek AM, Chapnik JS: Canadian J Otolaryngol, supp. No. 1, 3:1,'74

515. The weakest border of the frontal sinus and displaced first by a mucocele is:
A. anterior
B. lateral
C. medial or intersinus septum
D. posterior
E. floor (or roof of the orbit)
REF. Zizmor J, Noyek AM, Chapnik JS: Canadian J Otolaryngol, supp. No. 1, 3:1,'74

516. An air-fluid level in the ethmoid labyrinth in association with a mucocele invariably indicates:
A. decalcification of the intra-sinus septae
B. destruction of the lamina papyracea
C. obstruction of the lacrimal system
D. pyocele formation and rupture as a result of infection
E. early opacification of the ethmoid labyrinth
REF. Zizmor J. Noyek AM, Chapnik JS: Canadian J Otolaryngol, supp. No. 1, 3:1, '74

517. Which of the following cranial nerves may be involved in exophthalmos and ophthalmoplegia due to a sphenoid sinus mucocele?
A. second
B. third
C. fourth
D. fifth
E. sixth
REF. Zizmor J, Noyek AM, Chapnik JS: Canadian J Otolaryngol, supp. No. 1, 3:1,'74

518. A sphenoid mucocele with opacification and erosion extends initially into:
A. intersinus septum
B. posterior ethmoid cells
C. pterygoid (well pneumatized process)
D. petrous portion temporal bone
E. nasopharynx
REF. Zizmor J, Noyek AM, Chapnik JS: Canadian J Otolaryngol, supp. No. 1, 3:1,'74

519. The optic foramen and the superior orbital fissure are encroached upon when a sphenoid mucocele invades the:
A. petrous portion of the temporal bone
B. pterygoid process
C. posterior ethmoid cells
D. nasopharynx
E. intersinus septum
REF. Zizmor J, Noyek AM, Chapnik JS: Canadian J Otolaryngol, supp. No. 1, 3:1,'74

520. Which of the following are radiographic signs of infrasellar disease due to destruction by a sphenoid sinus mucocele?
A. erosion of the superior orbital fissure
B. destruction of the medial wall of the optic canal
C. undercutting of the anterior clinoid processes

D. bulging into the posterior ethmoid labyrinth
E. erosion of the sellar floor
REF. Zizmor J, Noyek AM, Chapnik JS: Canadian J Otolaryngol, supp. No. 1, 3:1,'74

521. With radiographic evidence of destruction of the sellar floor, which of the following lesions must be considered in the differential diagnosis?
A. sphenoid sinus mucocele
B. cholesteatoma
C. pituitary adenoma
D. juvenile angiofibroma
E. posterior ethmoiditis
REF. Zizmor J, Noyek AM, Chapnik JS: Canadian J Otolaryngol, supp. No. 1, 3:1,'74

522. Which of the following is true of maxillary sinus mucoceles?
A. uncommon
B. common
C. post-surgical
D. usually presents as a painless cheek and facial deformity with displacement of dentition
E. occasional unilateral nasal obstruction or exophthalmos
REF. Zizmor J, Noyek AM, Chapnik JS: Canadian J Otolaryngol, supp. No. 1, 3:1,'74

523. Although all of the following does occur, the maxillary sinus mucocele as an erosive, expanding, bone-destructive cyst usually destroys initially which one part of the sinus?
A. lateral antral wall with bony dehiscence
B. expansion of the alveolar process with displacement of the teeth
C. displacement of the naso-antral wall with shifting of the interior turbinate medially
D. erosion of the floor of the orbit
E. erosion of the posterior wall of the maxillary antrum into the pterygomaxillary space
REF. Zizmor J, Noyek AM, Chapnik JS: Canadian J Otolaryngol, supp. No. 1, 3:1,'74

524. It is virtually impossible to differentiate maxillary sinus mucocele from which of the following because maxillary mucocele always produces an opaque sinus (except for occasional aeration)?
A. secretory retention cyst
B. malignancy
C. cholesteatoma
D. serous cyst
E. dentigerous cyst
REF. Zizmor J, Noyek AM, Chapnik JS: Canadian J Otolaryngol, supp. No. 1, 3:1,'74

525. In carcinoma of the maxilla which of the following symptoms seems to indicate an ominous prognosis?
A. dental pain
B. drainage from a fistulous opening into the buccal cavity
C. swelling of the hard palate
D. unilateral numbness of the upper cheek due to involvement of the infraorbital nerve
E. trismus
REF. Som ML: Arch Otolaryngol, 99:270, Apr'74

526. In carcinoma of the maxilla only 10 percent with maxillectomy and orbital exenteration survive while with maxillectomy alone 43 percent are alive (all had a preoperative cancericidal dose of cobalt followed in four to six weeks by extirpative surgery). In order to determine which patients should have maxillectomy alone or maxillectomy with orbital exenteration, the most important single point to stress is:
A. routine x-rays
B. tomograms
C. Caldwell-Luc with exploration
D. biopsy ethmoids
E. exploration of the floor of the orbit immediately after raising of the skin flaps
REF. Som ML: Arch Otolaryngol, 99:270 Apr'74

527. Bacteriological findings in healthy noses commonly consist mainly of which of the following?
A. sterile
B. staphylococci
C. diphtheroid rods
D. pneumococci
E. haemophilus influenzae
REF. Axelsson A, Brorson JE: The Laryngoscope, 83:2003, Dec'73

528. Bacteriological nasal findings in acute maxillary sinusitis consist of which of the following?
A. no growth
B. pneumococci
C. haemophilus influenzae
D. staphylococci
E. diphtheroid rods
REF. Axelsson A, Brorson JE: The Laryngoscope, 83:2003, Dec'73

529. Bacteriological findings in aspirated sinus secretions in acute maxillary sinusitis showed which of the following?
A. no growth
B. pneumococci
C. haemophilus influenzae
D. staphylococci
E. diphtheroid rods
REF. Axelsson A, Brorson JE: The Laryngoscope, 83:2003, Dec'73

530. Which one of the following when found in the nose is considered to be of no harm to the carrier and in fact may indicate a healthy sinus?
A. no growth
B. pneumococcus
C. haemophilus influenzae
D. staphylococci
E. diphtheroid rods
REF. Axelsson A, Brorson JE: The Laryngoscope, 83:2003, Dec'73

531. The orbital apex syndrome may be due to an expanding mass including tumors in the sphenoid sinus and is characterized by which of the following?
A disturbances of vision
B. paresis of eye muscles
C. disorders of sympathetic nervous system
D. exophthalmos
E. pain
REF. Blum ME, Larson A: The Laryngoscope, 83:2042, Dec'73

532. Probably the most common surgical approach to the sphenoid sinus is:
A. transseptal
B. Cushing's subnasal midline rhinoseptal sphenoidotomy
C. Doyle's transpalatal operation
D. transantral - transethmoid approach
E. enlargement natural ostium by retraction septum laterally
REF. Blum ME, Larson A: The Laryngoscope, 83:2042 Dec'73

533. The most frequent complaints of patients with mucoceles and/or pyoceles in the frontal sinus are:
A. frontal headaches
B. eye problems
C. post-nasal discharge
D. frontal sinus tenderness
E. fluctuant swelling of the forehead
REF. Bordley JE, Bosley WR: Ann Otol, 82:696, Oct '73

534. The most frequent predisposing factors to mucocele formation in the frontal sinus are:
A. previous frontal sinus infection
B. previous frontal sinus surgery including neurosurgical procedures that violated the sinus
C. external trauma to the sinus
D. nasal allergy of long duration
E. osteomas in the nasofrontal duct area
REF. Bordley JE, Bosley WR: Ann Otol, 82:696, Oct '73

535. The most frequent presenting complaint in mucocele of the frontal sinus is:
A. frontal sinus tenderness
B. external frontal swelling
C. headaches localized to the frontal sinus region
D. visual complaints
E. post-nasal discharge
REF. Bordley JE, Bosley WR: Ann Otol, 82:696, Oct '73

536. The most frequent presenting sign in mucocele of the frontal sinus is:
A. ocular involvement including either periorbital swelling, proptosis, or diplopia
B. post-nasal discharge with or without cerebrospinal fluid leaks
C. frontal sinus tenderness
D. external frontal sinus mass or frontal cutaneous fistula
E. intranasal pathology
REF. Bordley JE, Bosley WR: Ann Otol, 82:696, Oct '73

537. Septal perforations appear to be most successfully closed by:
A. sliding flap techniques
B. composite graft from posterior aspect of the auricle
C. composite flap from the post-auricular area to repair one side of septal perforation and a sliding bipedicle flap from the floor of the nose to close the opposite side of the perforation
D. free buccal mucosal graft
E. pedicle buccal mucosal graft
REF. Kratz RC: Arch Otolaryngol, 98:380, Dec '73 (See Fig. 14)

538. Previously undiagnosed acute leukemia can initially precede other evidence of leukemia by months by which of the following?
A. persistent epistaxis
B. recurrent upper respiratory infections
C. chloromata (granulocytic sarcoma)
D. reticulum cell sarcoma
E. Ramsay Hunt syndrome
REF. Sklansky BD, Jafek BW, Wiernik PH: The Laryngoscope 84, 210, Feb '74

539. Epistaxis can be controlled in acute leukemia if which of the following is performed?
A. local pressure with anterior and if needed posterior nasal packing
B. topical vasoconstriction
C. whole blood transfusion

D. premarin
E. platelet transfusions
REF. Sklansky BD, Jafek BW, Wiernik PH: The Laryngoscope 84, 210, Feb '74

540. Although all of the following occur, the most common hemorrhagic complication in acute leukemia is in the:
A. skin and mucous membranes of the nose, mouth, pharynx, etc.
B. paranasal sinuses
C. middle ear (hemotympanum)
D. esophageal varices
E. alveolus with prolonged bleeding after dental extraction
REF. Sklansky BD, Jafek BW, Wiernik PH: The Laryngoscope, 84, 210, Feb '74

541. In acute leukemia there is an increasing incidence of local disseminated fungal infections with candida albicans frequently not diagnosed premortem. The most common site of local candida infections is in the:
A. nose
B. nasopharynx
C. oropharynx
D. trachea and bronchi
E. esophagus
REF. Sklansky BD, Jafek BW, Wiernik PH: The Laryngoscope, 84, 210, Feb '74

542. In acute leukemia which one of the following drugs deserves special attention in relation to neurotoxicity with cranial nerve palsies, especially bilateral ptosis and vocal cord paralysis?
A. kanamycin
B. polymyxin
C. methicillin
D. vincristine
E. cephalothin
REF. Sklansky BD, Jafek BW, Wiernik PH: The Laryngoscope, 84, 210, Feb '74

543. The trans-antral approach with microscopy may be used in which of the following procedures?
A. vidian neurectomy
B. external carotid artery ligation
C. maxillary neurectomy
D. spheno-palatine ganglionectomy
E. maxillary artery ligation
REF. Golding-Wood PH: The Laryngoscope, 83, 1673, Oct '73

544. The most serious complication of vidian neurectomy by the trans-antral route appears to be:
A. ophthalmoplegia
B. post-operative antral infection
C. secondary hemorrhage from the maxillary artery
D. loss of sensation in the lip
E. undue sensitivity of the face to temperature changes, such as exposure to cold weather
REF. Golding-Wood PH: The Laryngoscope, 83, 1673, Oct '73

545. Vidian neurectomy appears to be most useful in which of the following conditions?
A. atopic rhinitis
B. chronic epiphora
C. crocodile tears
D. senile nasal drip
E. cholinergic (non-atopic) chronic vasomotor rhinitis
REF. Golding-Wood PH: The Laryngoscope, 83, 1673, Oct '73

546. Which of the following are advantages of a transpalatine vidian neurectomy over other procedures?
A. more direct approach
B. avoidance of pterygo-palatine fat
C. avoidance of internal maxillary artery

D. avoidance of maxillary nerve
E. easy identification of the sphenopalatine artery
REF. Williams JD: Canadian J Otolaryngol, 2:4:337, '73

547. Epistaxis and serous otitis may be the presenting symptoms in patients with extracranial extension of a tumor from the middle cranial fossa. Neoplasms of neurogenic origin encountered in the nose or throat are uncommon but which of the following do occur?
A. meningocele
B. meningioma
C. neurofibroma
D. ganglioneuroma
E. encephalocele
REF. Smith EJ, El-Deiry A: Canadian J Otolaryngol, 2:4:362, '73

548. Neurogenic tumors can protrude into the nose through a developmental defect in the bones of the skull and these consist of which of the following?
A. meningocele
B. meningioma
C. ganglioneuroma
D. neurofibroma
E. hydro-encephalocele
REF. Smith EJ, El-Deiry A: Canadian J Otolaryngol, 2:4:362, '73

549. The titers of anti-Epstein virus precipitating antibodies using an indirect immunofluorescence antibody technique show the highest titer in which of the following conditions?
A. tonsillitis
B. paranasal sinusitis
C. nasopharyngeal carcinoma
D. leukemia
E. reticulum cell sarcoma
REF. Hsu M-M, Chiou J-F, McCabe BF: Ann Otol 83:19, Jan-Feb'74

550. The anti-Epstein titers of precipitating antibodies are stable and prolonged in which of the following conditions?
A. leukemia
B. sinusitis
C. Burkitt's lymphoma
D. infectious mononucleosis
E. nasopharyngeal carcinoma
REF. Hsu M-M, Chiou J-F, McCabe BF: Ann Otol 83:19, Jan-Feb'74

551. The anti-Epstein titer of precipitation antibodies is highest in nasopharyngeal carcinoma during which of the following?
A. stage I
B. stage II
C. stage III
D. stage IV
E. recurrence
REF. Hsu M-M, Chiou J-F, McCabe BF: Ann Otol 83:19, Jan-Feb'74

552. In describing the clinical extent of carcinoma of the maxillary antrum, Ohngren's line is:
A. horizontal line through the floor of the orbit
B. horizontal line through the floor of the maxillary sinus
C. line extending from the outer canthus of the orbit to the angle of the mandible
D. line extending from the inner canthus of the orbit to the mid-portion of the ramus of the mandible
E. line extending from the inner canthus of the orbit to the angle of the mandible
REF. Pearlman AW, Abadir R: The Laryngoscope 84:400, Mar'74

553. Which of the following is the major symptom or sign in patients with carcinoma of the maxillary antrum on admission for treatment?
A. long history nasal polyps
B. hemorrhage
C. nasal obstruction
D. nasal discharge
E. swelling affected cheek
REF. Pearlman AW, Abadir R: The Laryngoscope 84:400, Mar'74

554. In the treatment of orbital apex syndrome due to sinus infection, which one of the following drugs is considered hazardous?
A. heparin
B. glucocorticosteroids
C. chloramphenicol
D. crystallin penicillin
E. cephalexin
REF. Kronschnabel EF: The Laryngoscope, 84:353, Mar'74

555. In sphenoidal sinus mucoceles which of the following observations appear to be true?
A. optic atrophy occurs only when the mucocele encroaches on the optic nerve
B. exophthalmos occurs when the mucocele involves the ethmoidal sinus and displaces the medial orbital wall
C. elevation of the optic chiasm does not always produce the expected visual defects
D. encroachment by the mucocele on the superior orbital fissure does not always produce paresis of the extraocular muscles
E. as the mucocele expands and becomes larger, its density increases roentgenographically
REF. Valvassori GE, Putterman AM: Tr Am Acad Ophth & Otol, 77:op-703, Nov-Dec '73

556. Various viruses suspected of causing birth defects such as fetal brain damage and mental retardation include the cytomegaloviruses. In acute leukemia there is which of the following?
A. increased incidence of cytomegalic inclusion disease
B. decreased incidence of A above
C. increased incidence of cytomegalovirus in the saliva
D. increased incidence of cytomegalovirus in the urine
E. decreased incidence of C and D
REF. Sklansky BD, Jafek BW, Wiernik PH: The Laryngoscope 84:210, Feb '74

557. Adenocarcinoma of the nasal septum has which of the following features?
A. rare
B. predilection for ethmoid sinuses
C. excessive risk in occurrence among wood workers in the furniture industry
D. radiosensitive
E. occurs also in nickel refinery workers
REF. Tawashy K: Canadian J Otolaryngol, 3:1, 93, '74

558. Although all of the following are true, the orifice of the nasofrontal duct at the nasal end is found most often in which one of the following positions? (See Fig. 15)
A. above the anterior pole of the middle nasal concha
B. below the anterior pole of the middle concha, opening directly into the common meatus
C. on the lateral wall of the anterior third of the middle meatus in the form of an elbow pipe
D. in the middle third of the middle meatus together with the orifice of the maxillary sinus and a few ethmoid cells
E. at the top of the anterior third of the middle meatus, opening into the fornix
REF. Laszlo I: Tr Am Acad Ophth & Otol, 78:ORL-64, Mar-Apr '74

559. Sinus x-ray tomography is focusing on a predetermined plane blurring all other planes and if the x-ray tube moves in a single plane it is called which of the following?
A. linear or unidirectional tomography
B. laminagraphy
C. planigraphy
D. stratigraphy
E. polytomography
REF. Saunders WH, Kelley DR, Klosterman HD: Tr Am Acad Ophth & Otol, 78: ORL-68, Mar-Apr '74

560. Tomography in sinus x-rays with the x-ray tube traversing multiple planes is known as multidirectional tomography or polytomography and the movement of the tube is most frequently:
A. circular
B. elliptic
C. spiral
D. hypocycloidal
E. none of the above
REF. Saunders WH, Kelley DR, Klosterman HD: Tr Am Acad Ophth & Otol, 78:ORL-64, Mar-Apr'74

561. In sinus x-rays one of the chief advantages of polytomography over unidirectional tomography is sections thinner than:
A. 1 mm
B. 5 mm
C. 1 cm
D. 1.5 cm
E. 2 cm
REF. Saunders WH, Kelley DR, Klosterman HD: Tr Am Acad Ophth & Otol, 78:ORL-64, Mar-Apr'74

562. When routine sinus roentgenograms are interpreted as normal or near normal, polytomographic studies can show: (See Fig. 16)
A. specific extent of soft tissue masses
B. bony destruction
C. delineation of clinically undiscovered fractures
D. differentiation between benign tumors and neoplasms
E. differentiation between infection and malignancies
REF. Saunders WH, Kelley DR, Klosterman HD: Tr Am Acad Ophth & Otol, 78:ORL-64, Mar-Apr'74

563. In nasal hemangiopericytoma which of the following appear true?
A. rare with only eleven cases reported in the literature
B. epistaxis is the primary symptom
C. nasal obstruction does not occur but pain is common
D. may be benign or malignant but histologic difference cannot be determined
E. wide surgical resection is the treatment of choice but cryosurgery with minimal blood loss has been successful
REF. Benveniste RJ, Harris HE: Arch Otolaryngol, 98:358, Nov'73

564. Congenital hemangiopericytoma of the nasopharynx has which of the following features?
A. clinically and histologically may be confused with capillary hemangioma unless suspected
B. may be confused clinically with organoid glomus tumor
C. Gomori's reticulum stain is diagnostic
D. radio-resistant
E. bleeding is not common
REF. Abdalla AM: Canadian J Otolaryngol, 2:4:357, 1973

565. In chronic nasopharyngeal obstruction with adenotonsillar hypertrophy which of the following can occur?
A. 50% increase in PCO_2 above normal (pulmonary)
B. CO_2 retention (pulmonary)
C. bronchoconstriction
D. cardiac hypertrophy and failure
E. pulmonary edema
REF. Luke MJ, Mehrizi A, Folger GM Jr., Rowe RD: Pediatrics, 37:762, May'66

566. Changing experimental dogs from primarily a nose breather to a mouth breather by surgically creating a bilateral nasal obstruction produced after a 30 day adjustment period which of the following?
A. arterial hypoxemia
B. mild hypercapnia
C. increased inspiratory laryngeal resistance

D. increased expiratory laryngeal resistance
E. decreased pulmonary compliance
F. increase in total pulmonary resistance
REF. Ogura JH, Suemitsu M, Nelson JR, Kawamoto W: Ann Otol, 82:668, Sept-Oct'73

567. The enzyme acetylcholinesterase (AChE) is found in the olfactory mucosa of guinea pigs and rabbits. Which of the following has been found to be responsible for olfactory transduction?
A. stereochemistry
B. molecular vibration
C. charge transfer
D. membrane puncture
E. functional groups
F. membrane pores
G. enzymatically mediated chemical reactions
H. cholinesterase inhibition
I. unknown
REF. Nadol JB, Delorenzo AJD: Ann Otol, 83:55, Jan-Feb'74

568. Ultrastructure studies of olfactory epithelia in mice exposed once or twice daily to 10% cigarette smoke for six to nine days showed which of the following?
A. olfactory epithelium under conditions of the above experiment is not affected by cigarette smoke
B. olfactory epithelium is affected
C. reduction in size of olfactory vesicles and sensory cilia
D. reduction in microvilli of supporting cells
E. olfactory epithelia in all mice are not affected equally by acute smoke exposures and there is considerable strain differences in reaction to smoke insult indicating that susceptibility is genetically determined and any or all of the above (A, B, C, D) may or may not occur
REF. Matulionis DH: Ann Otol, 83:192, Mar-Apr'74

569. Which of the following systemic effects occur in patients with anterior and posterior packing for epistaxis?
A. mild to moderate decrease in arterial po_2 with hypoxia probably on basis of a nasal-pulmonary reflex and occurs with any nasal obstruction
B. increased arterial pco_2 with hypoventilation
C. increased respiratory rate
D. bradycardia due to increased vagal tone
E. insomnia or convulsions due to cerebral cortex activity
REF. Cook TA, Komorn RM: The Laryngoscope, 83:1802, Nov'73

570. Of the following tumors which have occurred in the maxillary sinus, which one is most rare?
A. epidermoid carcinoma
B. adenocarcinoma
C. lymphoepithelioma
D. mucoepidermoid carcinoma
E. leiomyoangioma
REF. Schwartzman J: The Laryngoscope 83:1856, Nov'73

571. Nasal deformities in the pediatric age group requiring surgery are the result of which of the following?
A. hereditary
B. trauma
C. trauma with increased or decreased nasal growth
D. development in cleft palate or cleft lip patients
REF. Crysdale WS: Canadian J Otolaryngol, 2:3:211, '73

572. Cosmetic surgery of deformities in symmetrical noses with good nasal function should be delayed in females until the age in years of:
A. 3 to 5
B. 6 to 9
C. 10 to 13
D. 15 to 17
E. 19 to 21
REF. Crysdale WS: Canadian J Otolarynagol, 2:3:211, '73

573. Cosmetic surgery of deformities in symmetrical noses with good nasal function should be delayed in males until the age in years of:
A. 3 to 5
B. 6 to 9
C. 10 to 13
D. 16 to 18
E. 19 to 21
REF. Crysdale WS: Canadian J Otolaryngol 2:3:211, '73

574. In the typical ipsilateral deformity in unilateral cleft patient, which of the following statement is incorrect?
A. nasal tip deviated to the abnormal side
B. upper lateral cartilage flatter
C. dome of lower lateral cartilage lower, retroposed, and less well developed
D. nasal floor wider
E. columella and cartilaginous septum deviated to the normal side
REF. Crysdale WS: Canadian J Otolaryngol, 2:3:211, '73

575. Late septal perforations may be prevented at the time of the septoplasty by following which of the following principles? (See fig. 17)
A. perfect hemostasis
B. recognization of fracture lines and duplication
C. periodic checks in the nasal cavity itself
D. care in cases with mucosal atrophy
E. stopping short of sharp summits in the septum so they can be fractured free from their base, then later dissected from the mucosa
REF. Pearson BW, Goodman WS: Canadian J Laryngol, 2:3:238, '73

576. The human inferior turbinate appears to have which of the following functions?
A. inspiratory air even in extreme environmental conditions is adequately warmed
B. inspiratory air is adequately humidified
C. warming and humidification of inspiratory air are dependent upon the presence of large complex turbinates
D. on expiration air is cooled and water is returned to the mucosal surface
E. on expiration air is cooled and heat is returned to the mucosal surface
REF. Cole P: Canadian J Otolaryngol, 2:3:238, '73

577. Which of the following are considered indications for the transsphenoidal approach to the hypophyseal fossa?
A. exeresis of pituitary tumors of regular shape
B. craniopharyngioma
C. "empty sella" combined with disorders of vision
D. trans-sphenoidal rhinorrhea
E. functional hypophysectomy for diabetic retinopathy or breast cancer metastases
REF. Guiot G: Rhinology, 11 (No. 4):137, Dec'73

578. Which of the following are considered contraindications for the trans-sphenoidal surgery to the hypophyseal fossa and should be approached by the intracranial method?
A. pituitary adenomas of regular shape fully enclosed by the dural envelope of the hypophyseal fossa
B. A with considerable supra-sellar expansion
C. pituitary adenomas with sphenoidal expansion
D. secreting pituitary adenoma (which may cause acromegaly, Cushing's disease, or galactorrhea)
E. irregular shaped adenomas
F. intra-cranial invasive adenomas
REF. Guiot G: Rhinology, 11 (No. 4):137, Dec'73

579. Which of the following are considered absolute indications for the trans-sphenoidal approach to the hypophyseal fossa?
A. pituitary adenoma invading the sinus sphenoidalis
B. A invading the squamosphenoid itself
C. pituitary adenoma in patients of advanced years
D. acute intra-sellar hypertension
E. intra-cranial invasive adenomas
REF. Guiot G: Rhinology 11 (No. 4):137, Dec '73 (See Fig. 18)

580. Which of the following are features of acute intra-sellar hypertension?
A. violent headaches
B. abrupt diminution of sight
C. oculomotor paralysis (frequently)
D. meningitic syndrome (sometimes)
E. acute suprarenal insufficiency syndrome (occasionally)
F. history of earlier amenorrhea
G. enlarged sella turcica
H. acute intra-sellar hypertensive syndrome may be induced by estrogens prescribed for amenorrhea whose cause (adenoma) was overlooked
REF. Guiot G: Rhinology 11 (No. 4):137, Dec '73

581. Children with cystic fibrosis have which of the following symptoms more often than normal children?
A. obstructive nasal symptoms
B. otitis media
C. deafness
D. tonsillitis
E. nasal polyps
REF. Taylor B, Evans JNG, Hope GA: Arch Dis Child 49:133, Feb '74

582. Although all of the following occur, apart from the pituitary adenoma, the most frequent intra-sellar tumor is:
A. craniopharyngioma
B. tetratoma
C. fibromyoma
D. ganglioneuroma
E. angioreticuloma
F. intra-sellar sub-diaphragmatic meningioma
REF. Guiot G: Rhinology 11 (No. 4):137, Dec '73

583. Sincipital encephalomeningoceles may appear as benign cystic swellings in the glabella area of noses. Indications for surgery are:
A. rapid enlargement
B. risk of rupture
C. hydrocephalus
D. encroachment on the eyes, nose or mouth
REF. Whatmore WJ: Br J Surg 60:261, Apr '73

584. Good nasal health is guaranteed by:
A. adequate airway alone - the size of the nasal airway is directly related to an improvement in nasal physiology
B. sufficient resistance to inspired air currents
C. sufficient resistance to expired air currents
D. B plus C
REF. Vanio-Mattila J: Acta Otolaryngol (Suppl.) 318:13, No month '74

585. Nasal malformations may produce a great variety of symptoms referable to the nose itself such as:
A. nasal obstruction
B. referred pain
C. considerable postnasal discharge
D. recurrent sore throat
E. cough
REF. Vainio-Mattila J: Acta Otolaryngol (Suppl.) 318:14, No month '74

586. Craniopharyngioma has which of the following characteristics?
A. usually attached to the pituitary stalk
B. usually supra-sellar
C. usually in contact with vital vasculo-neural elements and close to the hypothalamus
D. may be exclusively intra-sellar
E. never an indication for a trans-sphenoidal approach
F. usually can only be adequately extirpated by the intra-cranial route
REF. Guiot G: Rhinology 11 (No. 4):137, Dec '73

587. The following symptoms occur most frequently in the abnormally wide nose:
A. crusting and occasional bleeding
B. stuffiness
C. changes in ability to smell and taste
D. vague facial pains
E. headache
F. postnasal discharge
G. chronic sore throat
H. persistent cough
I. recurrent stuffy ears
J. chronic fatigue
REF. Vainio-Mattila J: Acta Otolaryngol (Suppl.) 318:14, No month '74

588. Following ablation of a large pituitary adenoma, an "empty sella" may result with which of the following complications and treatment?
A. drop of the dural sheath carrying with it the optochiasmatic system with a decrease in visual acuity and a new field defect
B. drop of the dural sheath carrying with it the third ventricle to the floor of the emptied sella
C. sphenoidal meningocele with rhinorrhea
D. trans-sphenoidal intervention indicated with extra-dural filling of lower half of the sella with particles of bone and muscle
E. intra-cranial surgical reconstruction of the dura indicated
REF. Guiot G: Rhinology 11 (No. 4):137, Dec '73 (See Fig. 19)

589. The second most common malignant tumor of the paranasal sinuses is:
A. squamous cell carcinoma
B. adenocarcinoma
C. sarcoma
D. melanoma
E. plasma cell cytoma
F. primary lymphoma
REF. Adams G, Duvall AJ III, Smith D, Pollak K: Minn Med 57:562, July '74

590. The most effective forms of treatment for epistaxis in cardiac or cardiac surgical patients on coumadin are:
A. cleansing of the bleeding point and cover with vaseline or vaseline packing
B. cover bleeding point with thin silastic sheeting (adheres to the bleeding point)
C. avoid use of nasal catheter, nasal oxygen tubing, etc.
D. cauterization of bleeding points and use ointment of 10 percent liquid petroleum, 40 percent anhydrous lanolin, 50 percent vaseline with one drop rose oil to every 10 grams
E. stop coumadin since anti-coagulant effects will continue 3-4 days
F. injection of 0.2 cc of 0.5 percent sodium morrhuate under the mucoperichondrium of the bleeding point with 25 gauge 1 1/2 inch needle
G. peroxide packs in the nose with pressure on the nasal tip (alae) for 10-15 minutes
H. gelfoam, oxycel or surgicel packs on the bleeding points
I. topical thrombin spray
J. packed erythrocytes
K. whole blood transfusion
REF. Gottschlak GH, McDonald TJ, Ipolyi FX, Irvine DW, Baer S, Clemons JE, Chonkich GD: I.C.S. of O and O 20:77, May '75

591. In postnasal packing with inflatable balloons, pressure necrosis of the nasal alae by the catheters of the balloons is common but alae necrosis can be prevented by:
A. protection of the alae by interposing several layers of gauze
B. use of postnasal ointment impregnated gauze without balloons
C. vaseline or iodoform gauze between the alae and rubber catheter
D. use of ragmop without balloons
E. injection of bleeding sites with two percent xylocaine with epinephrine 1:100,000 followed by cauterization and then the cauterized points covered with compressed gelfoam followed by special tampons made of vaseline gauze sutured with 0 silk (without balloons)
REF. Gottschlak GH, McDonald TJ, Ipolyi FX, Irvine DW, Baer S, Clemons JE, Chonkich GD: I.C.S. of O and O 20:77, May '75

592. Which one of the following drugs being more frequently used in drug abuse may cause acute psychotic reaction and expecially chronic nasal congestion not relieved by the usual decongestants?
A. marijuana
B. hallucinogens
C. Demerol
D. alcohol
E. cocaine
REF. Schnoll S: JAMA 232:706, May '75

593. All arteries within the vascular anatomy of the nasal mucosa communicate frequently with one another. Which of the following arteries can at times communicate with each other in Kiesselbach's or Little's area?
A. distal branches of the greater palatine
B. superior labial
C. sphenopalatine
D. posterior ethmoidal
E. anterior ethmoidal
REF. Petruson B: Acta Otolaryngol (Suppl.) 317:9, No month '74

594. Which of the following predisposing factors appears to cause epistaxis?
A. inflammatory reactions - upper respiratory infections, chemicals such as gentian violet (an epidemic occupational disease)
B. arteriosclerosis, varicose veins, and a family history of epistaxis such as patients with familial hemorrhagic telangiectasia
C. changes due to blood flow and pressure such as in patients with macroglobulinemia Waldenström
D. temporary increase in blood pressure
E. essential hypertension
F. impaired hemostasis due to von Willebrand's syndrome, acquired thrombocytopenia, any inherited defects of coagulation factors, treatment with drugs such as acetylsalicylic acid, dicumarol, heparin, streptokinase
REF. Petruson B: Acta Otolaryngol (Suppl.) 317:62, No month '74

595. Which one of the following sinuses is most commonly infected?
A. maxillary
B. ethmoid
C. sphenoid
D. frontal
REF. McCabe BF, Dolan KD, Harker LA, Abramson M: Ann Otol Rhinol Laryngol 84:859, Nov '75

596. Which of the following malignant tumors occur in the paranasal sinuses?
A. squamous cell carcinoma
B. adenocarcinoma
C. sarcoma
D. melanoma
E. plasma cell cytoma
F. primary lymphoma
REF. Adams G, Duvall AJ III, Smith D, Pollak K: Minn Med 57:562, July '74

597. The most common presenting signs of malignant tumors of the paranasal sinuses are:
A. epistaxis
B. swelling over the cheek
C. chronic sinusitis
D. sneezing
E. mass depressing the palate
REF. Adams G, Duvall AJ III, Smith D, Pollak K: Minn Med 57:562, July '74

598. The most common malignant tumor of the paranasal sinuses is:
A. squamous cell carcinoma
B. adenocarcinoma
C. sarcoma
D. melanoma
E. plasma cell cytoma
F. primary lymphoma
REF. Adams G, Duvall AJ III, Smith D, Pollak K: Minn Med 57:562, July '74

599. Selective internal carotid arteriography indicating the presence of a tumor stain in a lesion destroying the floor of the sella should raise the possibility of:
A. primary carcinoma of the sphenoid sinus
B. mucocele
C. meningioma
D. chromophobe adenoma
E. osteoma
REF. McCarthy DP, Gold L: Arch Otolaryngol 101:512, Aug '75

600. Which one of the following drugs commonly used to treat asthma (and sometimes sinusitis) may produce fetal goitre?
A. saturated solution of potassium iodide
B. hydroxyzine
C. tetracycline
D. corticosteroids
E. phenobarbital
REF. Graf MW: Modern Med 43:134, Mar '75; Patterson R: Allergy Diseases, 1st Ed., J.B. Lippincott Co., Philadelphia, pp. 285-286, 1972

601. The technique of trans-sphenoidal hypophysectomy over the intra-cranial approach has which of the following advantages?
A. little loss of blood even under general anesthesia
B. larger access area
C. bilateral approach and may be enlarged even further by resection of the piriform opening and by mobilization of the nasal septum
D. strictly median approach since the septum leads to the rostrum and the sphenoid sinus without danger to the sinus cavernosus area
E. extra-nasal (safe) method since the sella is reached through the mucosal sheath of the septum and thus isolating the cavity in which the operation is performed
REF. Bouche J: Rhinology 11 (No. 4):153, Dec '73

602. The following percent of patients given irradiation for recurrent tonsillitis require surgical tonsillectomy a few months or years later:
A. 0
B. 1-10
C. 15-25
D. 30-40
E. 50
REF. Refetoff S, Harrison J, Karanfilski BT, Kaplan EL, DeGroot LJ, Bekerman C: N Engl J Med 292:171, Jan '75

603. In a significant number of intrinsic asthmatics with nasal polyps, bronchospasm may be triggered by:
A. sinusitis
B. Tylenol
C. over-the-counter medications
D. acetylsalicylic acid
E. FDC yellow No. 5 tartrazine dye used in foods and medications
REF. ACA Course: Allergy News Bull 4:6, Issue 9, No month '75

604. When a physician is presented with an infant with a unilateral polypoid, reddish smooth non-pulsatile submucosal mass involving the upper anterior portion of the nasal cavity, which one of the following should be considered?
A. encephalocele
B. glioma
C. dermoid cyst
D. allergic polyps
E. hypertrophy of the middle turbinate
REF. Mallen RW, Kudryk WH: Can J Otolaryngol 3:2:187, '74

605. When a physician is presented with an infant with a unilateral polypoid, reddish smooth, pulsating submucosal mass involving the upper anterior portion of the nasal cavity (or entire nasal passage), which one of the following should be considered?
A. encephalocele
B. glioma
C. dermoid cyst
D. allergic polyps
E. hypertrophy of the middle turbinate
REF. Mallen RW, Kudryk WH: Can J Otolaryngol 3:2:187, '74

606. Nasal gliomas are uncommon lesions which present in young patients. Although all of the following surgical approaches have been successful, the procedure of choice appears to be:
A. primary transfrontal craniotomy
B. intranasal removal
C. lateral rhinotomy
D. inferior nasal approach
E. transnasal approach via a dorsal rhinotomy
REF. Mallen RW, Kudryk WH: Can J Otolaryngol 3:2:187, '74

607. A review of the literature shows which of the following conditions have been listed as etiologic factors in epistaxis?
A. upper respiratory infections
B. use of acetylsalicylic acid
C. systolic hypertension
D. diastolic hypertension
E. hematological diseases such as malignant hematopoietic tumors and defects in hemostasis
REF. Petruson B: Acta Otolaryngol (Suppl.) 317:7, No month '74

608. A solid tumor in the glabella of the nose may be a glioma which originates because of:
A. origin from the terminal nerve
B. malformation in closure of the anterior neuropore
C. deficiency of the mesoblast
D. disturbance in closure of the cecal foramen and of the nasofrontal fontanel
E. an encephalocele cut off from its origin
REF. Baran R, Kopf A, Schnitzler L: Ann Dermatol Syphiligr, 100:395-407, No month '73

609. Which of the following conditions may cause hyposmia?
A. pregnancy
B. smoking
C. allergy
D. head trauma
REF. Vainio-Mattila J: Acta Otolaryngol (Suppl.) 318:13, No month '74

610. The normal nose secretes one liter of water per day into the air passing through it with a resulting humidity expressed in percent of:
A. 50
B. 60
C. 70
D. 80
E. 90
REF. Vainio-Mattila J: Acta Otolaryngol (Suppl.) 318:12, No month '74

611. Physiological relationship between nasal obstruction and pulmonary function is shown by:
A. pulmonary resistance increasing and compliance decreasing with advancing degrees of nasal obstruction and these findings are observed during oral as well as nasal breathing (Ogura)
B. A abnormal pre-operative values reverting to normal range four to six months following successful nasal surgery in most patients
C. nasopulmonary and nasobronchial reflexes appearing to give increased bronchial tone in cases of nasal obstruction which explains the reversibility of pulmonary changes after nasal surgery
D. blowing air into one nostril causes an expansion of the corresponding side of the thorax but is absent when the nasal mucosa is anesthetized
E. a disturbance in the acid-base balance of the blood in patients with nasal obstruction suggesting that this finding may be due to reduced pulmonary ventilation
REF. Vainio-Mattila J: Acta Otolaryngol (Suppl.) 318:12, No month '74

612. Tolosa - Hunt syndrome is:
A. spasm of the internal carotid artery in the parasellar segment
B. obstruction of the internal carotid artery
C. sphenoid sinusitis with headaches
D. intracranial aneurysm in the 15-30 year age group
E. occlusion of the superior ophthalmic vein in cases of the superior orbital fissure syndrome
REF. Whitehead E, De Souza FM: Can J Otolaryngol 3:2:216, '74

613. Well-known functions of the nose are:
A. sense of smell
B. warming, moistening and cleansing of air before entering the lungs
C. defense and reflex functions
D. resonance chamber in the formation of speech and sound
E. pulmonary resistance increases and compliance decreases with advancing degrees of nasal obstruction and these findings are observed during oral as well as nasal breathing (Ogura)
REF. Vainio-Mattila J: Acta Otolaryngol (Suppl.) 318, No month '74

614. The following test substances for olfactory acuity include both weak and strong odors which are familiar and easily identifiable. Name the following test substances in their proper sequence progressing from weak odors to strong:
A. peppermint extract
B. rose water
C. spirits of camphor
D. cinnamon
E. oil of cloves
F. lavender oil
G. coffee
REF. Vainio-Mattila J: Acta Otolaryngol (Suppl.) 318:12, No month '74

615. A patient who denies any nasal sensation from which one of the following substances is suspicious of having a psychological or malingering problem?
A. spirits of camphor
B. lavender oil
C. oil of cloves
D. household ammonia
E. rose water
F. coffee
G. cinnamon
H. peppermint extract
REF. Vainio-Mattila J: Acta Otolaryngol (Suppl.) 318:12, No month '74

616. Which one of the following substances tests the trigeminal sensation of the nose?
A. rose water
B. coffee
C. cinnamon
D. spirits of camphor
E. lavender oil
F. oil of cloves
G. peppermint extract
H. household ammonia
REF. Vainio-Mattila J: Acta Otolaryngol (Suppl.) 318:12, No month '74

617. Chandler's classification of the pathogenesis of orbital inflammation secondary to sinusitis consists of:
A. inflammatory edema (of eyelids with or without edema of the orbital contents)
B. orbital cellulitis
C. subperiosteal abscess
D. orbital abscess
E. cavernous sinus thrombosis
REF. Rounthwaite EJ: Can J Otolaryngol 3:2:219, '74

618. The earliest symptom in superior orbital fissure syndrome is usually:
A. ptosis
B. diplopia
C. exophthalmos
D. ophthalmoplegia
E. pain
REF. Rounthwaite EJ: Can J Otolaryngol 3:2:219, '74

619. Inverted papillomas of the nasal and sinus cavities are:
A. most commonly localized on the lateral nasal wall
B. frequently found in the maxillary and ethmoid sinuses
C. consistent with opacification of nasal cavities and sinuses
D. diagnosed by polycycloid tomography and histologic examination
E. associated with osseous destruction
REF. Förste H-W: Fortschr Geb Roentgenstr Nuklearmed 121:1, July '74

620. A patient with severe headaches especially with eye symptoms with absent rhinoscopic findings with normal plain paranasal sinus films should alert the physician to which one of the following conditions?
A. subarachnoid hemorrhage
B. cavernous sinus thrombosis
C. spasm internal carotid artery (carotid arteriogram) in the parasellar segment
D. intracranial aneurysm
E. occlusion superior ophthalmic vein (orbital venograms)
F. mucocele of sphenoid sinus
G. early acute sphenoid sinusitis
REF. Whitehead E, De Souza FM: Can J Otolaryngol 3:2:216, '74

621. All of the following findings occur in both the superior orbital fissure syndrome and the orbital apex syndrome but the orbital apex syndrome has, in addition, which one of the following signs?
A. ptosis
B. diplopia
C. impairment of vision and contraction of the visual fields
D. ophthalmoplegia
E. wide pupil with loss of accommodation
REF. Rounthwaite EJ: Can J Otolaryngol 3:2:219, '74

622. The most common bacterial pathogens causing acute maxillary sinusitis are:
A. pneumococci
B. haemophilus influenzae
C. streptococci
D. staphylococci
E. pseudomonas
REF. Axelsson A, Brorson J-E: Ann Otol 83:323, May-June '74

623. Significant correlation appears to occur between nasal symptoms and which of the following indoor or outdoor working conditions?
A. high humidity
B. temperature variations
C. impurities in air (dust)
D. chemicals (gaseous)
E. draught
REF. Vainio-Mattila J: Acta Otolaryngol (Suppl.) 318:25, No month '74

624. Investigations of antibiotic concentrations in sinus mucosa and secretions in acute maxillary sinusitis have shown conflicting results. One study showed ampicillin achieved the highest concentration and other studies showed low antibiotic concentration with ampicillin. Which one of the following antibiotics gave the highest concentration in acute maxillary sinusitis excluding the ampicillin controversy?
A. cephadine (velosef) 0.25 gm four times daily for 10 days
B. erythromycinestolate (Ilosone) 0.5 gm twice daily for 10 days
C. tetracycline 250 mg four times daily
D. doxycycline 200 mg initially, 100 mg daily for nine days
E. spiramycin 1.5 gm twice daily for 10 days
REF. Axelsson A, Brorson J-E: Ann Otol 83:323, May-June '74

625. All of the following symptoms are considered significant in disturbances of nasal functions of structures but by correlation analyses which five symptoms appear to represent a nasal symptom complex?
A. nasal pains
B. cheek pains
C. swallowing pains
D. dryness of throat
E. sneezing
F. crusting of nose
G. hyposmia
H. epistaxis
I. postnasal discharge
J. snoring
K. mouth breathing
REF. Vainio-Mattila J: Acta Otolaryngol (Suppl.) 318:31, No month '74

626. There appears to be significant positive correlations between nasal disturbances and which of the following conditions?
A. chronic rhinitis
B. septal deviation
C. prominent nose
D. allergy
E. coronary arterial disease
F. smoking
G. severe head injury
H. asthma
I. heart disease
J. outdoor work
REF. Vainio-Mattila J: Acta Otolaryngol (Suppl.) 318:42, No month '74

627. All of the following symptoms appear to be more frequent in patients with septal obstruction but the symptoms which appear to reach the level of significance are:
A. chronic rhinitis
B. snoring
C. heart
D. mouth breathing
D. sinusitis
F. sneezing
G. trigeminal sensitivity
REF. Vainio-Mattila J: Acta Otolaryngol (Suppl.) 318:43, No month '74

628. Which two of the following are known to contain substances with animicrobial activity?
A. cerumen external auditory canal
B. middle ear effusions
C. saliva
D. maxillary sinus contents
E. esophageal secretions
REF. Axelsson A, Brorson J-E: Ann Otol 83:323, May-June '74

629. Rhinorrhea is an unusual postoperative complication following maxillectomy and although all of the following occur, the most common cause is probably:
A. poorly fitting prosthesis
B. Velo-pharyngeal incompetence
C. opening of the ipsilateral parotid duct above the level of the prosthesis
D. allergy
E. infection
F. recurrent malignant neoplasm
G. cerebral spinal fluid leak
REF. Clark C, Weaver AW, Smith DB: Arch Otolaryngol 101:492, Aug '75

630. Connective tissue disorders are among the least understood pathological entities which confront the otolaryngologist but one consistent pathological finding appears to be the presence of a vasculitis. In Wegener's granulomatosis, therapy which may prove promising is:
A. steroids
B. erythromycin
C. tetracycline
D. ampicillin
E. antimetabolites
REF. Lucente FE: Ann Otol 83:314, May-June '74

631. Failure to differentiate benign from malignant lesions of the sphenoid sinuses preoperatively has led to needless craniotomies in cases of benign neoplasms. Benign tumors and mucoceles closely mimic malignant tumors but malignant tumors can be diagnosed by:
A. bone destruction of the base of the skull, floor of the sella, and posterior wall of the orbit
B. third, fourth, sixth cranial nerve palsies and involvement of the ophthalmic division of the fifth cranial nerve
C. sinus radiographs
D. skull and sinus laminography and radionuclide brain scanning
E. internal carotid arteriography with numerous hypertrophied branches of the cavernous portion of the internal carotid artery and a dense tumor stain within the sphenoid sinus
REF. McCarthy DP, Gold L: Arch Otolaryngol 101:512, Aug '75

632. Selective carotid arteriography or angiography is not limited to the diagnosis of bleeding sites but indeed the same catheter can be used in a therapeutic fashion to thrombose bleeding vessels or false aneurysm in epistaxis. All of the following agents have been used but the agent of choice since it is non-allergenic, prepared easily and passes readily through a small (No. 5F) catheter is:
A. autologous clot
B. absorbable gelatine sponge (gelfoam)
C. polyvinyl alcohol
D. isobutyl 2-cyanoacrylate
REF. Miller FJ, Entzminger LB, Coleman LL, Conner GH, Weidner WA: Arch Otolaryngol 101:517, Aug '75

633. The effect of nasal obstruction on the pulmonary mechanics of dogs and patients shows:
A. unilateral nasal obstruction is compensated (pulmonary)
B. unilateral nasal obstruction is not compensated (pulmonary)
C. bilateral obstruction induces increased pulmonary airway resistance
D. bilateral obstruction does not induce increased pulmonary airway resistance
E. nasal obstruction alters the total pulmonary resistance in human and animal experiments
REF. Ogura JH: Ann Otol Rhinol Laryngol 84 (Suppl. 19):49, Mar '75

634. Humans with nasal packing for epistaxis:
A. die suddently without any apparent reason
B. reveal arterial blood gas changes with an elevated Pco_2
C. B with decreased Pco_2
D. B with elevated Po_2
E. B with decreased Po_2
REF. Ogura JH: Ann Otol Rhinol Laryngol 84 (Suppl. 19:49, Mar '75

635. The criteria for successful resection of a malignant tumor of the paranasal sinuses require that there be no:
A. invasion of the nasopharynx
B. invasion of the base of the skull
C. invasion of the posterior ethmoids
D. definite erosion of the posterior wall of the maxillary sinus
E. erosion of the pterygoid plates
REF. Adams G, Duvall AJ III, Smith D, Pollak K: Minn Med 57:562, July '74

636. Migraine is a vascular constriction of extracranial vessels followed by extreme vasodilation. A migraine headache is relieved by which of the following vasoconstrictors?
A. methysergide
B. betahistine hydrochloride
C. nicotinic acid
D. ergotamine suppository taken at bedtime for one week
E. elixir 50 mg nicotinyl alcohol per teaspoonful at 15 drops three times daily, increasing the dosage one drop daily until headache develops and then if no headache, two teaspoonfuls (100 mg) three times daily or 150 mg nicotinyl alcohol timespan twice daily
F. biofeedback temperature training by raising the temperature of the hands
REF. Grossan M: ORL Digest 37:17, Mar '75

637. Steroids supposedly reduce bleeding by:
A. suppressing phagocytosis of platelets in the spleen
B. reducing platelet antibody production
C. affecting vascular permeability
D. all of the above
E. none of the above
REF. McClure PD: Emergency Med 7:84, June '75

638. Which of the following lesions should be considered in the differential diagnosis of a mass within the sphenoid sinus?
A. mucocele
B. pyocele
C. pituitary tumor
D. meningioma
E. sarcoma of various types
F. aneurysm of internal carotid artery
G. F of the external carotid artery
H. chordoma
I. angiofibroma
J. metastatic tumors
K. primary carcinoma of the sphenoid sinus
REF. McCarthy DP, Gold L: Arch Otolaryngol 101:512, Aug '75

639. There is a significant correlation between decreased olfactory acuity and:
A. septal deviation
B. earlier head injury
C. advancing age
D. allergy
E. decreased nasal tip index
REF. Vainio-Mattila J: Acta Otolaryngol (Suppl.) 318:42, No month '74

640. The resistance in the nose to air currents is provided by:
A. free ends of the medial crura
B. free ends of the lateral crura
C. cul-de-sac
D. upper lateral valve
E. floor of the pyriform aperture
REF. Vainio-Mattila J: Acta Otolaryngol (Suppl.) 318:13, No month '74

641. Specimens obtained during Lynch or Caldwell-Luc procedures cultured for aerobes, anaerobes and fungi show:
A. mixed infections
B. sterile specimens
C. microaerophilic and anaerobic streptococci
D. anaerobic bacteroides
E. absence of fungi
REF. Frederick J, Braude AI: N Engl J Med 290:135, Jan '74

642. Patients less than 15 years of age usually have epistaxis from:
A. Kiesselbach's (Little's) area in the anterior part of the septum
B. anterior ethmoidal artery
C. posterior ethmoidal artery
D. sphenopalatine artery
E. posterior and lateral parts of the nasal cavity
REF. Petruson B: Acta Otolaryngol (Suppl.) 317:7, No month '74

643. Local treatment of a visible vessel in epistaxis consists of:
A. cauterization with silver nitrate, chromic acid, trichloracetic acid, electrical current
B. submucosal injection below the bleeding area with three percent water soluble Phlebocid to arrest bleeding by pressure and to cause an inflammatory thrombophlebitis in the vessels
C. submucosal injection of adrenalin 1:1000 with or without surface cauterization
D. spraying of a thin layer of plastic over the bleeding area
E. absorbable hemostatic sponge (spongostan, surgicel) over the bleeding point
REF. Petruson B: Acta Otolaryngol (Suppl.) 317:8, No month '74

644. Intranasal freezing at -20° C for one hour using a Steven's balloon for the control of invisible bleeding vessel epistaxis has the following permanent disadvantage:
A. severe inflammatory reaction
B. vascular thrombophlebitis
C. septal perforations
D. nasal adhesions
E. damaged medium sized vessels
REF. Petruson B: Acta Otolaryngol (Suppl.) 317:8, No month '74

645. It is a well known clinical observation that epistaxis can be arrested by:
A. sedation with morphine, tranquilizing drugs, etc.
B. hypnosis
C. vitamin C and K
D. drugs and/or transfusion in hematological diseases
E. oestrogen hormones
F. antifibrinolytic drugs such as epsilon-amino-caprionic acid, para-aminomethylbenzoic acid and tranexamic acid
REF. Petruson B: Acta Otolaryngol (Suppl.) 317:9, No month '74

646. The vascular anatomy of the nasal mucosa is supplied by the following branches of the internal carotid artery:
A. sphenopalatine
B. greater palatine
C. internal maxillary artery
D. anterior ethmoidal artery
E. posterior ethmoidal artery
REF. Petruson B: Acta Otolaryngol (Suppl.) 317:9, No month '74

647. Which one of the following arteries supplies the anterior third of the lateral wall of the nasal cavity and a similar portion of the septum?
A. sphenopalatine
B. superior labial
C. anterior ethmoidal
D. greater palatine
E. posterior ethmoidal
REF. Petruson B: Acta Otolaryngol (Suppl.) 317:9, No month '74

648. Which one of the following arteries supplies the superior concha and the corresponding portions of the septum?
A. sphenopalatine
B. anterior ethmoidal
C. greater palatine
D. internal maxillary
E. posterior ethmoidal
REF. Petruson B: Acta Otolaryngol (Suppl.) 317:9, No month '74

649. Which one of the following arteries supplies the posterior and lower parts of the lateral wall and of the septum?
A. anterior ethmoidal
B. posterior ethmoidal
C. distal branches of the greater palatine artery
D. external maxillary artery
E. sphenopalatine artery
REF. Petruson B: Acta Otolaryngol (Suppl.) 317:9, No month '74

650. All of the following symptoms occur in inverted papilloma of the nasal and sinus cavities but the predominant symptoms are:
A. nasal stenosis
B. bloody nasal secretions
C. headaches
D. watery or purulent nasal secretion
E. distention of the nasal cavity
REF. Förste H-W: Fortschr Geb Roentgenstr Nuklearmed 121:1, July '74

651. Recently intractable spontaneous epistaxis has been controlled by a new method which appears to be effective:
A. posterior and anterior surgical packing
B. external carotid ligation
C. ligation internal maxillary artery through the posterior wall of the maxillary sinus using microscopic techniques
D. balloon catherization
E. electrocoagulation
F. transcatheter gelfoam embolization
REF. Sokoloff J, Wickbom I, McDonald D, Brahme F, Goergen G, Goldberger LE: Radiology 111:285, May '74

652. The treatment of choice for intractable vasomotor rhinitis or allergic rhinitis resistant to conservative therapy appears to be:
A. vidian neurectomy (Golding-Wood)
B. transantral subperiosteal vidian neurectomy
C. steroids
D. provocative tests
E. septoplasty with or without partial turbinectomy
REF. Nomura Y: The Laryngoscope 84:578, Apr '74

653. One of the most distressing aspects of thyroid disease is malignant exophthalmos which may result in loss of vision. Numerous surgical procedures have been described but the procedure of choice appears to be:
A. Kronlein lateral decompression into the region of the temporalis muscle by removal of part of the zygoma
B. Naffziger removal of the orbital roof
C. transantral decompression of the orbital contents into the ethmoid and maxillary sinuses
D. Sewall decompression of the orbital contents mesially into the anterior ethmoid sinuses
E. Hirsch removal of the orbital floor for decompression of the orbital contents
REF. Ogura JH, Lucente FE: The Laryngoscope 84:637, Apr '74

FIGURES FOR SECTION II

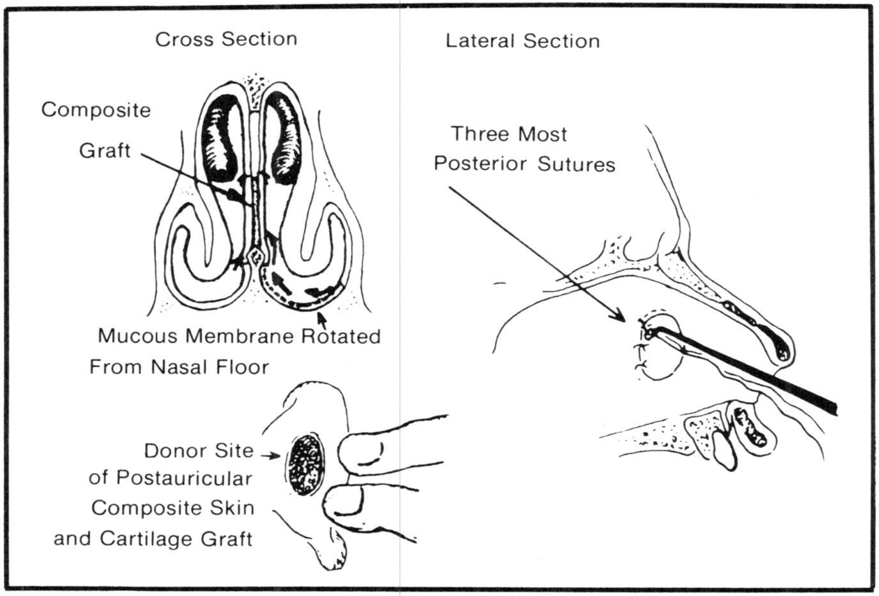

Fig. 14. At the left below, postauricular area from which composite graft is removed. At right, technique for suturing graft in place using a Buck ear curette. At the left above, graft sutured in position with nasal mucous membrane closing septal perforation opposite graft. (Courtesy of Kratz, RC: Arch Otolaryng 98:380, Dec '73)

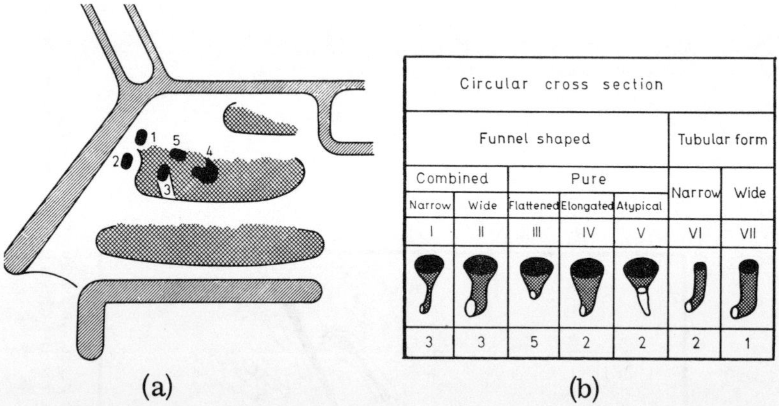

Fig. 15. (a) Possible positions of orifice of nasofrontal duct. (b) Classification of first main group of circular ducts. (Courtesy of Laszlo, I : Tr Am Acad Ophth & Otol 78:ORL-64, Mar-Apr'74)

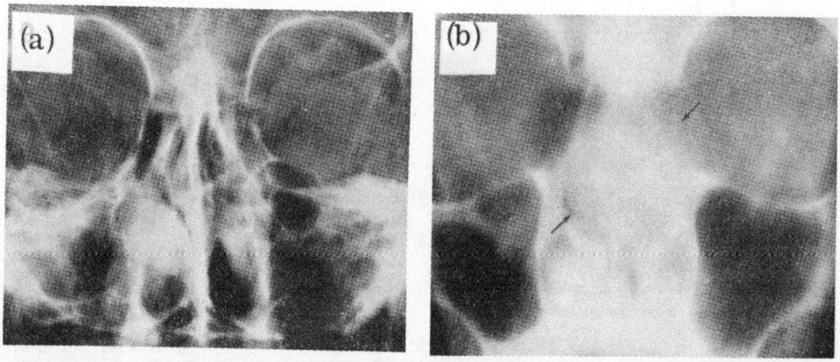

Fig. 16. (a) Normal Caldwell sinus projection. (b) Frontal polytomogram showing destruction of entire upper septum and erosion of left lamina papyracea (arrow). (Courtesy of Saunders, WH; Kelley, DR; Klosterman, HD: Tr Am Acad Ophth & Otol 78:ORL-64, Mar-Apr'74)

1.

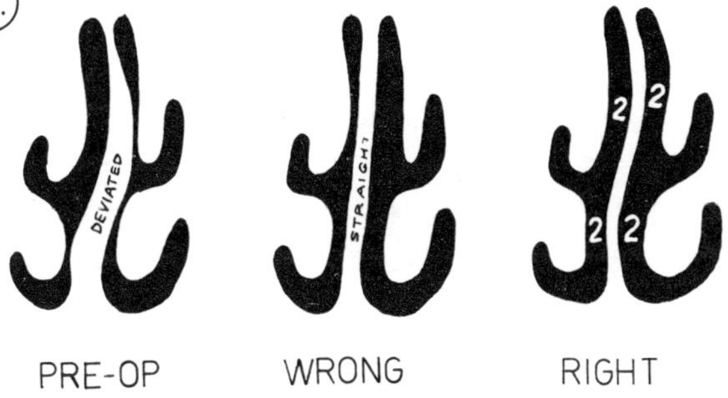

2.

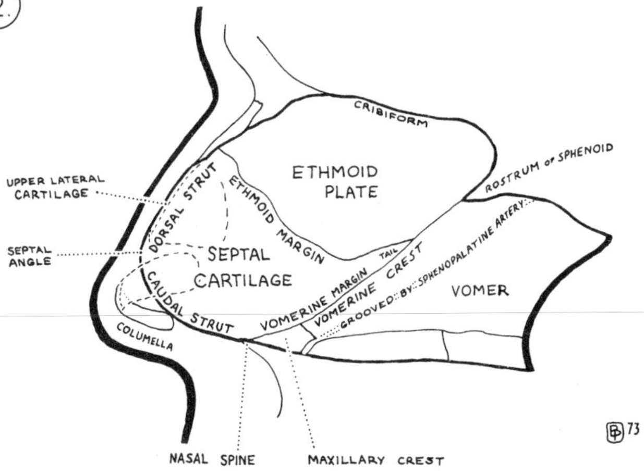

Fig. 17. (1) The aim of septal surgery is a 2 mm airway bilaterally.
(2) Terminology for surgical anatomy of the septum.

FIGURE 17, numbers 1 through 16 through the courtesy of Pearson, BW; Goodman, WS: Canadian J Laryngol 2:3:238, '73

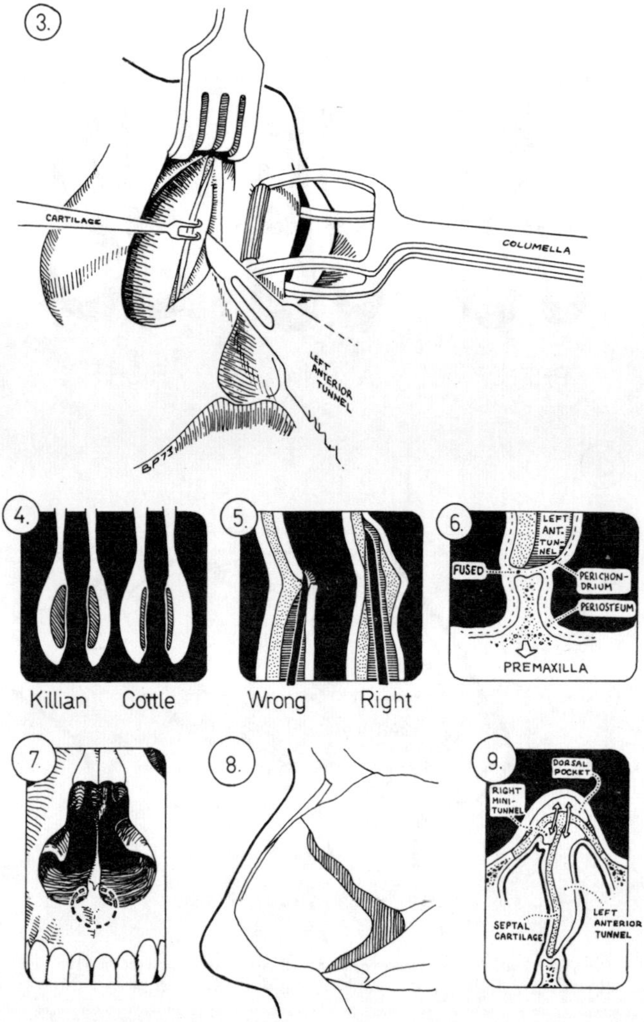

Fig. 17. (3) The right hemitransfixion incision. The stage is set for development of the left anterior tunnel. (4) The Killian speculum blades are thick, using up much more room in the nose than the Cottle blades. (5) Dealing with a sharp angulation by transecting the base of the angle and elevating the muco-perichondrium beyond it. The summit can be teased away from the mobile flap later. (6) Exposing the maxillary and vomerine crests will require a sharp incision into the interior periosteal compartment in which they live. The approach can be made from the left anterior tunnel above or from the premaxilla in front. (7) The area of bone exposed initially in the Cottle maxilla-premaxilla approach. This exposure affords subsequent passage into the right-left inferior tunnels. (8) the minimum cartilaginous resection removes the vomerine and the ethmoid margins. The septal cartilage is still attached to its muco-perichondrium on the right, but becomes mobile on two of its three fixed sides. (9) Submucosal detachment of the upper lateral cartilages from the dorsal strut in the nose with cartilaginous scoliosis.

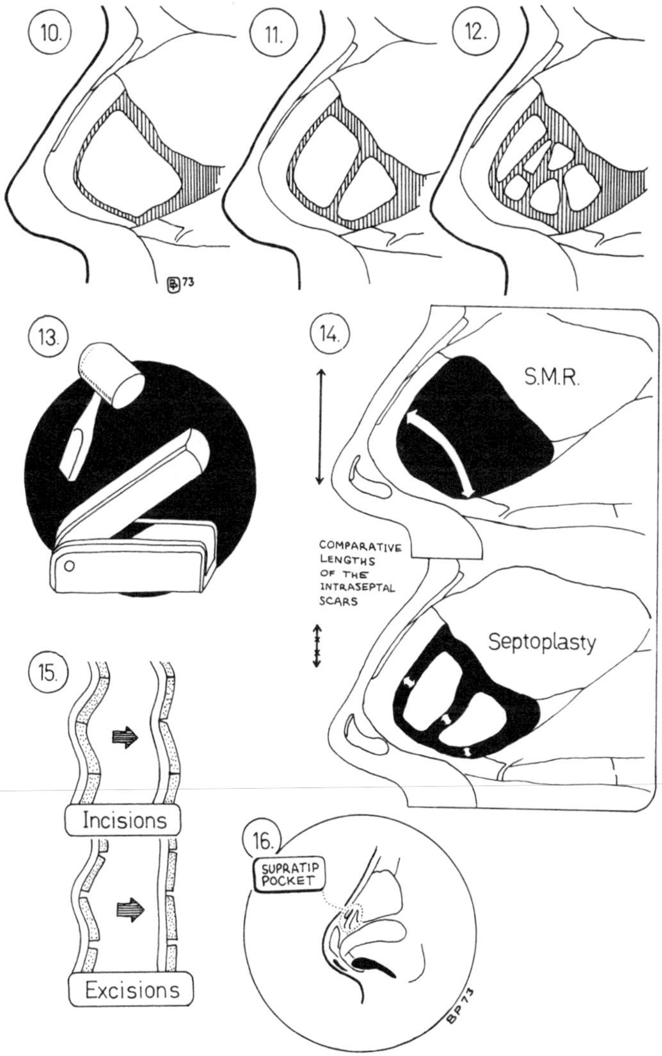

Fig. 17. (10) The central part of the septum cartilage can be freed from the caudal and dorsal struts by boomerang shaped excision as shown. Subsequent processing of compound cartilaginous curves can be undertaken in safety. (11) Simple angulations of the central area can be flattened with excision of a strip at the site of the bend. (12) The central area can be reduced to a number of islands, or facets, to allow flattening of a spherical surface. (13) Crushing box. The cartilage is placed under the hinged bar. (14) Supratip depression is secondary to scar contraction. Conservation of septal cartilage reduces intraseptal scar contraction to a minimum. (15) Since the cartilage that remains is attached to mucosa on one side, cartilage strip excisions are required to secure mobility. (16) The supratip will collapse slightly as the angle of the septum retracts. A pocket made through the anterior end of the hemitransfixion incision will accept morcelized cartilage to prevent deformity.

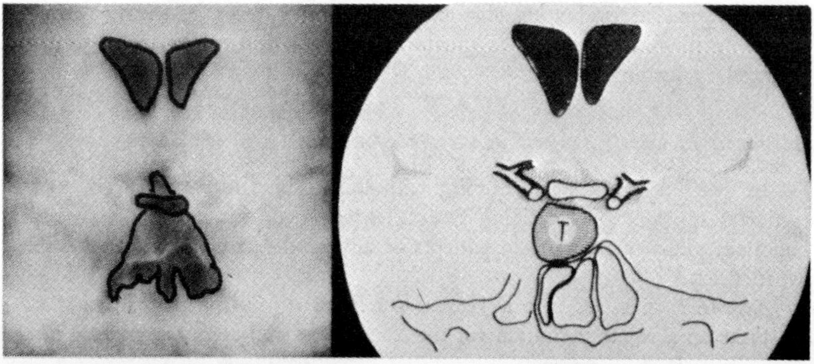

Fig. 18. A so-called micro-adenoma developed within the basal and lateral wing of the hypophysis. It lowers the floor of the sella on the right and it does not elevate the diaphragm. The chiasma is free within the chiasmatic cisterna and clearly seen here with its dumb-bell shape above the sella. A good indication for micro-transsphenoidal surgery. (Courtesy of Guiot, G. : Rhinology, 11: No. 4, 137, Dec'73)

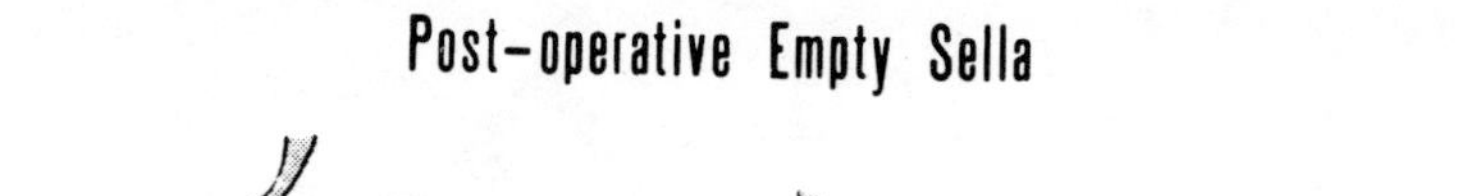

Fig. 19A. The three mechanisms of an empty sella following the ablation of a large pituitary adenoma.

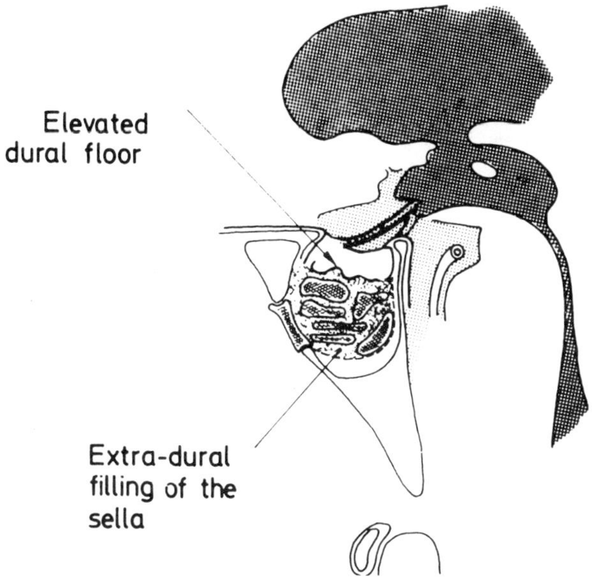

Empty sella may be the cause of two complications which justify the choice of a transsphenoidal intervention; impaired sight and rhinorrhoea.

Fig. 19B. Diagram of the operation proposed (with D. Olson) in order to alleviate a symptomatic empty sella. (Figs. 19A and 19B courtesy of Guiot, G. : Rhinology, 11:No. 4, 137, Dec '73. Paper presented at the Symposium on Transnasal Hypophysectomy, V Congress of the European Rhinologic Society, Barcelona, June 1972.

654. Iatrogenic injury to the hypopharynx and cervical esophagus can result from a nasogastric tube after 48 hours of intubation. An "iced nasogastric tube" converts a flexible instrument into a rigid tube capable of penetrating lumen walls. Although all of the following may occur, the most serious injury is:
A. nasal (mucosa) tear with epistaxis
B. penetration posterior wall of the nasopharynx
C. ulceration of the posterior wall of the oropharynx
D. laceration base of the tongue
E. postcricoid ulceration
REF. Wolff AP, Kessler S: Ann Otol, 82:778, Nov-Dec'73

655. The most frequent and dangerous complication of adenotonsillectomy is:
A. hemorrhage
B. infection
C. damage to the lingual nerve
D. damage to the glossopharyngeal nerve
E. damage to the hypoglossal nerve
REF. Williams JD, Pope TH: Arch Otolaryng, 98:306, Nov'73

656. The most important arterial blood supply and probably the only one that pierces the capsule of the tonsil is the tonsillar branch of the:
A. palatine artery
B. ascending pharyngeal artery
C. ascending palatine artery
D. dorsal lingual artery
E. facial (external maxillary) artery
REF. Williams JD, Pope TH: Arch Otolaryng, 98:306, Nov'73 (See Fig. 20)

657. In the prevention of primary tonsillectomy bleeding which of the following techniques appear to have the least morbidity and mortality?
A. dissection-snare with sponge pressure alone
B. ligation of bleeding vessels only
C. ligation of bleeding vessels followed by suturing faucial pillars
D. spot cauterization of bleeding vessels without suturing faucial pillars
E. routine cauterization of the entire midfossa region plus the upper and lower poles regardless of active bleeding and without suturing
REF. Williams JD, Pope TH: Arch Otolaryng, 98:306, Nov'73 (See Fig. 21)

658. The most common tumor arising in the parotid salivary gland is:
A. adenocarcinoma
B. squamous cell carcinoma
C. pleomorphic adenoma (mixed tumor)
D. reticulum cell sarcoma
E. lymphosarcoma
REF. Boles R, Johns ME, Batsakis JG: Ann Otol, 82:684, Sept-Oct'73

659. Which of the following methods are adequate in diagnosing carcinoma in pleomorphic adenomas in the parotid gland?
A. needle biopsy
B. skin incision with limited tissue biopsy
C. total excision of the tumor but without margin and frozen section
D. total excision of the tumor with wide margin with frozen section
E. total excision of the tumor with wide margin and numerous permanent sections
REF. Boles R, Johns ME, Batsakis JG: Ann Otol, 82:684, Sept-Oct'73

660. Sebaceous carcinoma of the parotid gland is rare and may represent aggressive variants or derivatives of mixed tumors or mucoepidermoid tumors with the malignant sebaceous cells dominating the histologic picture. Adequate therapy consists of:
A. radiotherapy
B. cyclophosphamide, 50 mg orally twice daily with weekly injections of methotrexate, 25 mg intramuscularly
C. B with vincristine, 1.0 mg given intravenously

D. B with 5-fluorouracil 500 mg intravenously
E. wide local excision with partial or total parotidectomy with or without neck dissection
REF. Shulman J, Waisman J, Morledge D: Arch Otolaryng, 98:417, Dec'73

661. Primary tonsillar bleeding includes all bleeding requiring attention within 24 to 48 hours after surgery and is in most instances related to surgical technique. The mortality rate is around 1.03 per 10,000 operations. The primary cause of death is:
A. too heavy sedation
B. laryngeal edema due to intratracheal anesthesia
C. prolonged recovery from anesthetic agents
D. aspiration of blood and vomitus with hypoventilation
E. cardiac arrest
REF. Williams JD, Pope TH: Arch Otolaryng, 98:306, Nov'73

662. Psychological problems associated with an adenotonsillectomy or tubomyringotomy may involve which one or more of the following:
A. a previously healthy child may be impressed with the idea that he is different or "something is wrong" with him
B. parents may actually give the impression that the child is being punished
C. general anesthesia and child's first "trip" with unconsciousness and fear of "no return"
D. overemphasis by parent on an insignificant small (or even large) dorsal nasal hump, but viewing a draining ear for which an adenotonsillectomy and/or tubomyringotomy is scheduled with nonchalance and negating in the child's mind the true purpose of the operation and resulting also in social ostracism
E. depersonalization especially in a university hospital
REF. Lucente FE: The Laryngoscope, 83:1684, Oct'73

663. In unilateral massive tonsillar hemorrhage, bleeding can always be controlled by:
A. suturing faucial pillars
B. suturing tonsillar pillars over surgicel
C. ligation external carotid artery
D. ligation both external carotid arteries
E. not always any of the above
REF. Maguire AJ, Briant TDR, Wortzman G: Canadian J Otolaryng, 3:1:86, '74

664. In unilateral massive tonsillar hemorrhage which of the following arteries may be involved?
A. external carotid
B. occipital
C. ascending deep cervical
D. vertebral
E. facial
REF. Maguire AJ, Briant TDR, Wortzman G: Canadian J Otolaryng, 3:1:86, '74 (See Fig. 22)

665. The site of predilection for malignant minor salivary gland tumors is:
A. palate
B. tongue
C. buccal mucosa
D. alveolar ridge
E. floor of mouth
REF. Gross CW, Nakamura T, Maguda TA, Gros JC: Canadian J Otolaryng, 3:1:56,'74

666. The most common malignant minor salivary gland tumor is:
A. adenocarcinoma
B. mucoepidermoid carcinoma
C. malignant mixed tumor
D. squamous cell carcinoma
E. adenoid cystic adenocarcinoma
REF. Gross CW, Nakamura T, Maguda TA, Gros JC: Canadian J Otolaryng, 3:1:56,'74

667. Distant metastases in malignant minor salivary gland tumors occur most commonly in:
A. brain
B. lungs
C. bone
D. liver
E. generalized
REF. Gross CW, Nakamura T, Maguda TA, Gros JC: Canadian J Otolaryng, 3:1:56,'74

668. In malignant minor salivary gland tumors initial surgery with wide tumor margin is the important determinant of cure but which of the following is most sensitive to radiation?
A. adenoid cystic adenocarcinoma
B. mucoepidermoid carcinoma
C. adenocarcinoma
D. malignant mixed tumor
E. acinic cell adenocarcinoma
REF. Gross CW, Nakamura T, Maguda TA, Gros JC: Canadian J Otolaryngol, 3:1:56,'74

669. Which of the following tumors are inadequately excised most frequently?
A. oral
B. hypopharyngeal
C. oropharynx
D. supraglottic larynx
E. glottic larynx
REF. Lee JG: Tr Am Acad Ophth & Otol, 78:ORL-49, Jan-Feb'74

670. Which of the following medications will solve the problem of indirect laryngoscopy in a severe "gaggy" patient?
A. pontocaine pharyngeal spray
B. lidocaine pharyngeal spray
C. A or B plus nasal spray
D. lidocaine injection through cricothyroid membrane
E. intravenous diazepam (Valium)
REF. Saunders WH: Tr Am Acad Ophth & Otol, 77:ORL-411, Nov-Dec'73

671. Failure to adequately drain a peritonsillar abscess may lead to which of the following conditions?
A. parapharyngeal abscess
B. pharyngomaxillary space abscess
C. laryngeal edema with epiglottitis and mediastinitis
D. generalized sepsis
E. spontaneous hemorrhage from major vessels
REF. Brandow EC: Tr Am Acad Ophth & Oto, 77:ORL-412, Nov-Dec'73

672. Peritonsillar abscess or "quinsy" is an abscess forming between the palatine tonsillar capsule and which of the following muscles?
A. glossopalatinus
B. palatinopharyngeus
C. middle pharyngeal constrictor
D. tensor veli palatinus
E. superior pharyngeal constrictor
REF. Brandow EC: Tr Am Acad Ophth & Oto, 77:ORL-412, Nov-Dec'73

673. The surgical procedure of choice for acute peritonsillar abscess is:
A. incision and drainage
B. immediate tonsillectomy on involved side
C. A above with removal upper half of involved tonsil
D. partial dissection upper pole with luxation and removal entire tonsil after a few days
E. complete immediate bilateral tonsillectomy
REF. Brandow EC: Tr Am Acad Ophth & Oto, 77:ORL-412, Nov-Dec'73

674. The pus in peritonsillar abscess is usually located:
A. behind upper pole
B. behind midportion palatine tonsil
C. behind lower pole
D. multiloculated
E. diffuse without localization
REF. Brandow EC: Tr Am Acad Ophth & Oto, 77:ORL-412, Nov-Dec'73

675. The classic symptoms of peritonsillar abscess are a toxic appearing individual with which of the following symptoms?
A. pyrexia
B. trismus
C. dysphagia
D. odynophagia
E. drooling of saliva
REF. Keat-Jin L, Traxler JH, Smith HW: Tr Am Acad Ophth & Otol, 77:ORL-417, Nov-Dec'73

676. In peritonsillar abscess there is usually:
A. leukocytosis
B. shift to the left in blood count
C. may be no elevation in leukocytes
D. lymphocytosis
E. positive "mono spot test" or Paul-Bunnell test
REF. Keat-Jin L, Traxler JH, Smith HW: Tr Am Acad Ophth & Oto, 77:ORL-417, Nov-Dec'73

677. Patients with peritonsillar abscess or infectious mononucleosis may have the same symptoms. In infectious mononucleosis there is usually:
A. leukocytosis
B. may be no elevation in leukocytes
C. shift to the left in the blood count
D. lymphocytosis
E. positive "mono spot test" or the Paul-Bunnell test
REF. Keat-Jin L, Traxler JH, Smith HW: Tr Am Acad Ophth & Oto, 77:ORL-417, Nov-Dec'73

678. Complications from peritonsillar abscess are rare but which of the following have been recorded?
A. spontaneous rupture with aspiration and pulmonary abscesses
B. dissection into the posterior compartment of the parapharyngeal space involving vital vascular and neural structures
C. involvement retropharyngeal space with mediastinitis
D. endocranial involvement with edema, cavernous sinus thrombosis, brain abscess and meningitis
E. osteomyelitis of sella turcica
REF. Keat-Jin L, Traxler JH, Smith HW: Tr Am Acad Ophth & Oto, 77:ORL-417, Nov-Dec'73

679. Which of the following have a definite effect on deglutition in man?
A. anesthesia of the oral cavity
B. anesthesia of the pharynx
C. anesthesia of the esophagus
D. simultaneous anesthesia of an area consisting of the soft palate, tonsillar pillars, tonsils, base of tongue and pharynx
E. hypopharyngeal diverticulum
REF. Mansson I, Sandberg N: The Laryngoscope, 84:427, Mar'74

680. Oncocytic tumors in the salivary glands have a low incidence and there is a continuing debate over whether the tumors are the result of hyperplasia or neoplasia. To qualify for the designation of oncocyte, a cell should have which of the following standards?
A. cell appears only in an organ with histological maturity
B. cell manifests a high level of oxidative activity in histochemical preparations
C. cells possess an unusually large number of mitochondria preparations which may show increased size, pleomorphism, and contain glycogen and/or dense analogous matrical inclusions

D. mitochondrial matrix do not contain intramitochondrial dense granules
E. special cyto-architectural features such as basal infolding, brush borders, etc., are in a stage of regression or absent
REF. Johns ME, Batsakis JG, Short CD: The Laryngoscope 83:1940, Dec'73

681. Hemangiopericytoma has which of the following features:
A. rare vascular tumor featuring Zimmerman's pericytes
B. potentially malignant with at least half metastasizing
C. intimate association with formed blood vessels and best demonstrated with a reticulum stain (Gomori) which is a necessary feature in the diagnosis
D. lack organoid features of glomus tumors but may have features of fibrosarcoma and other mesenchymal tumors
E. treatment of choice is wide local excision since adjunctive radiotherapy and irradiation alone have been disappointing
REF. Neal TF, Starke WR: The Laryngoscope, 83:1953, Dec'73

682. Oropharyngeal microflora subsequent to tonsillectomy and adenoidectomy has which of the following characteristics?
A. from an abnormal (pathologic) oropharyngeal microflora toward a more physiologic state
B. a significant rise in the anti-streptolysin-o titer
C. marked decrease in number of the bacterial pathogen streptococcus pyogenes
D. marked decrease in streptococcus groups A, B, C, and D
E. reduction in Hemophilus influenzae
REF. Sprinkle PM, Veltri RW: Tr Am Acad Ophth & Otol, 78:ORL-60, Mar-Apr'74

683. Routine prophylactic antibiotics in routine surgery other than oral or pharyngeal demonstrate which of the following?
A. prevent sepsis
B. do not prevent sepsis
C. may decrease wound infection
D. may increase wound infection
E. may decrease pulmonary infection
REF. Dor P, Klastersky J: The Laryngoscope, 83:1992, Dec'73

684. Prophylactic ampicillin and cloxacillin antibiotics in oral and pharyngeal surgery for cancer indicate which of the following statements are true?
A. frequency of postoperative wound infection is significantly lower in antibiotic treated patients
B. frequency of respiratory infections is significantly lower in antibiotic treated patients
C. gram-negative rods cause most infections
D. antibiotic therapy does not increase the rate of pharyngeal asymptomatic colonization by bacteria
E. antibiotic therapy does not increase the rate of wound asymptomatic colonization by bacteria
REF. Dor P, Klastersky J: The Laryngoscope, 83:1992, Dec'73

685. In injection of the greater palatine foramen with xylocaine one percent with epinephrine 1:100,000 (in a hypertensive patient with epistaxis from the posterior portion of the inferior meatus), 3 to 4 ml should be inserted into the canal at a depth from the palate no greater in mm than:
A. 8
B. 13
C. 19
D. 27
E. 32
REF. Hetter GP: Coll Ltrs Int Corr Soc Oph Otolaryngol 19:81, Feb '75

686. In patients after treatment for chronic tonsillitis, ordinary throat cultures:
A. when negative, are the criterion of adequate antibiotic treatment
B. are less likely to reveal pathogenic bacteria than cultures taken from the surface of tonsils in the anesthetized patient
C. A reveals same bacteria under conditions of B
D. are less likely to reveal organisms than cultures from the parenchyma of the excised tonsils
E. A reveals same bacteria under conditions of D
REF. Lotter AM, Allen GW: EENT Monthly 54:97, Mar '75

687. Adenoidectomy for recurrent acute otitis media and chronic middle ear effusions results in:
A. a definite lower incidence of purulent otorrhea
B. an increased incidence of severe ear disease in most patients
C. more severe ear disease in some children
D. improvement in most children with large adenoids
E. improvement in most children with small adenoids
F. high failure rate when associated with allergic rhinitis
REF. Bluestone CD: Ann Otol Rhinol Laryngol 84 (Suppl. 19):44, Mar '75

688. Obstructive adenoids in relation to otitis media indicate:
A. efficacy of adenoidectomy has yet to be shown
B. some children develop more severe ear disease following adenoidectomy
C. adenoidectomy in children with retrograde obstruction (preadenoidectomy roentgenogram) is usually successful
D. C with normal retrograde function and reflux is usually a failure
E. most children with large adenoids have retrograde obstruction
REF. Bluestone CD: Ann Otol Rhinol Laryngol 84 (Suppl. 19):44, Mar '75

689. Serial cephalometric radiographs taken on the same individuals indicate that the peak mass (greatest bulk) of adenoids is attained during which of the following age-in-years period?
A. birth-three
B. three-five
C. six-seven
D. eight-nine
E. ten-fifteen
REF. Subtelny JD: Ann Otol Rhinol Laryngol 84 (Suppl. 19):50, Mar '75

690. Serial cephalometric x-rays taken on the same individuals indicate that the growth potential of nasopharyngeal lymphatic tissue (adenoids) is most rapid during which of the following age-in-years period?
A. birth-one
B. birth-three
C. three-five
D. six-eight
E. nine-twelve
REF. Subtelny JD: Ann Otol Rhinol Laryngol 84 (Suppl. 19):50, Mar '75

691. During the early years, growth of adenoid tissue, nasopharyngeal area and upper face remain in a state of equilibrium permitting the maintenance of an adequate airway space in the nasopharynx. When the adenoid tissue increases, as a reaction to infection or allergy at a faster rate than increase in the dimensions of the nasopharyngeal cavity, which of the following conditions result?
A. mouth-breathing habit
B. tongue moves downward and forward away from the soft palate
C. depression in the posture of the mandible
D. longer and narrow face "adenoid facies"
E. narrow upper arch and malocclusion
REF. Subtelny JD: Ann Otol Rhinol Laryngol 84 (Suppl. 19):50, Mar '75

692. The "functional matrix theory" of craniofacial development hypothesizes which of the following:
A. closely associated with the functional activities of the head and neck areas
B. direction of growth of the skeletal structures of the face can be influenced by disproportional increase in growth of adenoids
C. B in growth of tonsils
D. adenoid tissue may reach its peak mass prior to timing of prepubertal growth in craniofacial growth in individuals
REF. Subtelny JD: Ann Otol Rhinol Laryngol 84 (Suppl. 19):50, Mar '75

693. Cephalometric films in children indicate:
A. sparse development of adenoid tissue is always associated with overt signs of immunologic deficiency
B. size of the palatine tonsil always mimics the size of the adenoid in the same individual
C. hypertrophied adenoids may involute before puberty
D. palatine tonsils never regress
E. Waldeyer's ring is not a unitary organ but the adenoids and tonsils have disparate embryonic origins, cytology and immunocompetence
REF. Pruzansky S: Ann Otol Rhinol Laryngol 84 (Suppl. 19):55, Mar '75

694. Roentgenographic visualization of nasopharyngeal lymphoid tissue in adults varying in age from 16 to 80 years with an equal number of each sex suggests that complete involution of the adenoids occur by age of:
A. 15 years
B. 20 years
C. 25 years
D. 30 years
E. throughout life
REF. Pruzansky S: Ann Otol Rhinol Laryngol 84 (Suppl. 19):55, Mar '75

695. Recurrent exudative tonsillitis in children is characterized by the persistent presence of which of the following bacterial and/or fungal species?
A. streptococcus pyogenes
B. pneumococcus sp
C. staphylococcus aureus
D. hemophilus influenzae
E. Candida albicans
F. gram negative aerobes and anaerobes
REF. Sprinkle PM: Ann Otol Rhinol Laryngol 84 (Suppl. 19):25, Mar '75

696. Following adenotonsillectomy for recurrent exudative tonsillitis in children:
A. IgG increases
B. IgG decreases to a normal level
C. IgA increases
D. IgA decreases to a normal level
E. No change in IgG or IgA levels
REF. Sprinkle PM: Ann Otol Rhinol Laryngol 84 (Suppl. 19):25, Mar '75

697. Immunologically, children with recurrent exudative tonsillitis have statistically significant presence of:
A. hypergammaglobulinemia
B. adult or higher than adult levels of IgG
C. reduced levels of IgG
D. adult or higher than adult levels of IgA
E. reduced levels of IgA
REF. Sprinkle PM: Ann Otol Rhinol Laryngol 84 (Suppl. 19):25, Mar '75

698. The results of throat cultures in tonsillitis as routinely used in clinical practice are:
A. sophisticated enough for adequate treatment
B. not accurate enough for adequate therapy
C. adequate for diagnosis of the etiological agent or agents
D. not adequate for proper diagnosis of etiological agents
E. determining factor in a decision about indication for a tonsillectomy
REF. Sprinkle PM: Ann Otol Rhinol Laryngol 84 (Suppl. 19):25, Mar '75

699. The term sore throat is:
A. a diagnosis
B. a symptom
C. limited to infection with streptococcus pyogenes
D. C with pneumococcus sp
E. C with Hemophilus influenzae
REF. Sprinkle PM: Ann Otol Rhinol Laryngol 84 (Suppl. 19):25, Mar '75

700. The production of rheumatic fever by streptococcus pyogenes:
A. meets Koch's postulates
B. does not meet Koch's postulates
C. involves complement
D. does not involve complement
E, may be a bacterial-viral relationship
REF. Sprinkle PM: Ann Otol Rhinol Laryngol 84 (Suppl. 19):25, Mar '75

701. Which of the following intrinsic factors may affect or modify the ecological system (oral microflora) in the upper respiratory tract in the human host?
A. secretory IgA
B. secretory IgE
C. adenotonsillectomy
D. salivary enzymes
E. interferon
F. antibiotics
G. antibiosis
H. aging
I. dentition
REF. Sprinkle PM: Ann Otol Rhinol Laryngol 84 (Suppl. 19):25, Mar '75

702. All of the following complications and conditions are associated with diseases of the tonsils and adenoids but which one condition is uncommon?
A. peritonsillar cellulitis
B. peritonsillar abscess
C. retropharyngeal abscess
D. parapharyngeal abscess
E. tonsillar abscess
REF. Bluestone CD, et al.: Ann Otol Rhinol Laryngol 84 (Suppl. 19):11, Mar '75

703. Exudative tonsillitis with a syndrome of pharyngoconjunctival fever is most likely due to:
A. streptococcus pyogenes
B. haemophilus influenzae
C. staphylococcus aureus
D. M. pneumoniae
E. adenoviruses
REF. Klein JO: Ann Otol Rhinol Laryngol 84 (Suppl. 19):30, Mar '75

704. The predominant bacterial cause of pharyngotonsillitis and exudative tonsillitis is:
A. staphylococcus aureus
B. A beta hemolytic streptococci
C. anaerobic bacteria
D. diplococcus pneumoniae
E. bacterial variants (L-forms)
REF. Klein JO: Ann Otol Rhinol Laryngol 84 (Suppl. 19):30, Mar '75

705. Which one of the following forms of therapy is definitely contraindicated in the treatment of a ranula?
A. marsupialization
B. ligation of the duct
C. instillation of a mild corrosive chemical into the cyst
D. aspiration
E. extirpation of the gland (sublingual)
REF. Schwartz SI: Principles of Surgery, McGraw-Hill Book Co., New York City, p. 565, 1974

706. A cystic swelling in the floor of the mouth caused by obstruction of the sublingual duct (ranula) is best treated by:
A. aspiration
B. marsupialization
C. ligation of Wharton's duct
D. extirpation of the gland (sublingual)
E. instillation of a mild corrosive chemical into the cyst
REF. Frazier W: Mod Med 43:81, Sept '75; Schwartz SI: Principles of Surgery, McGraw-Hill Book Co., New York City, p. 565, 1974

707. Which one of the following forms of therapy is not indicated for any parotid tumors?
A. superficial lobectomy
B. radical parotidectomy
C. simple excision
D. chemotherapy
E. irradiation without tissue biopsy
REF. Gaisford JC, et al.: Plast Reconstr Surg 43:504, No. 5, No month '69

708. The appropriate initial therapy for a mass in the parotid gland is:
A. incisional biopsy with frozen section
B. superficial lobectomy with frozen section
C. radical parotidectomy with frozen section
D. radiotherapy
E. chemotherapy
REF. Frazier W: Mod Med 43:81, Sept '75

709. What percent of parotid tumors are benign and mostly mixed tumors?
A. 10
B. 20
C. 30
D. 50
E. 80
REF. Gaisford JC, et al.: Plast Reconstr Surg 43:504, No. 5, No month '69

710. What percent of all salivary gland tumors arise in the parotid?
A. 10
B. 20
C. 30
D. 50
E. 80
REF. Gaisford JC, et al.: Plast Reconstr Surg 43:504, No. 5, No month '69

711. In a small suspicious neoplastic lesion of the tongue with a small ipsilateral neck node, which of the following initial procedures are contraindicated?
A. biopsy of the tongue (primary) lesion
B. open neck biopsy of the cervical node with possible seeding of the skin and subcutaneous tissue
C, irradiation without prior diagnosis
D. radical surgery without prior diagnosis
E. neck dissection before control of the primary lesion
REF. MacComb, WS, Fletcher GH: Cancer of the Head and Neck, Williams & Wilkins Co., Baltimore, p. 91, 1967

712. The initial treatment for a suspicious neoplastic lesion of the tongue with a small ipsilateral neck node is:
A. biopsy of the tongue lesion to confirm histologically the diagnosis
B. surgical removal of the primary and neck node with frozen section
C. biopsy of the neck mass
D. irradiation simultaneously of the primary and neck lesion
E. irradiation of the neck prior to removal of the primary lesion
REF. MacComb WS, Fletcher GH: Cancer of the Head and Neck, Williams & Wilkins Co., Baltimore, p. 91, 1967

713. A patient with extensive ulcerations of the mouth, nose, throat (and vagina) diagnosed as pemphigus vulgaris by biopsy is most effectively treated by:
A. steroids
B. combined immunosuppressive and corticosteroid therapy
C. methotrexate
D. cyclophosphamide
E. gold salts
F. antibiotics
G. smallpox immunizations
REF. Felice FM, Gutherie MB: Consultant 15:15, Sept '75

714. A patient with clinical leukoplakia of the oral mucosa (white patch-like lesions that do not wipe off) with a biopsy showing dyskeratosis should be treated by:
A. early surgical removal
B. freezing nitrogen solutions
C. elimination of sources of irritation (dental caries, ill-fitting dentures)
D. restriction of excessive alcohol consumption, smoking, and biting cheeks
E. vitamins in high dosage
REF. Fox WF: Consultant 15:(Brief Consultation), Sept '75

715. A patient with clinical leukoplakia of the oral mucosa (white patch-like lesions that do not wipe off and with a benign biopsy) should be treated by:
A. elimination of sources of irritation (dental consultation about jagged teeth, ill-fitting dentures)
B. restriction of smoking
C. B of excessive alcohol consumption
D. discontinuation of the habit of biting cheeks
E. regular examination every 6 to 12 months
F. vitamins in high dosage
REF. Fox WF: Consultant 15:(Brief Consultation), Sept '75

716. Parotid sialocele as a result of trauma to Stensen's duct is most effectively treated by:
A. radiation (1,800 rads)
B. duct ligation
C. parasympathetic denervation by the transtympanic sectioning of Jacobson's nerve over the promontory (exploratory tympanotomy)
D. anticholinergic drugs - atropine sulfate, methantheline bromide
E. superficial parotidectomy
F. needle aspiration
REF. Langenbrunner DJ: Trans Am Acad Ophthalmol Otolaryngol 80:ORL-375, July '75

717. The most common malignant tumor in the parotid in children is:
A. mucoepidermoid cancer
B. undifferentiated cancer
C. adenocarcinoma
D. undifferentiated sarcoma
E. adenocystic carcinoma
F. acinic cell carcinoma
G. squamous cell carcinoma
REF. Fechner RE: Arch Otolaryngol 101:520, Aug '75

718. The most common benign tumor in the parotid in children is:
A. lymphangioma
B. mixed (pleomorphic adenoma)
C. Warthin tumor (papillary cystadenoma lymphomastosum) or adenolymphoma
D. hemangioma
E. neurinoma
REF. Fechner RE: Arch Otolaryngol 101:520, Aug '75

719. Infectious mononucleosis (glandular fever) may have all of the following neurological symptoms preceding the full clinical syndrome. The most common symptom is:
A. lymphocytic meningitis
B. encephalomyelitis
C. polyneuritis
D. mononeuritis
REF. Michel RG, Pope TH, Jr., Patterson CN: Arch Otolaryngol 101:486, Aug '75

720. Teratogenic anomalies such as cleft palate and tracheoesophageal fistula or atresia can occur (during the first trimester of pregnancy) from:
A. the pill
B. hormonal pregnancy tests
C. medroxy - progesterone
D. progesterone
E. thalidomide
F. rubella
G. lithium
H. exogenous thyroid
I. diphenylhydantoin
J. penicillin
K. dextroamphetamine
L. LSD
M. "speed"
N. hashish
O. marijuana
P. estrogen
REF. Nora AH, Nora JJ: Emergency Med 7:187, June '75

721. Sialography or x-ray visualization of the salivary glands and their ducts for the injection of a radiopaque contrast medium include all of the following but preference is usually given to the use of:
A. lacrimal dilators or tapered probes
B. polyethylene tubing
C. 20-gauge 3 inch needle
D. lipiodol (Fougera) a fat-soluble agent
E. salpix (Ortho), a water-soluble substance
REF. Fordham SD, Schatz CJ: Emergency Med 7:101, June '75

722. The incidence of Ampicillin rashes is:
A. greater with intramuscular or intravenous injection
B. greater when given orally
C. greater with increased dosage
D. varies with specific commercial preparations
E. in general not related to administration, dosage or commercial preparation
REF. Jegasothy BV: Mod Med 43:113, Aug '75

723. Ampicillin rashes occur usually after the following day of therapy:
A. 3rd
B. 5th
C. 9th
D. 14th
E. 21st
REF. Jegasothy BV: Mod Med 43:113, Aug '75

724. Ampicillin rashes resemble drug eruptions in general and their incidence is higher in patients with:
A. pneumonia
B. pharyngitis
C. tonsillitis
D. rhinosinusitis
E. infectious mononucleosis
REF. Jegasothy BV: Mod Med 43:113, Aug '75

725. Serum copper levels are elevated in which of the following conditions:
A. viral infections
B. chronic inflammation
C. acute inflammation
D. thyroid hormones
E. exacerbation of Hodgkin's disease
REF. Hrgovcic MJ, Tessmer CF, Mumford DM, Ong PS, Gamble JF, Shullenberger CC: Tex Med 71:53, Feb '75

726. Cicatricial pemphigoid (benign mucosal pemphigoid) may be related to bullous pemphigoid and predominantly affects the mucosa, pharynx, larynx, esophagus, genitalia, eyes and also skin. Cicatricial pemphigoid is:
A. autoimmune
B. hereditary
C. blistering (tense vesicles)
D. characterized in most patients by the deposition of IgG in the basement membrane zone of the mucosa (direct immunofluorescence)
E. usually diagnosed by biopsy and cytologic smears
REF. Bean SF: South Med J 67:1187, Oct '74

727. Herpangia with sudden fever of short duration and vesicular or ulcerated lesions in the faucial area and/or soft palate with acute lymphonodular pharyngitis occurring in epidemic patterns in the Summer and Fall is associated with:
A. coxsackie virus A
B. adenovirus
C. rhinovirus
D. parainfluenza viruses
E. Epstein-Barr virus
REF. Klein JO: Ann Otol Rhinol Laryngol 84 (Suppl. 19):30, Mar '75

728. Candida albicans appears in:
A. exudative tonsillitis in an immuno-competent patient without antibody therapy
B. young infant as thrush
C. immuno-compromised host
D. patient receiving Ampicillin for short duration
E. patient receiving broad spectrum antimicrobial therapy for a prolonged period
REF. Klein JO: Ann Otol Rhinol Laryngol 84 (Suppl. 19):30, Mar '75

729. Primary herpetic infection with lesions in the anterior mouth but which may spread extensively to involve the oropharynx is usually associated with:
A. adenovirus
B. herpesvirus hominus
C. rhinovirus
D. parainfluenza virus
E. respiratory syncytial virus
REF. Klein JO: Ann Otol Rhinol Laryngol 84 (Suppl. 19):30, Mar '75

730. A cause of pharyngitis which is becoming more common and may be easily overlooked is that due to:
A. M. hominis
B. hperpesvirus hominis
C. treponema pallidum
D. bacterial variants (L-forms)
E. Neisseria gonorrhoeae
REF. Klein JO: Ann Otol Rhinol Laryngol 84 (Suppl. 19):30, Mar '75

731. A patient with prolonged and undetected (or detected) fever with or without cervical adenitis with normal nasal passages, normal middle ears-mouth-pharynx-larynx, and normal sinus x-rays has most likely if due to an upper respiratory lesion:
A. haemophilus influenzae infection
B. influenza
C. parainfluenza
D. suppurative adenoiditis or nasopharyngitis
E. anaerobic bacterial infection
REF. Klein JO: Ann Otol Rhinol Laryngol 84 (Suppl. 19):30, Mar '75

732. Suppurative adenoiditis or nasopharyngitis with or without cervical adenitis is due usually to:
A. staphylococcus aureus
B. streptococcus pyogenes
C. haemophilus influenzae
D. diplococcus pneumoniae
E. anaerobic bacteria
REF. Klein JO: Ann Otol Rhinol Laryngol 84 (Suppl. 19):30, Mar '75

733. Which of the following microorganisms occur infrequently in the United States in association with tonsillitis and adenoiditis but must be considered?
A. diphtheria
B. tuberculosis
C. syphilis
D. anaerobic bacteria
E. diplococcus pneumoniae
REF. Klein JO: Ann Otol Rhinol Laryngol 84 (Suppl. 19):30, Mar '75

734. Which of the following diseases of the oral cavity usually do not involve the tonsils or adenoids?
A. streptococcus infection
B. Vincent's infection associated with fusiform bacilli and oral spirochetes
C. haemophilus influenzae
D. noma due to fuso-spirochetes and possibly oral streptococci and staphylococci
E. aphthous stomatitis
REF. Klein JO: Ann Otol Rhinol Laryngol 84 (Suppl. 19):30, Mar '75

735. The etiology of aphthous stomatitis is due to:
A. adenovirus
B. rhinovirus
C. herpesvirus hominis
D. parainfluenza virus
E. uncertain
REF. Klein JO: Ann Otol Rhinol Laryngol 84 (Suppl. 19):30, Mar '75

736. Microorganism responsible for systemic disease which may include inflammation of the tonsils and pharynx are:
A. Neissseria meningococcus
B. toxoplasma gondi
C. listeria monocytogenes
D. echoviruses
E. measles
REF. Klein JO: Ann Otol Rhinol Laryngol 84 (Suppl. 19):30, Mar '75

737. Which of the following microorganisms have been suggested as causes of pharyngotonsillitis but whose relationship to disease is equivocal?
A. mycoplasma hominis
B. streptococcus pyogenes
C. staphylococcus aureus
D. adenovirus
E. bacterial variants (L-forms)
REF. Klein JO: Ann Otol Rhinol Laryngol 84 (Suppl. 19):30, Mar '75

738. Which of the following organisms have proven to be responsible for various upper respiratory signs and symptoms including pharyngotonsillitis?
A. mycoplasma pneumoniae
B. rhinoviruses
C. syncytial virus
D. parainfluenza virus
E. influenzae virus
REF. Klein JO: Ann Otol Rhinol Laryngol 84 (Suppl. 19):30, Mar '75

739. A major cause of acute pharyngitis or exudative tonsillitis in adolescents and young adults is:
A. Neisseria gonorrhoeae
B. Epstein-Barr virus
C. treponema pallidum
D. anaerobic bacteria
E. Candida albicans
REF. Klein JO: Ann Otol Rhinol Laryngol 84 (Suppl. 19):30, Mar '75

740. Herpetic gingivostomatitis occurs in intravenously used marihuana and may be caused by:
A. drug impairment of the patient's immune response
B. cannabinols in marihuana
C. phenols in marihuana
D. leukopenia
E. needle transmission of virus
REF. Payne RJ: JAMA 233:351, July '75

741. A patient with an upper respiratory illness caused by hemophilus influenzae and not responding to ampicillin should be treated as an outpatient with which one of the following drugs?
A. chloramphenicol
B. keflex
C. tetracycline
D. lincomycin
E. clindamycin
REF. Kitto W: JAMA 233:325, July '75

742. Strains of haemophilus influenzae have shown increasing resistance to which one of the following drugs?
A. chloramphenicol
B. ampicillin
C. tetracycline
D. lincomycin
E. clindamycin
REF. Kitto W: JAMA 233:325, July '75

743. Although useful in herpes simplex and herpes zoster, idoxuridine (stoxil) interferes with DNA synthesis and cell division and should not be used in:
A. children
B. females of any age
C. males of any age
D. elderly persons
E. pregnant women
REF. Dawber R: Br Med J 2:526, June '74

744. A physician must remember that in the treatment of severe haemophilus influenzae infection, resistant to Ampicillin and not responding to tetracyclines, chloramphenicol is useful and safe if which of the following rules are observed?
A. hospital medication only with daily blood studies to warn of the development of aplastic anemia
B. adequate dosage
C. adjunct to penicillin where it is useful in breached bacterial defenses
D. clinically valuable where bone marrow depression led to the initial infection
E. outpatient medication on a limited time basis
REF. Kitto W: JAMA 233:325, July '75

745. A variety of microorganisms may be etiologically involved in acute tonsillitis, adenoiditis, or adenotonsillitis and most of these are:
A. staphylococcus aureus
B. group A, B-hemolytic streptococcus
C. streptococcus pyogens
D. C diphtheria
E. viruses
REF. Bluestone CD, et al.: Ann Otol Rhinol Laryngol 84 (Suppl. 19):11, Mar '75

746. When the palatine tonsils are severely hypertrophied, a tonsillectomy is certainly indicated in:
A. dysphagia with obstruction of the digestive tract for six or more months
B. weight loss for six or more months
C. failure to gain weight for six or more months
D. cor pulmonale
E. altered speech or dental abnormalities
REF. Bluestone CD, et al.: Ann Otol Rhinol Laryngol 84 (Suppl. 19):11, Mar '75

747. Adenoidectomy is usually contraindicated in:
A. velopharyngeal insufficiency
B. blood dyscrasias (certain types)
C. allergy (nasal, severe, acute) without treatment
D. acute inflammatory rhinosinusitis or acute upper respiratory infection
E. immunologic deficiencies
REF. Bluestone CD, et al.: Ann Otol Rhinol Laryngol 84 (Suppl. 19):11, Mar '75

748. When the adenoids are severely hypertrophied, an adenoidectomy is certainly indicated in:
A. abnormalities of breathing
B. abnormalities of speech
C. dental malocclusion
D. recurrent or chronic rhinitis or sinusitis
E. obstruction to the eustachian tube with associated middle ear disease
REF. Bluestone CD, et al.: Ann Otol Rhinol Laryngol 84 (Suppl. 19):11, Mar '75

749. The mortality of tonsillectomies in the United States is an average of one death per number of tonsillectomies of?
A. 9,000
B. 11,000
C. 16,000
D. 42,000
E. 63,000
REF. Bluestone CD, et al.: Ann Otol Rhinol Laryngol 84 (Suppl. 19):11, Mar '75

750. The cause of death in adenotonsillectomy is due to:
A. anesthetic chemicals
B. cardiac arrest
C. hemorrhage
D. infection
E. dehydration (severe)
REF. Bluestone CD, et al.: Ann Otol Rhinol Laryngol 84 (Suppl. 19):11, Mar '75

751. All of the following complications and conditions are associated with diseases of the tonsils and adenoids but which one condition is uncommon?
A. fetor oris
B. rhinitis
C. weight loss or failure to gain weight
D. congestive heart failure
E. paranasal sinusitis
REF. Bluestone CD, et al.: Ann Otol Rhinol Laryngol 84 (Suppl. 19):11, Mar '75

752. Obstruction due to hypertrophied adenoids or tonsils or both may cause abnormalities of:
A. breathing
B. speaking
C. feeding
D. hearing
E. facial development
REF. Bluestone CD, et al.: Ann Otol Rhinol Laryngol 84 (Suppl. 19):11, Mar '75

753. In the pathogenesis of acute tonsillitis and adenoiditis or adenotonsillitis, a variety of microorganisms may be etiologically involved but among bacteria which two of the following are recognized as important agents?
A. streptococcus pyogenes
B. staphylococcus aureus
C. escherichia coli
D. proteus vulgaris
E. C diphtheria
REF. Bluestone CD, et al.: Ann Otol Rhinol Laryngol 84 (Suppl. 19):11, Mar '75

754. The treatment of acute tonsillitis, adenoiditis and pharyngotonsillitis should be guided mainly by the results of the culture and in bacteriologically confirmed infections due to group A, B-hemolytic streptococcus, the therapy of choice is:
A. penicillin G
B. penicillin V
C. A or B
D. erythromycin
E. clindamycin
REF. Bluestone CD, et al.: Ann Otol Rhinol Laryngol 84 (Suppl. 19):11, Mar '75

755. In patients allergic to penicillin with acute tonsillitis, adenoiditis or pharyngotonsillitis due to proven group A, B-hemolytic streptococcus, the medication should be:
A. erythromycin
B. sulfacetamide
C. tetracyline
D. clindamycin
E. oral cephalosporin
REF. Bluestone CD, et al.: Ann Otol Rhinol Laryngol 84 (Suppl. 19):11, Mar '75

756. When the culture is negative, the treatment of chronic tonsillitis, adenoiditis and pharyngotonsillitis should consist of a trial period of prophylactic:
A. erythromycin
B. clindamycin
C. oral cephalosporin
D. sulfacetamide
E. penicillin
REF. Bluestone CD, et al.: Ann Otol Rhinol Laryngol 84 (Suppl. 19):11, Mar '75

757. Contraindications to adenoidectomy are:
A. congenital palatopharyngeal incompetence
B. bifid or missing uvula
C. zona pellucida of the soft palate
D. submucous defect of the muscle in the midline of the soft palate
E. submucous cleft of the hard palate from notching of the posterior nasal spine to extensive absence of the bony palatal shelves
REF. Pruzansky S: Ann Otol Rhinol Laryngol 84 (Suppl. 19):55, Mar '75

758. Seriatim roentgencephalometry (cephalometric radiograph) in a study of tonsils and adenoids shows:
A. soft palate at rest is extended to lay on the upper pole of the tonsil
B. A on the dorsum of the tongue
C. enlarged (hypertrophied) palatine tonsil contributes to alteration in respiratory pattern
D. C affects kinesiology of the tongue and circumoral musculature with deleterious effects on developing dental occlusion
E. snoring noise when patient is asleep
REF. Pruzansky S: Ann Otol Rhinol Laryngol 84 (Suppl. 19):55, Mar '75

759. Which of the following can occur in the Waldeyer lymphoid ring?
A. lymphosarcoma
B. lymphoepithelioma
C. epidermoid carcinoma
D. Hodgkin's disease
E. all of these
REF. Todd GB, Michaels L: Cancer 34:1769, Nov '74

760. The relationship between tonsils and speech production indicate that:
A. very little information is available about the effect of hypertrophied tonsils on speech production
B. enlarged palatine tonsils usually have no noticeable effect on speech
C. very large palatine tonsils obstructing the oral airway affect speech production (voice quality and speech articulation)
D. very large palatine tonsils may aid speech production in congenital palatopharyngeal incompetence
E. there is absolutely no relationship
REF. Morris HL: Ann Otol Rhinol Laryngol 84 (Suppl. 19):63, Mar '75

761. All of the following complications and conditions are associated with diseases of the tonsils and adenoids but which one condition is uncommon?
A. hemorrhage
B. cervical lymphadentitis
C. rhinitis
D. paranasal sinusitis
E. otitis media
REF. Bluestone CD, et al.: Ann Otol Rhinol Laryngol 84 (Suppl. 19):11, Mar '75

762. All of the following complications and conditions are associated with diseases of the tonsils and adenoids but which one condition is uncommon?
A. abnormalities of dentition
B. abnormalities of speech
C. gangrene of tonsils
D. impairment of hearing
E. disorders of olfaction
REF. Bluestone CD, et al.: Ann Otol Rhinol Laryngol 84 (Suppl. 19):11, Mar '75

763. The most common surgical procedure in otolaryngology is tonsillectomy and the most frequent complication is hemorrhage. Zonal electrocoagulation results in:
A. shortened operating time
B. more postoperative morbidity than from spot electrocoagulation
C. B less morbidity
D. more postoperative morbidity than from ligation
E. D less morbidity
REF. Roy A, Rosa CDL, Vecchio A: Arch Otolaryngol 102:9, Jan '76

764. Mixed tumors of the parotid:
A. are the most common benign tumors of salivary origin
B. occur rarely as synchronous or simultaneous bilateral tumors
C. B occur commonly
D. are treated by superficial parotidectomy
E. are resected without facial nerve dissection
REF. Brill AH, Fitz-Hugh S: Arch Otolaryngol 101:751, Dec '75

FIGURES FOR SECTION III

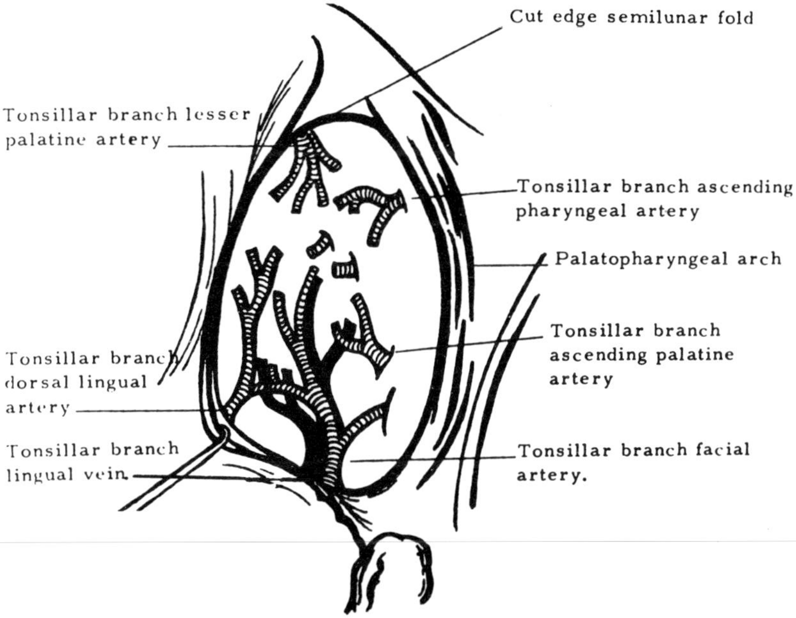

Fig. 20. Primary blood supply to tonsil. Tonsillar branch of lingual vein probably chief drain. Tonsillar branch of facial artery probably only one that pierces capsule of tonsil. (Courtesy of Williams, J. D.; Pope, T. H.: Arch Otolaryng, 98:306, Nov'73)

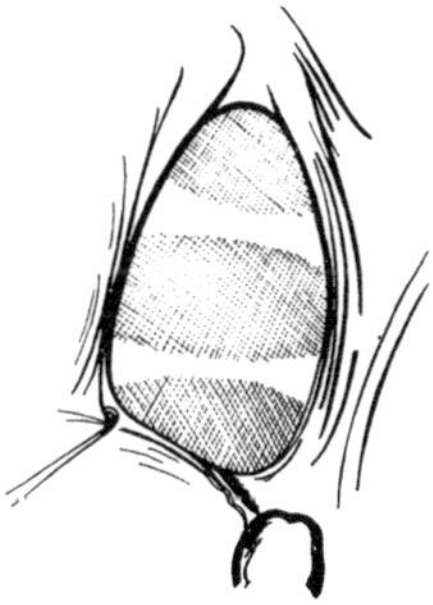

← Fig. 21. Cauterized areas (cross-hatched areas) in tonsillar fossa. (Courtesy of Williams, J. D.; Pope, T. H.: Arch Otolaryng, 98:306, Nov'73)

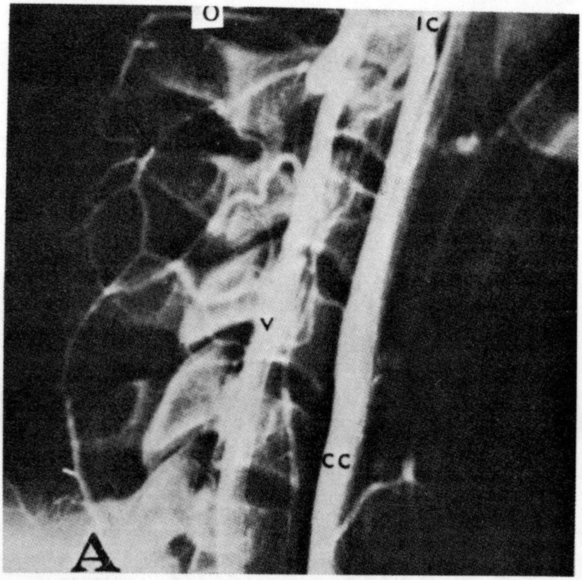

Fig. 22A. (A) R Brachial Arteriogram: shows filling of the vertebral (V), common carotid (CC) arteries, and right internal carotid (IC). (There is some filling left IC also). The external carotid branches do not fill due to their previous ligation. Note occipital artery (O) opacified via ascending deep cervical vessels and from muscular branches of the vertebral artery.

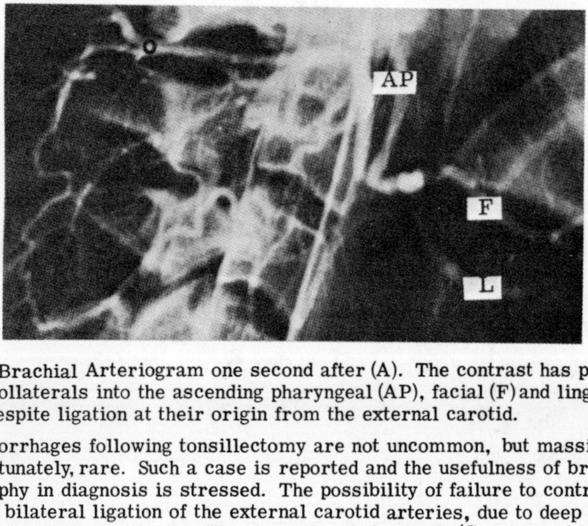

Fig. 22B. Brachial Arteriogram one second after (A). The contrast has passed from the collaterals into the ascending pharyngeal (AP), facial (F) and lingual (L) arteries despite ligation at their origin from the external carotid.

Slight hemorrhages following tonsillectomy are not uncommon, but massive bleeding is, fortunately, rare. Such a case is reported and the usefulness of brachial arteriography in diagnosis is stressed. The possibility of failure to control hemorrhage with bilateral ligation of the external carotid arteries, due to deep cervical collateral circulation to the tonsillar fossa is emphasized. (Courtesy of Maguire, A. J.; Briant, T. D. R.; Wortzman, G.: Canadian J Otolaryng, 3:1:86, '74)

765. Which of the following appear to be true of tuberculous cervical lymphadenitis?
A. uncommon in United States
B. number of cases of scrofula are increasing
C. localized process without active pulmonary tuberculosis does occur
D. radical surgery is the treatment of choice
E. antituberculous chemotherapy is the treatment of choice
REF. Ord RJ, Matz GJ: Arch Otolaryngol, 99:327, May'74

766. The initial symptom in 90% of patients with tuberculous cervical lymphadenitis is:
A. enlarging neck mass
B. draining sinus tract
C. neck mass with draining sinus tract
D. generalized inflammation without fever
E. generalized inflammation with fever
REF. Ord RJ, Matz GJ: Arch Otolaryngol, 99:327, May'74

767. Tuberculous cervical lymphadenitis is found in all of the following locations but less frequently in which two of the following areas?
A. anterior cervical area
B. submandibular
C. posterior triangle
D. supraclavicular
E. parotid
REF. Ord RJ, Matz GJ: Arch Otolaryngol, 99:327, May'74 (See Fig. 23)

768. Intradermal skin testing with purified protein derivative (PPD) in patients with typical cervical lymphadenitis due to mycobacteria tuberculosis gives a positive reaction greater in mm in diameter than:
A. 2
B. 5
C. 10
D. 15
E. 20
REF. Ord RJ, Matz GJ: Arch Otolaryngol, 99:327, May'74

769. In atypical mycobacteria tuberculous cervical lymphadenitis, which of the following statements are true?
A. 10% of patients fall in this category
B. histological appearance indistinguishable from typical Mycobacteria Tuberculosis
C. weakly positive or negative reaction to first strength or intermediate strength tests with PPD
D. normal pulmonary x-ray films
E. causes progressive disease when inoculated in guinea pigs
REF. Ord RJ, Matz GJ: Arch Otolaryngol, 99:327, May'74

770. Atypical mycobacteria usually involve which of the following cervical nodes?
A. submental
B. submandibular
C. tonsillar
D. posterior triangle
E. supraclavicular
REF. Ord RJ, Matz GJ: Arch Otolaryngol, 99:327, May'74

771. Sodium iodine I-131 given in thyroid - ablative doses to pregnant women during the third or fourth month of pregnancy can result in the fetus in:
A. iodine crossing the placental barrier
B. (fetal thyroid has a specific affinity for iodine) a much greater concentration of iodine in the fetal thyroid compared with the maternal thyroid
C. local radiation damage to the embryonic tracheal cartilage with resultant hypoplasia
D. later stridor in the newborn infant
E. later infant thyroid hypoplasia
REF. Jafek BW, Small R, Lillina DL: Arch Otolaryngol, 99:369, May'74

772. Oat cell carcinoma of the larynx is an extremely rare neoplasm but may be mistaken for which one of the following tumors?
A. epidermoid carcinoma
B. adenocarcinoma
C. melanoma
D. glomus tumor
E. lymphosarcoma
REF. Ferlito A: Ann Otol, 83:254, Mar-Apr'74

773. One of the most dramatic complications of tracheostomy or endotracheal intubation is a fistula between the trachea and the innominate artery and usually occurs under which of the following conditions and signs?
A. patients requiring ventilatory assistance with cuffed tracheostomy tube placed below the level of the fourth tracheal ring
B. occurs with cuffed tubes
C. occurs with non-cuffed tubes
D. visible pulsations of the tracheostomy tube is a warning sign
E. earliest sign is bright red bleeding from the tracheostomy tube and massive hemorrhage usually occurs as the tracheostomy tube is changed
REF. Weissman BW: The Laryngoscope, 84:205, Feb'74

774. The best emergency procedures for control of a massive hemorrhage from a tracheo-innominate fistula, secondary to tracheostomy tube or endotracheal intubation tube, is:
A. re-inflation of the tracheostomy tube cuff
B. insertion of a cuffed tracheotomy tube with inflation
C. make a small suprasternal incision and compress the innominate artery between the surgeon's finger and the sternum
D. median sternotomy with ligation innominate artery
E. median sternotomy with ligation of the innominate, subclavian and carotid arteries
REF. Weissman BW: The Laryngoscope, 84:205, Feb'74

775. Following median sternotomy for massive hemorrhage from a tracheo-innominate fistula secondary to tracheostomy or endotracheal intubation, the procedure of choice to prevent a subclavian-steal type syndrome is:
A. ligation of the innominate artery above and below the ruptured site
B. repair of the innominate artery by a graft
C. complete excision of the ruptured arterial site with over-sewing of the cut ends
D. C with ligation of the subclavian artery
E. C with ligation of the subclavian and carotid arteries
REF. Weissman BW: The Laryngoscope, 84:205, Feb'74

776. Unilateral or bilateral vocal cord paralysis unrelated to any known cause should have which of the following in a diagnostic profile?
A. CBC and VDRL
B. blood sugar
C. latex fixation
D. serum sampling for toxic heavy metals
E. radiologic and endoscopic evaluation
REF. Maisel RH, Ogura JH: The Laryngoscope, 84:302, Feb'74

777. Vocal cord paralysis is usually a symptom of a disease related to the vagus nerve and the cause may be found in the thorax, mediastinum, neck or cranium. CNS disease causes the following percent of all paralysis:
A. 5
B. 10
C. 15
D. 20
E. 30
REF. Maisel RH, Ogura JH: The Laryngoscope, 84:302, Feb'74

778. Cortical representation of the laryngeal muscles has which of the following features?
A. anterior central gyrus localization
B. occasional post central gyrus activity

C. frontal lobe localization within the longitudinal fissure
D. unilateral cortical representation with cortical paralysis common
E. bilateral cortical representation with cortical paralysis very rare
REF. Maisel RH, Ogura JH: The Laryngoscope, 84:302, Feb'74

779. The nucleus ambiguus is the motor nucleus to the larynx and this $1\frac{1}{2}$ to 2 cm. long nucleus is topographically represented as follows:
A. abductors cephalad to the superior laryngeal nerve
B. abductors most caudad
C. superior laryngeal nerve cephalad to the abductors
D. adductor muscles most caudad
E. adductors cephalad to the superior laryngeal nerve
REF. Maisel RH, Ogura JH: The Laryngoscope, 84:302, Feb'74

780. The cricothyroid muscle is innervated by:
A. recurrent laryngeal nerve
B. XIth cranial nerve
C. internal branch superior laryngeal nerve
D. external branch superior laryngeal nerve
E. branch hypoglossal nerve
REF. Maisel RH, Ogura JH: The Laryngoscope 84:302, Feb '74

781. Excepting the cricothyroid muscle, motor fibers to all other intrinsic laryngeal muscles is by:
A. recurrent laryngeal nerve
B. XIth cranial nerve
C. internal branch superior laryngeal nerve
D. external branch superior laryngeal nerve
E. branch hypoglossal nerve
REF. Maisel RH, Ogura JH: The Laryngoscope, 84:320 Feb'74

782. Sensation to the mucous membrane of the larynx is through the:
A. recurrent laryngeal nerve
B. XIth cranial nerve
C. internal branch superior laryngeal nerve
D. external branch superior laryngeal nerve
E. branch hypoglossal nerve
REF. Maisel RH, Ogura JH: The Laryngoscope, 84:302, Feb'74

783. Paralysis affecting the recurrent laryngeal nerve produces paramedian or median position of the vocal cord due to:
A. paralysis of the thyroarytenoideus
B. paralysis of the interarytenoideus
C. paralysis of A with cricothyroid functioning as a tensor of the vocal cords
D. paralysis of B with cricothyroid functioning as a tensor of the vocal cords
E. paralysis of all muscles of the intrinsic larynx except the cricothyroid which tenses the vocal cords and whose only antagonist is the abducting posterior cricothyroid muscle
REF. Maisel RH, Ogura JH: The Laryngoscope, 84:302,Feb'74

784. Combined unilateral paralysis of both vagus branches (superior laryngeal and recurrent laryngeal) to the laryngeal muscles usually produces a vocal cord in the position of:
A. extreme abduction
B. abduction
C. intermediate
D. paramedian
E. median or adduction
REF. Maisel RH, Ogura JH: The Laryngoscope, 84:302, Feb'74

785. Thyromegaly with vocal cord paralysis is usually due to:
A. Hashimoto's disease
B. toxic goiter
C. benign hypertrophy of the thyroid due to iodine or thyroxin deficiency
D. nodular thyroid
E. malignancy
REF. Maisel RH, Ogura JH: The Laryngoscope, 84:302, Feb'74

786. In evaluating vocal cord paralysis of undetermined etiology which of the following special tests should be considered?
A. neck and chest x-rays, particularly with left-sided paralysis and when a small lesion cannot be palpated in the neck
B. endoscopy including nasopharynx, esophagus, and bronchoscopy with aspiration for determination of possible malignancy of the lower respiratory tract
C. barium swallow
D. T_4, thyroid scan and uptake especially in short, fat or well-muscled necks
E. skull x-rays particularly of the jugular foramen
F. angiography
REF. Maisel RH, Ogura JH: The Laryngoscope, 84:302, Feb'74

787. Lung cancer with vocal cord paralysis is very unfavorable and is evidence of cancer in the:
A. right upper lobe
B. right lower lobe
C. left upper lobe
D. left lower lobe
E. mediastinum
REF. Maisel RH, Ogura JH: The Laryngoscope, 84:302, Feb'74

788. In pulmonary cancer, thoracic inlet syndrome has a poor prognosis and consists of paralysis of which of the following nerves?
A. vagus
B. phrenic
C. spinal accessory
D. vagus and phrenic
E. vagus and spinal accessory
REF. Maisel RH, Ogura JH: The Laryngoscope, 84:302, Feb'74

789. Vocal cord paralysis with x-ray evidence of a mediastinal mass may be curable because etiology may be:
A. cancer
B. lymph node masses
C. cardiac disease
D. bacterial mediastinitis
E. acute tuberculous mediastinitis
REF. Maisel RH, Ogura JH: The Laryngoscope, 84:302, Feb'74

790. Inflammatory conditions which should be considered in vocal cord paralysis are:
A. tuberculosis
B. viral - "shingles"
C. polio
D. arthritis (fixation cricoarytenoid joint)
E. diphtheria
REF. Maisel RH, Ogura JH: The Laryngoscope, 84:302, Feb'74

791. Central nervous system (CNS) conditions which should be considered in vocal cord paralysis are:
A. vascular and degenerative diseases
B. tumors - myelomeningocele, etc.
C. syringomyelia
D. trisomy 18
E. Arnold-Chiari malformation
REF. Maisel RH, Ogura JH: The Laryngoscope, 84:302, Feb'74

792. Vocal cord paralysis with x-ray evidence of lymph node masses in the mediastinum may indicate:
A. tuberculosis
B. histoplasmosis
C. metastatic cancer
D. metastatic lymphoma
E. bacterial infection
REF. Maisel RH, Ogura JH: The Laryngoscope, 84:302, Feb '74

793. Neoplasms which should be considered in vocal cord paralysis are:
A. Tapia's syndrome due to a large lymph node (metastatic) from cancer of tonsil
B. carotid body or Glomus tumor middle ear with extension
C. cancer nasopharynx, neck, trachea, esophagus, lung, thyroid
D. cancer or lymphoma metastatic mediastinal nodes
E. neurolemmoma
F. jugular foramen chordoma
REF. Maisel RH, Ogura JH: The Laryngoscope, 84:302, Feb'74

794. Traumatic lesions which should be considered in vocal cord paralysis are:
A. cardiomegaly and aortic aneurysm
B. blunt injury including gun shot (GSW) wounds
C. thyroid surgery, removal of neck tumors, and radical neck dissections
D. temporal bone resection
E. intubation for treatment and/or surgery (including adenotonsillectomy with bilateral paralysis due to irregular inflation of the endotracheal balloon pressing the recurrent laryngeal nerve against the thyroid cartilage)
F. acute local trauma to the larynx with or without flexion-extension injury to the spine
REF. Maisel RH, Ogura JH: The Laryngoscope, 84:302, Feb'74

795. The etiology of bilateral vocal cord paralysis is primarily due to which two of the following conditions?
A. tumors in the neck
B. tumors in the lung
C. thyroid surgery
D. blunt injury to the neck
E. central nervous system diseases (vascular and degenerative)
REF. Maisel RH, Ogura JH: The Laryngoscope, 84:302, Feb'74

796. Bilateral vocal cord paralysis can occur, though rarely, in which of the following conditions?
A. congenital arytenoid fixation
B. laryngeal manipulation or radiotherapy
C. neurologic diseases
D. metabolic and infectious diseases
E. neoplasms
REF. Maisel RH, Ogura JH: The Laryngoscope, 84:302, Feb'74

797. Which of the following procedures are successful in the treatment for symptomatic bilateral vocal cord paralysis?
A. external arytenoidectomy (Woodman)
B. King procedure
C. arytenoidectomy through suspension laryngoscope
D. open arytenoidectomy with skin grafting (laryngofissure)
E. open arytenoidectomy with primary suturing
REF. Maisel RH, Ogura JH: The Laryngoscope, 84:302, Feb'74

798. Most patients with recent vocal cord paralysis will acknowledge some dysphagia but a barium swallow is indicated in vocal cord paralysis primarily to determine:
A. presence of a hypopharyngeal tumor
B. presence of an esophageal tumor
C. globus

D. Zenker's diverticulum
E. demonstrate whether aspiration of food occurs and whether therapy of the paralysis is necessary
REF. Maisel RH: Ogura JH: The Laryngoscope, 84:302, Feb'74

799. The treatment for a permanent unilateral vocal cord paralysis is symptomatic because of a "breathy" voice due to incomplete glottic closure and at times because of aspiration. Which of the following is the procedure of choice at this time?
A. teflon injection (50 percent glycerin, 50 percent polyteflon - glycerin is absorbed over years) beneath the paralyzed cord
B. decompression of the recurrent laryngeal nerve
C. uncapping the cricothyroid joint to increase the distance between the anterior commissure and vocal process allowing a tighter glottic closure
D. laryngofissure with cartilage implant beneath the paralyzed cord
E. laryngofissure with injection of teflon beneath paralyzed cord
REF. Maisel RH, Ogura JH: The Laryngoscope, 84:302, Feb'74

800. Unilateral vocal cord paralysis immediately following a thyroidectomy is best treated by:
A. observation with expectation of spontaneous recovery or movement of the nonparalyzed cord beyond the midline to the paralyzed cord with symptomatic recovery
B. teflon injection into the usual space between the thyroid cartilage and paralyzed vocal cord
C. immediate decompression of the recurrent laryngeal nerve and suturing the nerve through reopening the thyroidectomy wound
D. B_{12} 1000 mcg daily
E. uncapping the cricothyroid joint
REF. Author's comment

801. Restoration of pharyngoesophageal continuity after resection of cancer of the base of the tongue, laryngopharynx and/or cervical esophagus may be accomplished by which of the following procedures?
A. skin graft reconstruction with split thickness skin graft sutured over a plastic stent (Conley)
B. skin pedicled flaps (Wookey), using a tube created from the skin and subcutaneous tissues (modified by Montgomery)
C. tube pedicle grafts
D. jejunal and colonic intestinal transplants and gastric antrum mobilized or as revascularized autografts
E. one stage reconstruction of Aviles
REF. Aviles E: The Laryngoscope 84:317, Feb'74

802. Juvenile papillomatosis is the most common benign tumor of the larynx in childhood, passing from a period of rapid growth to a self-limiting period at puberty. Which of the following medical treatment has appeared to be of value in children without laryngeal obstruction?
A. tetracycline (Holinger)
B. systemic hormones (Szpunar)
C. bovine wart vaccine (Moffit)
D. autogenous vaccine (Holinger)
E. careful observation since the disease is known to disappear spontaneously
REF. Giancarlo HR: The Laryngoscope, 84:169, Feb'74

803. The most recent procedure reported with promising results in the treatment of juvenile laryngeal papillomatosis is:
A. direct laryngoscopy with careful scalping of the individual tumor with cutting forceps-during surgery the tumors appear to have the ability to seed themselves into the epiglottis and into the trachea

B. electrocautery
C. x-ray and radium treatment
D. direct application of caustics, such as silver nitrate, podophylin, bismuth, etc.
E. direct application of ultrasound (Arslan:2. 5 watts cm^2 at a frequency of 3 megahertz for 30 to 40 minutes)
REF. Giancarlo HR: The Laryngoscope, 84:169, Feb'74

804. Which of the following techniques for the roentoenographic study of the larynx and hypopharynx appears to require the least patient cooperation, no topical anesthesia, no instillation of positive contrast material and yet produces significant diagnostic radiological information including paralysis of vocal cords and tumors?
A. conventional roentgenography
B. tomography
C. zonography
D. positive contrast larynogography
E. xeroradiographic zonography
REF. Woesner ME, Braun EJ, Sanders I: Ann Otol, 83:42, Jan-Feb'74

805. Osteophytes involving the cervical vertebra and intervertebral spaces are common in middle and older aged people and although usually asymptomatic can cause dysphagia and dysphonia. These osteophytes are described in the literature as cervical:
A. osteophytes
B. exostosis
C. arthritis
D. arthrosis
E. spondylosis
REF. Saffouri MH, Ward PH: Ann Otol, 83:65, Jan-Feb'74

806. The most common complaint in patients (usually 45 years of age or older) with cervical osteophytes is:
A. dysphagia
B. pain in the neck and arms secondary to nerve root compression
C. dysphonia with or without pain
D. dry cough with or without a sensation of a foreign body in the throat
E. otalgia
REF. Saffouri MH, Ward PH: Ann Otol, 83:65, Jan-Feb'74

807. Cervical osteophytes are believed due to degeneration of intervertebral discs but since the disease process occurs in the areas of maximal cervical movement, trauma cannot be dismissed as a possible etiologic factor. Which of the following conditions must be considered in the differential diagnosis?
A. benign and malignant tumors of the larynx, hypopharynx, and upper cervical esophagus
B. esophagitis including caustic strictures
C. Plummer-Vinson syndrome
D. diverticula (Zenker's)
E. globus hystericus
REF. Saffouri MH, Ward PH: Ann Otol, 83:65, Jan-Feb'74

808. Symptomatic osteophytes of the lower cervical spine (C-5, 6, 7) are most easily diagnosed by:
A. indirect laryngoscopy
B. roentgengrams
C. cineesophagrams
D. pharyngoscopy
E. esophagoscopy
REF. Saffouri MH, Ward PH: Ann Otol, 83:65, Jan-Feb'74

809. In the following question, each numbered item is to be matched with one lettered item. Each choice may be used more than once. In symptomatic cervical osteophytic lesions, the best surgical approach is:
A. transoral
B. external cervical

1. C-2
2. C-3
3. C-4
4. C-5
5. C-6
6. C-7

REF. Saffouri MH, Ward PH: Ann Otol, 83:65, Jan-Feb'74

810. In the lateral external approach to resection of cervical osteophytes below the C-4 level, which of the following anatomical structures may be injured?
A. common carotid artery
B. internal jugular vein
C. inferior thyroid artery
D. superior laryngeal nerve
E. recurrent laryngeal nerve
REF. Saffouri MH, Ward PH: Ann Otol, 83:65, Jan-Feb'74

811. In the lateral approach to resection of cervical osteophytes at the C-2, 3, 4, level, which of the following anatomical structures may be injured?
A. superior laryngeal nerve
B. hypoglossal nerve
C. external carotid artery and major branching vessels
D. thyrocervical trunk
E. inferior thyroid artery
REF. Saffouri MH, Ward PH: Ann Otol, 83:65, Jan-Feb'74

812. A silicone T-tube tracheal stent to support a repaired and reconstructed cervical trachea or end-to-end anastomosis of the trachea has which of the following advantages?
A. little or no tissue reaction to the silicone
B. mucus does not readily adhere to the surface of the tube
C. silicone does not harden after prolonged body contact as do most other plastic substances
D. T-tube can remain plugged, providing the airway is adequate, with normal phonation
E. never needs changing
REF. Montgomery WW: Ann Otol, 83:71, Jan-Feb'74

813. Examination of the anterior commissure of the larynx reveal which of the following facts?
A. anterior subglottic larynx has a midline embryological origin
B. vocal ligaments fuse to form a common anterior commissure tendon (Broyles)
C. ventricles fuse to form the most anterior portion of the laryngeal lumen
D. the conus elasticus penetrated by vessels is not an effective barrier to tumor spread
E. lateral subglottic portions of the larynx fuse to each other
REF. Tucker GF Jr., Alonso WA, Tucker JA, Cowan M, Druck N: Ann Otol, 82-625, Sept-Oct'73

814. Of the following unusual subglottic tumors in children which one is considered malignant?
A. capillary hemangioma
B. hemangiopericytoma
C. hemangioendothelioma
D. lymphangioma
REF. Jaffe BF: Ann Otol, 82:637, Sept-Oct'73

815. Following tracheal intubation for long anesthesia during cardiac surgery in a young child, with a tracheotomy tube, because the vocal cords appeared fixed in the midline position would make a surgeon consider which one of the following rare conditions?
A. bilateral abductor paralysis due to the intrathoracic operation
B. bilateral abductor paralysis due to the endotracheal balloon pressing the recurrent laryngeal nerves against the thyroid cartilage
C. congenital webs

D. vocal cord adhesions post intubation or pseudobilateral abductor cord paralysis
E. lymphoangioma
REF. Jaffe BF: Ann Otol, 82:637, Sept-Oct'73

816. Retrograde dilatation in benign esophageal strictures due to chemical burns is much safer than antegrade dilatation because the retrograde route "pulls" rather than "pushes" the dilator through the strictured area. Which of the following complications can occur when either method is used?
A. esophageal perforation due to the esophagoscope or dilators usually in the upper or lower one-thirds of the esophagus
B. strangulation of the bowel when a guide string is swallowed
C. mediastinitis
D. pyothorax
E. metastatic abscesses-brain, septic arthritis
REF. Rontal E, Meyerhoff W, Duvall AJ: Ann Otol, 82, 643, Sept-Oct'73

817. Although all of the following occur, the two primary sites of origin of metastatic brain abscesses are:
A. otologic
B. sinus
C. chronic lung disease (e.g. bronchiectasis)
D. skin lesions
E. infections of bone and heart
REF. Rontal E, Meyerhoff W, Duvall AJ: Ann Otol, 83:643, Sept-Oct'73

818. The time of greatest danger for gross perforation of the esophagus by esophagoscopy and/or dilatation in steroid treated patients for chemical strictures appear to be in the following week-period:
A. one
B. two
C. three
D. four
E. four to six or even greater
REF. Rontal E, Meyerhoff W, Duvall AJ: Ann Otol, 82:643, Sept-Oct'73

819. It appears from both electron microscopic examination and clinical association that laryngeal papilloma in children have which of the following in common:
A. related etiologically to skin warts (verruca vulgaris)
B. related etiologically to genital warts (condyloma acuminatum)
C. deficiencies in Mg++ and CA++ electrolyte metabolism in the serum may contribute to individual susceptibility
D. skin warts and genital warts are caused by the same viral agents
E. suspensions prepared from laryngeal papillomas show numerous virus particles
REF. Cook TA, Cohn AM, Brunschwig JP, Goepfert H, Butel JS, Rawls WE: Ann Otol, 82:649, Sept-Oct'73

820. Which of the following drugs have produced significant long-term successful results in the treatment of juvenile papillomatosis?
A. tetracyclines
B. corticosteroids
C. estrogens
D. podophylline
E. small pox inoculation into the lesions
F. bovine vaccination
G. inactivated autogenous vaccine
H. attenuated virus vaccines
I. indoxuridine (Stoxil)
J. all
K. none
REF. Cook TA, Cohn AM, Brunschwig JP, Goepfert H, Butel JS, Rawls WE: Ann Otol, 82:649, Sept-Oct'73

821. Which of the following physical modes of treatment of juvenile papillomatosis have been successful but long-term follow-up results must be evaluated to determine any side effects?
A. ultrasound
B. cryosurgery

C. microscopically controlled laser
D. electrocautery
E. radiation therapy
REF. Cook TA, Cohn AM, Brunschwig JP, Goepfert H, Butel JS, Rawls WE: Ann Otol, 82:649, Sept-Oct'73

822. The methods of treatment for juvenile laryngeal papillomatosis recommended by most otolaryngologists today are:
A. periodic observation in small lesions causing mild dysphonia
B. suspension endolaryngeal excision under microscopy without tracheotomy
C. B with tracheotomy when respiratory obstruction occurs
D. thyrotomy with tracheotomy in extensive involvement
E. electrocauterization of the local lesions with or without tracheotomy depending on airway obstruction
REF. Cook TA, Cohn AM, Brunschwig JP, Goepfert H, Butel JS, Rawls WE: Ann Otol, 82:649, Sept-Oct'73

823. Cryosurgery appears to be successful as a primary treatment for which of the following cancers of the larynx?
A. T_1
B. T_2
C. T_3
D. T_4
E. multicentric carinoma in situ
REF. Miller D: Ann Otol, 82:656, Sept-Oct'73

824. An apparent disadvantage to the use of cryosurgery to papillomatosis in a child's larynx is:
A. unable to obtain sufficient depth of tissue destruction (-20° C)
B. smoky cloud obscuring the field of vision
C. damage to tracheal mucosa
D. damage to arytenoid areas
E. tracheotomy always necessary
REF. Miller D: Ann Otol, 82:656, Sept-Oct'73

825. The material of choice for intracordal injection for correction of paralytic dysphonia is:
A. bone dust
B. tantalum
C. tantalum oxide
D. silicone
E. teflon particles in a glycerin base (polytef)
REF. Dedo HH, Urrea RD, Lawson L: Ann Otol, 82:661, Sept-Oct'73

826. Which of the following are necessary to evaluate the functional results of intracordal injection of teflon for correction of paralytic dysphonia?
A. vocal quality, pitch range and intensity
B. phonation time
C. ultra high speed photography of the vocal cord
D. voice spectrographs
E. aerodynamic studies
REF. Dedo HH, Urrea RD, Lawson L: Ann Otol, 82:661, Sept-Oct'73

827. All of the following are indications for intracordal injection of teflon for the relief of paralytic dysphonia except:
A. scar band pseudocord
B. unilateral vocal cord paralysis
C. vocal cord volume defects
D. glottic incompetence following arytenoidectomy, cordectomy, hemilaryngectomy, or blunt laryngeal trauma
E. congenital dysplastic dysphonia - bilateral bowed vocal cords
REF. Dedo HH, Urrea RD, Lawson L: Ann Otol, 82:661, Sept-Oct'73

828. All of the following are contraindications to intracordal injection of teflon for the relief of paralytic dysphonia except:
A. most bilateral vocal cord paralysis and scar band pseudocord
B. central nervous system lesions where dysphonia is caused by complex dysarthria
C. psychologically unstable patient
D. paralysis present less than six months unless caused by malignancy or surgery
E. congenital dysplastic dysphonia - bilateral bowed vocal cords
REF. Dedo HH, Urrea RD, Lawson L: Ann Otol, 82:661, Sept-Oct'73

829. The three most common operations responsible for vocal cord paralysis are:
A. surgical excision of cord substance
B. thyroidectomy
C. anterior cervical fusion
D. neck biopsy
E. heart surgery
REF. Dedo HH, Urrea RD, Lawson L: Ann Otol, 82:661, Sept-Oct'73

830. Vocal cord paralysis due to carotid artery endarterectomy may recover spontaneously as late as the following months after surgery:
A. one
B. two
C. three to four
D. four to five
E. six to eight
REF. Dedo HH, Urrea RD, Lawson L: Ann Otol, 82:661, Sept-Oct'73

831. An unusual contraindication to intracordal injection of teflon for the relief of paralytic dysphonia because the opposite cord may become paralyzed is:
A. idiopathic paralysis of less than six months' duration
B. laryngofissure
C. vocal cord biopsy
D. glottic incompetence following arytenoidectomy
E. carotid artery endarterectomy when the opposite carotid is scheduled for surgery
REF. Dedo HH, Urrea RD, Lawson L: Ann Otol, 82:661, Sept-Oct'73

832. Posttraumatic or postsurgical defects with vocal cord loss or replacement by a hard scar band have poor results from intracordal injection of teflon for correction of paralytic dysphonia unless which one of the following preliminary procedures is done?
A. laryngofissure with muscle implant
B. arytenoidectomy
C. cricopharyngeal myotomy
D. tracheotomy
E. steriod injection, Decadron 5cc IM at the time of surgery
REF. Dedo HH, Urrea RD, Lawson L: Ann Otol, 82:661, Sept-Oct'73

833. Which of the following facts about congenital cysts of the larynx appear to be true?
A. same as so-called lateral saccular cysts (Desanto)
B. variant of a laryngocele
C. derivatives of third visceral pouch
D. developmental abnormalities incurred during canalization of epithelial primordium of the laryngeal ventricle and saccule
E. form from epithelial buds sequestered during saccular development
REF. DeWater FWV: The Laryngoscope, 83:1185, Aug'73

834. In an infant with progressive symptoms of respiratory difficulty, dysphagia with choking on feeding, and a worsening cry not uncommonly relieved with the baby on its back in a hyperextended position most likely has which one of the following conditions?
A. laryngeal web or stenosis
B. vascular abnormalities
C. laryngomalacia
D. vocal cord paralysis
E. congenital laryngeal cyst
REF. DeWater FWV: The Laryngoscope, 83:1185, Aug'73

835. In the adult with a laryngeal cyst, the most common symptoms are:
A. hemoptysis
B. vocal change
C. mild deglutatory difficulties
D. occasional respiratory abnormalities, particularly shortness of breath on exertion
E. upper respiratory infection with precipitation of a sudden enlargement of the cyst with dysphonia, dysphagia and dyspnea
REF. DeWater FWV: The Laryngoscope, 83:1185, Aug'73

836. Although all of the following tests are of value, in an infant with a laryngeal cyst the most important diagnostic procedure is:
A. x-rays with a contrast agent
B. x-rays with air as the contrast material
C. chest x-ray
D. barium swallow
E. direct laryngoscopy
REF. DeWater FWV: The Laryngoscope, 83:1185, Aug'73
Author: Refer question 804

837. Although all of the following tests are of value, in an adult with a laryngeal cyst the most important diagnostic procedures are:
A. x-rays with a contrast agent
B. x-rays with air as the contrast material
C. chest x-ray
D. barium swallow
E. direct laryngoscopy
REF. DeWater FWV: The Laryngoscope, 83:1185, Aug'73
Author: Refer question 804

838. In infants with symptomatic laryngeal cysts which of the following treatments have been successful?
A. direct laryngoscopy with repeated needling and aspiration
B. suspension laryngoscopy with A above
C. A with partial excision of the cyst wall dome (marsupialization)
D. B with marsupialization
E. endoscopic marsupialization by removal of the cyst wall dome and stripping of the remaining cyst wall with laryngeal forceps
REF. DeWater FWV: The Laryngoscope, 83:1185, Aug'73

839. In infants with symptomatic laryngeal cysts which one of the following surgical procedures appear to be preferable?
A. direct laryngoscopy with repeated needling and aspiration
B. suspension laryngoscopy with A above
C. A with partial excision of the cyst wall dome (marsupialization)
D. B with marsupialization
E. endoscopic marsupialization by removal of the cyst wall dome and stripping of the remaining cyst wall with laryngeal cup forceps
REF. DeWater FWV: The Laryngoscope, 83:1185, Aug'73

840. In adults with symptomatic laryngeal cysts which one of the following surgical procedures appears to be preferable?
A. splitting the thyrohyoid membrane along the superior margin of the thyroid cartilage
B. midline laryngofissure
C. lateral thyrotomy with extra-lumenal approach to the pre-epiglottic and paraglottic space with tracheotomy
D. C with intra-lumenal approach without tracheotomy
E. endoscopic marsupialization by removal of the cyst wall dome and stripping of the remaining cyst wall with laryngeal cup forceps
REF. DeWater FWV: The Laryngoscope, 83:1185, Aug'73

841. Tracheal strictures should always be first treated by dilatations and have been successful when the stenosis is less in cm in length of:
A. one
B. two
C. three
D. four
E. five
REF. Dedo HH, Fishman NH: The Laryngoscope, 83:1204, Aug'73

842. Tracheal dilations for stricture will be unsuccessful if no improvement has resulted after the following number of dilatations?
A. two to three
B. six to seven
C. nine to twelve
D. fifteen to seventeen
E. twenty
REF. Dedo HH, Fishman NH: The Laryngoscope, 83:1204, Aug'73

843. Segmental resections can successfully repair tracheal stenosis up to cm in length of:
A. 1-2
B. 2-3
C. 3-4
D. 4-5
E. 5-7
REF. Dedo HH, Fishman NH: The Laryngoscope, 83:1204, Aug'73

844. The chief early problem after laryngeal release and tracheal mobilization for resection of tracheal stenosis is aspiration which can be avoided most easily by which one of the following procedures?
A. tracheotomy
B. esophageal feeding tube
C. intravenous fluids
D. swallowing practice (taking a deep breath, holding it while swallowing Jello rapidly)
E. gastrostomy
REF. Dedo HH, Fishman NH: The Laryngoscope, 83:1204, Aug'73

845. Partial incision of the membranes between the tracheal rings to permit anastomosis after segmental resection of a tracheal stenosis can result in:
A. excellent cure
B. tracheal fistula through the skin
C. chronic subcutaneous crepitation of air beneath the cervical skin with recurrent abscesses
D. immediate and recurring neck infections
E. tracheal necrosis
REF. Dedo HH, Fishman NH: The Laryngoscope, 83:1204, Aug'73

846. Subglottic (or tracheal) stenosis is in most instances successfully repaired by which of the following procedures?
A. multiple dilations
B. split-thickness skin grafts over stents
C. simple resection of the stenosis (not over two tracheal rings) or replacement of the damaged segments with plastic or metal prosthesis
D. all of the above
E. none of the above
REF. Dedo HH, Fishman NH: The Laryngoscope, 83:1204, Aug'73

847. Most, if not all, epiglottitis in children is caused by:
A. pneumococci
B. beta hemolytic streptococci
C. hemophilus influenzae, type B
D. staphylococcus
E. penicillin resistant staphylococcus
REF. Hawkins DB, Miller AH, Sachs GB, Benz RT: The Laryngoscope, 83: 1211, Aug'73

848. In acute epiglottitis which one of the following conditions is common in adults but rare in children?
A. almost always produces severe airway obstruction
B. abscess of the epiglottis
C. rapid onset and progression
D. tracheotomy
E. always, or almost always, caused by hemophilus influenzae, type B
REF. Hawkins DB, Miller AH, Sachs GB, Benz RT: The Laryngoscope, 83: 1211, Aug'73

849. In acute epiglottitis which of the following conditions are common in children?
A. almost always produces severe airway obstruction
B. abscess of the epiglottis
C. rapid onset and progression
D. tracheotomy is fairly common
E. almost always caused by hemophilus influenzae, type B
REF. Hawkins DB, Miller AH, Sachs GB, Benz RT: The Laryngoscope, 83: 1211, Aug'73

850. In acute epiglottitis in either children or adults the antibiotic of choice is:
A. ampicillin
B. tetracycline
C. streptomycin
D. keflin
E. erythromycin
REF. Hawkins DB, Miller AH, Sachs GB, Benz RT:The Laryngoscope, 83: 1211, Aug'73

851. Most epiglottitis in adults is caused by:
A. hemophilus influenzae, type B
B. pneumococci
C. beta hemolytic streptococci
D. staphylococci
E. monilia
REF. Hawkins DB, Miller AH, Sachs GB, Benz RT:The Laryngoscope, 83: 1211, Aug'73

852. Epiglottitis in adults is most severe when due to the following pathogen?
A. hemophilus influenzae, type B
B. pneumococci
C. beta hemolytic streptococci
D. staphylococci
E. monilia
REF. Hawkins DB, Miller AH, Sachs GB, Benz RT: The Laryngoscope, 83: 1211, Aug'73

853. In the therapy of acute epiglottitis in either children or adults which of the following should be considered?
A. mist tent
B. intravenous antibiotics
C. tracheostomy when indicated
D. steroids when indicated
E. blood and throat cultures
REF. Hawkins DB, Miller AH, Sachs GB, Benz RT: The Laryngoscope, 83: 1211, Aug'73

854. Apneic anesthesia for microlaryngeal surgery has which of the following advantages?
A. unlimited time for surgery
B. absence of any cardiac arrhythmias
C. unobstructed view of the endolarynx
D. avoid laryngeal trauma due to an endotracheal tube
E. precludes seeding of the larynx and trachea with malignant cells when the endotracheal tube is passed
REF. Nelson RA, Miller T: The Laryngoscope, 83:1228, Aug'73

855. The characteristic early symptoms of epiglottitis in adults are:
A. fever
B. sore throat
C. dysphonia
D. inspiratory stridor
E. acute painful dysphagia
REF. Hawkins DB, Miller AH, Sachs GB, Benz RT: The Laryngoscope, 83: 1211, Aug'73

856. Unilateral or bilateral laryngeal paralysis is not an uncommon cause for severe airway obstruction, aspiration syndromes and voice changes in children. Which of the following causes have been found?
A. central nervous system diseases including meningomyelocele with or without Arnold-Chiari malformation or hydrocephalus
B. trauma including head during the birth process because of breech or shoulder dystocia or face presentation
C. congenital mediastinal tumors such as cystic hygroma, cardiovascular anomalies, etc.
D. trauma to the recurrent laryngeal nerves during neck or chest surgery
E. neuromuscular disease
REF. Cohen SR: The Laryngoscope, 83:1293, Aug'73

857. Arytenoidectomy in children is different from that in adults because:
A. rare
B. preliminary tracheotomy in most cases becomes an absolute necessity to prevent severe brain damage from hypoxia or anoxia in the neonate
C. timing of the arytenoidectomy is of utmost importance since vocal cord recovery can occur in children after a period of two to three years (surgical etiology excluded)
D. around 5 years is the ideal time for surgery
E. adult techniques cannot be used
REF. Cohen SR: The Laryngoscope, 83:1293, Aug'73

858. All of the following have caused bilateral abductor paralysis of the larynx in children but a most unusual cause has been which one of the following?
A. surgical removal of thyroid carcinoma
B. birth trauma
C. arthrogryposis
D. congenital paralysis of neurological origin
E. cystic hygroma of the mediastinum
REF. Cohen SR: The Laryngoscope, 83:1293, Aug'73

859. In the diagnosis of bronchogenic carcinoma, the procedure of choice and significantly so is:
A. cytology
B. bronchoscopy
C. B plus A
D. scalene node biopsy
E. mediastinoscopy
REF. Preciado MC, Duvall III, AJ, Koop SH: The Laryngoscope, 83:1300, Aug'73

860. In the diagnosis of sarcoidosis, the procedure of choice is:
A. cytology
B. bronchoscopy
C. B plus A
D. scalene node biopsy
E. mediastinoscopy
REF. Preciado MC, Duvall III AJ, Koop SH: The Laryngoscope, 83:1300, Aug'73

861. Although all of the following are relative contraindications, the only absolute contraindication to mediastinoscopy is:
A. tracheal deviation
B. thoracic aortic aneurysms
C. increased superior vena cava pressure

D. peripheral malignant pulmonary lesions
E. previous mediastinoscopy
REF. Preciado MC, Duvall III AJ, Koop SH: The Laryngoscope, 83:1300, Aug'73

862. Mediastinoscopy is indicated in which of the following conditions?
A. bronchogenic carcinoma to predict resectability
B. sarcoidosis
C. mediastinal masses of undetermined origin (benign or metastatic)
D. active tuberculosis (atypical mycobacteria)
E. histoplasmosis
REF. Preciado MC, Duvall III AJ, Koop SH: The Laryngoscope, 83:1300, Aug'73

863. Which of the following conditions are in a development and evaluation stage as indications for mediastinoscopy?
A. insertion of atrial triggered pacemakers
B. performance of intrathoracic right vagotomy
C. insertion of mediastinal radon seeds
D. evaluation and staging of lymphomas
E. performance of thymectomies
REF. Preciado MC, Duvall III AJ, Koop SH: The Laryngoscope, 83:1300, Aug'73

864. In experienced "hands" the complication rate is around 1. 5 to 2. 0 percent and the mortality rate around 1. 0 percent in mediastinoscopy but a thorough knowledge of the mediastinal anatomy is necessary if the surgeon is to avoid catastrophe. Which of the following serious complications have occurred?
A. biopsy of pulmonary and innominate arteries, superior vena cava and azygos vein and myocardium
B. stroke secondary to innominate artery compression
C. vagus and recurrent nerve injuries
D. air embolism
E. pneumothorax and subcutaneous emphysema
REF. Preciado MC, Duvall III AJ, Koop SH: The Laryngoscope, 83:1300, Aug'73

865. In mediastinoscopy which of the following complications, though rare, occur with experienced surgeons?
A. significant temperature elevation on the evening of the procedure (antibiotics not necessary)
B. pneumothorax
C. vocal cord paralysis
D. hematoma
E. arrhythmia and transient hypotension
REF. Preciado MC, Duvall III AJ, Koop SH: The Laryngoscope, 83:1300, Aug'73

866. In the following question, match each numbered item with one lettered item.
A. right common carotid artery
B. left common carotid artery

1. branch of the innominate artery
2. emanates directly from the arch of the aorta
REF. Shumrick DA: The Laryngoscope, 83:1051, July'73

867. The common carotid artery bifurcates into the internal and external branches at the level of the:
A. suprasternal notch
B. cricoid
C. thyroid cartilage
D. hyoid bone
E. mastoid tip
REF. Shumrick DA: The Laryngoscope, 83:1051, July'73

IN THE FOLLOWING QUESTION MATCH EACH NUMBERED ITEM WITH ONE LETTERED ITEM. EACH CHOICE MAY BE USED MORE THAN ONCE:

868. The internal and external carotid arteries give rise to which of the following branches?
A. internal carotid
B. external carotid

1. superior thyroid
2. ascending pharyngeal
3. lingual
4. facial or external maxillary
5. occipital
6. postauricular
7. superficial temporal
8. internal maxillary

REF. Shumrick DA: The Laryngoscope, 83:1051, July'73

869. Which of the following factors increases the probability of carotid artery rupture in neck surgery for malignancy?
A. patient over 50 years of age with weight loss between 10 and 15 percent
B. pre-operative irradiation, especially a full therapeutic dose administered three months or more prior to definitive surgery
C. invasion of the carotid by tumor
D. invasion of the carotid by infection
E. patient in negative nitrogen balance and sustained A/G ratio reversal with below normal hemoglobin and blood volume
REF. Shumrick DA: The Laryngoscope, 83:1051, July'73

870. The three main contributing factors to carotid artery rupture in neck cancer surgery are:
A. surgical technique
B. type of malignancy
C. previous irradiation of either low or high dose magnitude
D. development of a fistula
E. combination of radiation and fistula
REF. Shumrick DA: The Laryngoscope, 83:1051, July'73

871. Which of the following procedures should be initiated at once to prevent carotid rupture following cancer surgery and wound breakdown?
A. culture and sensitivity tests with antibiotic therapy
B. "seat" the floating flaps by adequate drainage and firm but not strangulating pressure with dressings
C. remove sutures only as necessary
D. allow flaps to retract to their respective bases
E. surgical exposure of the carotid to determine its status
REF. Shumrick DA: The Laryngoscope, 83:1051, July'73

872. Which of the following procedures should be initiated at once if cervical wound breakdown occurs and the carotid artery is exposed following cancer surgery?
A. culture and sensitivity tests with antibiotic therapy
B. adequate drainage and firm but gentle pressure with dressings
C. remove sutures only as necessary and allow flaps to retract to their respective bases
D. return patient to the operating room immediately for a split thickness skin graft to cover the artery (if not done previously by a dermal graft)
E. immediate elevation and repositioning of another skin flap
REF. Shumrick DA: The Laryngoscope, 83:1051, July'73

873. The most sensitive site for carotid artery rupture is at the level of the:
A. superior thyroid artery
B. ascending pharyngeal artery
C. carotid bulb in the region of the bifurcation

D. external maxillary
E. occipital
REF. Shumrick DA: The Laryngoscope, 83:1051, July'73

874. In an apparent impending carotid artery rupture in a cervical wound breakdown after cancer surgery, the arterial rupture usually occurs during the following day-period:
A. 1 to 2
B. 4 to 5
C. 6 to 10
D. 12 to 14
E. 21 to 28
REF. Shumrick DA: The Laryngoscope, 83:1051, July'73

875. If the carotid artery reaches an aneurysmic state or ruptures, which of the following should be done?
A. patient taken to the operating room and the common carotid artery and its divisions ligated and sectioned
B. complications explained to the patient and family
C. angiograms in the preligation period are very helpful in predicting adequate cerebral crossover
D. ligate the carotid artery with no. 0 chromic suture (the proximal or inferior end) far enough away to prevent a secondary rupture and oversew the stump with no. 28 stainless steel wire and "bury" in the paraspinal muscles
E. stump of the common carotid artery and both the internal and external carotid arteries should be ligated and buried in the paraspinal muscles
REF. Shumrick DA: The Laryngoscope, 83:1051, July'73

876. Which of the following may be expected following ligation of the common carotid artery?
A. paresis including hemiplegia (permanent)
B. death
C. nothing
D. minimal neurologic changes which are quickly reversed
E. long-delayed stroke (due ascending thrombosis of cerebral portion of internal carotid artery)
REF. Shumrick DA: The Laryngoscope, 83:1051, July'73

877. Which of the following surgical procedures may be used to prevent carotid artery rupture?
A. Frazier "S" incision
B. dermal skin grafts with dermatome setting of 0.0015 inches and 3 cm wide but not including any epidermal tissue
C. levator scapulae muscle sectioned at its inferior border and rotated medially to cover the carotid artery
D. planned pharyngostome
E. B plus C
REF. Shumrick DA: The Laryngoscope, 83:1051, July'73

878. Studies indicate that with hematoporphyrin derivative bronchogenic carcinomas may be detected and localized by the use of violet light sources and flexible fiberoptic bronchoscopes to view the characteristic fluorescence. The most satisfactory method (but still experimental) for the treatment of these in situ carcinomas appear to be (in patients with inadequate respiratory reserve):
A. local excision through endoscopy
B. electrocoagulation
C. lobotomy with local excision
D. lobectomy
E. cryosurgery
REF. Neel III HB, Farrell KH, DeSanto LW, Payne WS, Sanderson DR: The Laryngoscope, 83:1062, July'73

879. In tracheal repair for avulsion, the most successful surgical procedure has been:
A. segmental replacement with marlex mesh
B. replacement with tantalum mesh
C. replacement with polyethylene or silastic tubing
D. porous tissue lining (stainless steel mesh tube, Dacron Velour)
E. mobilization of the larynx and trachea with end-to-end anastomosis of the cut ends of the trachea
REF. Wykoff TW: The Laryngoscope, 83:1072, July'73

880. Which of the following appears true of the cytomegalovirus?
A. has been isolated in tissue culture of a laryngeal papilloma
B. has not been isolated from a laryngeal papilloma
C. is a tumorgenic virus
D. is not a tumorgenic virus
E. is a passenger virus
REF. Boyle WF, Riggs JL, Oshiro LS, Lennettee EH: The Laryngoscope, 83:1102, July'73

881. Electron microscopic serial studies of adult laryngeal papilloma indicate:
A. transition of papilloma from a benign to a malignant lesion
B. papillomata never become malignant
C. presence of papova virus group
D. a papilloma virus has never been propagated in tissue culture
E. the papova virus in laryngeal papilloma is morphologically similar to the genital wart virus (electronic microscope)
REF. Boyle WF, Riggs JL, Oshiro LS, Lennettee EH: The Laryngoscope, 83:1102, July'73

882. The papova virus found in papillomas by electron microscopy are:
A. tumorigenic
B. not tumorigenic
C. "papova" is an acronym of papilloma and polyoma
D. can alter a whole cell so that normal restraints on its own multiplication are abolished
E. crystalline lattice assemblies are characteristic of papova group (intranuclear viral particles in the shape of an icosahedron, 45 mu in diameter, containing a densely staining core, generally scattered throughout the nucleus, and occasionally in crystalline arrays)
REF. Boyle WF, Riggs JL, Oshiro LS, Lennettee EH: The Laryngoscope, 83:1102, July'73

883. Tube feedings are frequently used by otolaryngologists in treating head and neck malignancies. Common side effects of these diets include:
A. borborygmi
B. meteorism
C. cramping
D. distention
E. diarrhea
REF. Walike BC, Walike JW: The Laryngoscope, 83:1109, July'73

884. The tube feeding syndrome in cancer of the head and neck may have which of the following dire complications?
A. dehydration
B. hypernatremia
C. hyperchloremia
D. azotemia
E. diarrhea
REF. Walike BC, Walike JW: The Laryngoscope, 83:1109, July'73

885. The suggested causes of diarrhea in tube feeding in head and neck cancer are:
A. rate of administration
B. temperature of liquid diet
C. location of tube tip
D. osmolality of the diet
E. contents of the diet
REF. Walike BC, Walike JW: The Laryngoscope, 83:1109, July'73

886. Lactose is known to cause diarrhea and lactose is the primary carbohydrate of milk, the basic ingredient of most tube feeding diets. Lactose intolerance occurs in:
A. congenital lactose intolerance or lactase deficiency with severe diarrhea in neonates due to insufficient amount of the enzyme lactase in the brush border of the mucosa of the jejunum
B. secondary lactase deficiency due to diseases affecting the small intestinal mucosa, particularly sprue and acute infectious diarrhea
C. acquired lactate deficiency (intolerance) in adults who were normal as infants
D. 90 - 95 percent of negroes and 5 - 10 percent of caucasians are lactase deficient
E. almost all adult non-humans
REF. Walike BC, Walike JW: The Laryngoscope, 83:1109, July '73

887. Which of the following methods are used to detect lactose intolerant patients?
A. blood fasting sugar
B. lactose tolerance test
C. post-prandial blood sugar
D. symptoms of intolerance following lactose tolerance test (LTT) or ingestion of milk
E. peroral or surgically obtained biopsy of the jejunal mucosa showing a deficiency of the lactase enzyme
REF. Walike BC, Walike JW: The Laryngoscope, 83:1109, July '73

888. The lactose tolerance test (LTT) consists of the oral administration of 50 or 100 gm lactose (or 2 gm kg) and monitoring blood glucose as in the glucose tolerance test. A rise of which of the following indicates lack of hydrolysis of lactose due to lactase deficiency?
A. less than 10-15 mg%
B. less than 20-25 mg%
C. less than 30-35 mg%
D. less than 40-45 mg%
E. less than 50-55 mg%
REF. Walike BC, Walike JW: The Laryngoscope, 83:1109, July '73

889. Which of the following are proper indications for frozen sections?
A. nature of disease (benign or malignant) to determine immediate surgical action
B. extent of disease to determine margins of resection
C. save hospitalization time
D. relatives demand an immediate diagnosis
E. Jehovah complex
REF. Saltzstein SL, Nahum AM: The Laryngoscope, 83:1128, July '73

890. Pain associated with cancer in the larynx is an ominous sign which can mean which of the following?
A. ulcerated growth with exposed nerve endings (with or without secondary infection) or deep infiltration of tumor to involve sensory nerves
B. invasion of cartilage framework of the larynx (with or without some degree of perichondritis)
C. spread outside the laryngeal framework into the cervical soft tissues or into the hypopharynx
D. all of the above
E. none of the above
REF. Mendonca DR, Bryce DP: Canadian J Otolaryngol, 2:3, 271, '73

891. The term transglottic tumor or cancer means:
A. large growth involving the supraglottic, glottic and subglottic regions of the larynx
B. growth involving the glottic laryngeal area
C. growth involving the subglottic area

D. growth involving any of the supraglottic areas of the larynx
E. large, deep growth occupying the tissues above and below the ventricle (McGavran, Beuer and Ogura-1961) characterized by invasion of the "paraglottic space"
REF. Mendonca DR, Bryce DP: Canadian J Otolaryngol, 2:3, 271, '73

892. The prognosis is poor in carcinoma invading the subglottic area and the extent of the tumor can probably be assessed (when possible) by which one of the following methods?
A. tomography and laryngography
B. direct anterior commissure laryngoscopy with multiple biopsies
C. use of right-angled telescope
D. microlaryngoscopy (and use of microlaryngeal mirrors)
E. transconioscopy under local anesthesia whereby a rhinopharyngoscope is introduced through the cricothyroid membrane
REF. Mendonca DR, Bryce DP: Canadian J Otolaryngol, 2:3, 271, '73

893. Transglottic cancer is characterized by:
A. invasion of paraglottic space (Tucker-1962)
B. aggressive growth patterns
C. does not directly infiltrate the laryngeal framework in most cases and extending outside the laryngeal confines
D. extends into the neck through the cricothyroid space laterally
E. non-aggressive and remains localized to the paraglottic space
REF. Mendonca DR, Bryce DP: Canadian J Otolaryngol, 2:3, 271, '73

894. A curative dose of irradiation (cobalt 60) can "cure" the following percent of T_3 laryngeal carcinomas:
A. 10
B. 25
C. 33
D. 50
E. 75
REF. Mendonca DR, Bryce DP: Canadian J Otolaryngol, 2:3, 271, '73

895. The delphian lymph nodes are characterized by:
A. primarily drains the larynx
B. primarily drains the thyroid
C. involvement in the metastatic spread of cancer of the larynx
D. involved by direct spread of cancer through the cricothyroid membrane
E. enlargement of the internal jugular chain
REF. Mendonca DR, Bryce DP: Canadian J Otolaryngol, 2:3, 271, '73

896. Glottic and supraglottic laryngeal webs are most effectively treated by:
A. endoscopic dilatations
B. endoscopic excision of the webs
C. laryngofissure with excision of the webs
D. tracheotomy under two percent xylocaine anesthesia followed by laryngofissure and use of a tantalum keel (McNaught)
E. D same with use of a silicone elastomer keel (Montgomery)
REF. Holinger LD, Wong HW, Hemenway WG: Arch Otolaryngol 101:496, Aug '75

897. The treatment of the hyoid syndrome consists of all of the following but the treatment of choice is:
A. heat applications
B. ultrasound
C. local infiltration of anesthetics
D. C with steroids
E. excision of the tip of the hyoid (greater cornu)
REF. Kopstein E: Arch Otolaryngol 101:484, Aug '75

898. Which of the following should be considered in the differential diagnosis of the hyoid syndrome?
A. temporomandibular joint syndrome (TM-Joint disease)
B. dental abnormalities
C. unerupted molars
D. cervical arthritis
E. esophageal diverticula
F. tumors
G. foreign bodies
H. chronic tonsillitis
I. neuralgias
REF. Kopstein E: Arch Otolaryngol 101:484, Aug '75

899. Which of the following cause the hyoid syndrome?
A. bursitis
B. insertion tendinosis
C. mechanical restriction due to excess bony growth or calcification
D. local pressures due to excess bony growth or calcification
E. obscure
REF. Kopstein E: Arch Otolaryngol 101:484, Aug '75

900. Although all of the following facts are true, the two commonest findings related to the hyoid syndrome are:
A. elongation of the styloid process (x-ray)
B. variants and abnormalities of the hyoid (x-ray)
C. normal x-ray findings of the hyoid bone and styloid process
D. an enlarged styloid process tender to intraoral palpation (so-called Eagle Syndrome)
E. marked tenderness at the tip of the greater cornu of the hyoid bone
REF. Kopstein E: Arch Otolaryngol 101:484, Aug '75

901. Symptoms of Hyoid Syndrome consist of:
A. pain in the lateral part of the neck with otalgia
B. chronic "sore throat"
C. dysphagia or sensation of a foreign body on swallowing
D. unpleasant sensations on protruding the tongue
E. pain along the internal and external carotid arteries and even impairment of a singing voice
REF. Kopstein E: Arch Otolaryngol 101:484, Aug '75

902. The retrostyloid space contains:
A. external carotid artery
B. internal carotid artery
C. cranial nerves 5, 6
D. cranial nerves 7, 9, 10, 11, 12
E. sympathetic chain
F. ascending pharyngeal artery
G. ascending palatine artery
REF. Stewart C, Passy V: Arch Otolaryngol 101:478, Aug '75

903. The superior part of the lateropharyngeal space (lateral to the pharyngeal constrictor muscles) contains the following structures:
A. internal carotid artery
B. external carotid artery
C. internal jugular vein
D. mandibular branch of the trigeminal nerve
E. internal maxillary artery (internal meningeal arterial branch)
F. cranial nerves 6, 7
G. auriculotemporal nerve
H. chorda tympani nerve
REF. Stewart C, Passy V: Arch Otolaryngol 101:478, Aug '75

904. Muscles attached to the stylohyoid process are:
A. palatoglossal
B. pterygoid
C. superior pharyngeal constrictor
D. middle pharyngeal constrictor
E. inferior pharyngeal constrictor
REF. Stewart C, Passy V: Arch Otolaryngol 101:478, Aug '75

905. Sequential serum copper levels in Hodgkin's disease are elevated in:
A. exacerbation of disease activity
B. impending relapse during remission
C. residual active disease with decrease in levels during therapy but failure to reach normal levels
D. terminal event in some patients
E. intercurrent infection
F. pregnancy, estrogen therapy (including contraceptive use), androgens
REF. Hrgovcic MJ, Tessmer CF, Mumford DM, Ong PS, Gamble JF, Shullenberger CC: Tex Med 71:53, Feb '75

906. The incidence of false-negative bronchial exfoliative cytologic findings in washings of patients with primary lung cancer ranges (depending on the size and location of the tumors) in percent from:
A. 1-3
B. 7-9
C. 5-10
D. 11-19
E. 20-50
REF. Dellon AL, Chu EW, Hall CA, Chretien PB: Arch Otolaryngol 101:465, Aug '75

907. Acute congestion and hemorrhage in many organs have been found in man after severe stress. Which of the following appear to be influenced by stress or steroids?
A. ulcers of the gastrointestinal tract
B. congestion and hemorrhage of the lungs
C. anatomic changes of the adrenal glands
D. sublaryngeal mucosal hemorrhage involving the entire circumference of the upper 2 to 3 cm of the trachea
E. loss of voice in frightened people (larynx)
REF. Payan HM: South Med J 68:81, Jan '75

908. When considering thyroid scan for cancer, the physician must consider which of the following facts?
A. clinically solitary cold nodules with malignancy is overemphasized because only a small percentage of these nodules are cancerous
B. do not scan any patient unless a palpable lump is present in the thyroid
C. irradiation in a thyroid scan exposes the thyroid to a radiation dose which may cause cancer
D. thyroid cancer has a low incidence and mortality rate even with distant metastases
E. careful physical examination with needle biopsy seems to be a logical alternative to surgery
REF. DeGroot LJ, Wang CA, Miller JM, Guansing AR, Leeper RD: Med World News 16:56, July '75

909. A patient with a very severe acute epiglottitis requiring an immediate tracheotomy should be treated with intravenous:
A. chloramphenicol
B. keflex
C. tetracycline
D. lincomycin
E. clindamycin
REF. Kitto W: JAMA 233:325, July '75

910. Bronchial brushing through transnasal flexible fiberoptic bronchoscopy in the diagnosis of localized peripheral pulmonary lesions down to the subsegmental level with absence of visible bronchial abnormalities proved to be very useful in the diagnosis of:
A. squamous cell carcinoma
B. adenocarcinoma
C. undifferentiated carcinoma
E. tuberculosis
REF. Kovnat DM, et al.: Chest 67:179, Feb '75

911. The preferred method of managing patients with life-threatening, massive hemoptysis is:
A. sedation with head-elevated bed rest
B. synkavite
C. premarin
D. identification of the bleeding site and electrocauterization by bronchoscopy
E. identification of the bleeding site by bronchoscopy followed by thoractomy with resection of the bleeding source
REF. McCollum WB, et al.: Chest 67:152, Feb '75

912. Following "difficult" esophagoscopy and bronchograms in children, it is imperative by taking a postoperative chest film to exclude the possibility of:
A. perforated esophagus
B. perforated hypopharynx
C. arytenoid injury
D. vocal cord injury
E. pneumothorax
REF. Salem MR, Bennett EJ, Schweiss JF, Baraka A, Dalal FY, Collins VJ: JAMA 233:238, July '75

913. Bradycardia or even cardiac arrest after even one dose of succinylcholine can be effectively blocked by a variety of drugs including:
A. morphine
B. demerol
C. codeine
D. phenobarbital
E. atropine
REF. Salem MR, Bennett EJ, Schweiss JR, Baraka A, Dalal FY, Collins VJ: JAMA 233:238, July '75

914. During anesthesia the accidental administration of potassium can be a contributing factor in the occurrence of cardiac arrest and has resulted from:
A. penicillin potassium
B. potassium drip
C. citrated cold blood
D. fresh frozen plasma
E. use of succinylcholine in injured patients with release of massive quantities of potassium from muscles
REF. Salem MR, Bennett EJ, Schweiss JR, Baraka A, Dalal FY, Collins VJ: JAMA 233:238, July '75

915. Succinylcholine should be avoided in patients with:
A. trauma including head and neck
B. burns including head and neck
C. paraplegia
D. acute neurological disease
E. high levels of serum potassium
REF. Salem MR, Bennett EJ, Schweiss JF, Baraka A, Dalal FY, Collins VJ: JAMA 233:238, July '75

916. The occurrence of cardiac arrest shortly after intubation in most patients while halothane and intermittent positive-pressure breathing (IPPB) is being given suggests the presence of:
A. airway obstruction due to endotracheal tube in the esophagus
B. aspiration with airway obstruction in a patient with elevated intragastric pressure (food, etc.)
C. incomplete muscular relaxation with active vomiting

D. absence of cricoid pressure by the anesthetist
E. associated hypovolemia
REF. Salem MR, Bennett EJ, Schweiss JF, Baraka A, Dalal FY, Collins VJ: JAMA 233:238, July '75

917. Cardiac arrest caused by anesthesia continues to occur. The majority of cardiac arrests are preventable. Which of the following facts appear to be true?
A. respiratory embarrassment precedes cardiac arrest in most cases
B. more than half of the deaths from anesthesia occur in healthy children
C. blood loss is a common cause of cessation of circulatory action during anesthesia
D. deliberate hypotension cannot be used safely and successfully in pediatric patients
E. certain anesthetic agents such as halothane should be avoided in anemic infants
REF. Salem MR, Bennett EJ, Schweiss JF, Baraka A, Dalal FY, Collins VJ: JAMA 233:238, July '75

918. In the following question each lettered item is to be matched with one or more numbered items. Recent nonendoscopic methods to remove foreign bodies have resulted in severe complications:
A. esophageal meat impaction dissolved with papain
B. coins extracted from the esophagus by using a distended Foley catheter
C. bronchial foreign bodies expelled by placing the patient in a head-down position and tapping the chest

1. deaths
2. possible aspiration
3. cardiorespiratory arrest
4. blindness (temporary)
REF. Ritter FN: Ann Otol Rhinol Laryngol 83:729, Nov '74

919. Death may result from major vessel erosion with hemorrhage, sepsis, or asphyxiation in pterygomaxillary space abscess. Symptoms include:
A. fever due to infection with group A stretococcus pyogenes but other organisms (due to antibiotic use) may be involved, including Bacteroides
B. sore throat and malaise
C. otalgia
D. cervical rigidity and trismus
E. bulging of the posterolateral wall and tonsillar region (anterior compartment) and/or posterior pharyngeal wall and parotid space (posterior compartment)
REF. Mattucci K, Samet C: NY State J Med 74:1409, July '74

920. Which of the following skin complications occurs in patients receiving immunosuppressive agents after homografts when the immunosuppressive regimen usually consists of azathioprine, prednisolone and antilymphocytic globulin?
A. Cushingoid changes
B. facial erythema and telangiectasis, steroid acne, striae, atrophic and friable, dry skin, keratosis pilaris
C. purpura
D. altered fat distribution
E. extensive areas of gangrene resulting from secondary hyperparathyroidism and severe calcification of cutaneous blood vessels with death
F. hirsutism
G. cytotoxic scalp hair loss
H. cutaneous infections: warts, herpes simplex, herpes zoster, tinea versicolor
I. de novo skin cancer
J. erythromelanosis
K. acanthosis nigricans

L. cold intolerance (front teeth)
M. metastatic calcification
N. red lunulae
O. hyperpigmentation of exposed skin
REF. Koranda FC, Dehmel EM, Kahn G, Penn I: JAMA 229:419, July '74

921. Major factors causing the greatest immediate threat to life in patients with carotid artery injuries are:
A. massive hemothorax
B. severe shock due to hemorrhage which may appear innocuous at first
C. bleeding, obstructing the patient's airway
D. cerebral ischemia with irreversible brain damage
E. cerebral ischemia with death
REF. DiVincenti FC, Weber BB: Am Surg 40:277, May '74

922. Arteriograms in suspected carotid arterial injuries:
A. avoids needless surgery in about one-third of patients
B. always demonstrates extravasation of contrast material in injury
C. may be negative in injury and cause harm due to delay in initiating surgery
D. should always be performed before surgery
E. indicate no extreme position on arteriography is tenable for proper treatment
REF. Smith RF, Elliott JP, Hageman JH, Szilagy DE, Xavier AO: Arch Surg 109:198, Aug '74

923. Patients with no cellular immunity, are hypocalcemic, and have no thymus or parathyroid glands have:
A. Hodgkin's disease
B. systemic sarcoidosis
C. leprosy
D. chronic lymphatic leukemia
E. Di George's syndrome
REF. Graf MW: Modern Med 43:134, Mar '75; Samter M (Editor): Immunology Diseases, 2nd Ed., Little, Brown & Co., Boston, p. 239, 1971

924. A variable depression of cell-mediated immunity often related to the activity of the disease is observed in:
A. Hodgkin's disease
B. systemic sarcoidosis
C. leprosy
D. chronic lymphatic leukemia
E. DiGeorge's syndrome
REF. Graft MW: Modern Med 43:134, Mar '75; Samter M (Editor): Immunologic Diseases, 2nd Ed., Little, Brown & Co., Boston, p. 239, 1971

925. Anteriorly, both the supraglottic and subglottic structures are embryologically derived from wedge-shaped, midline cell masses whereas the glottic structures are derived from two laterally placed cell masses which fuse at the anterior commissure (Tucker's x-shaped concept). Which of the following tumors often remain ipsilateral even after reaching the anterior commissure?
A. supraglottic
B. glottic
C. subglottic
REF. Nostrand AWP V: Can J Otolaryngol 3 (No. 4):408, No month '74

926. Which of the following statements appear to be true in laryngeal carcinomas?
A. Fixation of the vocal cord in glottic cancer is a poor prognostic sign
B. A is not a poor prognostic sign
C. main cause of cord fixation is invasion of the thryoarytenoid muscle
D. C of the cricoarytenoid joint
E. glottic tumors tend to spread vertically into the subglottic and supraglottic regions long before they spread horizontally to the opposite hemilarynx
REF. Nostrand AWP V: Can J Otolaryngol 3 (No. 4):408, No month '74

927. The supraglottic laryngeal structures are embroyologically largely derived from which of the following arches?
A. I
B. II
C. III
D. IV
E. V
F. VI
REF. Nostrand AWP V: Can J Otolaryngol 3 (No. 4):408, No month '74

928. Which of the following structures may be invaded in a glottic carcinoma with a fixed vocal cord?
A. thyroarytenoid muscle
B. lateral cricoarytenoid muscle
C. interarytenoid muscle
D. posterior cricoarytenoid muscle
E. cricoarytenoid joint
F. perineural invasion
G. thyroid cartilage
H. extension outside of the larynx
REF. Olofsson J: Can J Otolaryngol 3 (No. 4):446, No month '74

929. Partial laryngectomy with voice conservation surgery should be practiced with extreme caution in which of the following patients with laryngeal carcinoma?
A. non-irradiated glottic primary carcinomas with mucosal invasion
B. supraglottic primaries
C. tumors extending more than one cm below the free margin of the vocal cord
D. extension of cancer from a vocal cord upward onto the base of the epiglottis
E. extension of a vocal cord cancer across the ventricle to the false cord
REF. Nostrand AWP V: Can J Otolaryngol 3 (No. 4):408, No month '74; Kirchner JA: Can J Otolaryngol 3 (No. 4):460, No month '74

930. Primary cancers arising in the subglottic region:
A. are rare - four to five percent of laryngeal carcinomas
B. tend to spread circumferentially
C. are usually associated with vocal cord paralysis
D. present palpable cervical lymph nodes in the majority of patients
E. have a poor prognosis with metastasis to the paratracheal nodes in 50 percent of all larynges examined by serial section
REF. Nostrand AWP: Can J Otolaryngol 3 (No. 4):408, No month '74; Lund WS: Can J Otolaryngol 3 (No. 4):469, No month '74

931. A study of metastatic routes in the neck from squamous cell carcinomas arising in the mucosal surfaces of the upper air and food passages reveal:
A. separated groups of involved nodes are a poor prognostic sign
B. palpable nodes may not be involved with cancer
C. B always involved with cancer
D. small nodes with or without cancer survive radiotherapy very poorly
E. growth of a neoplasm within a node is often explosive
REF. Nostrand AWP: Can J Otolaryngol 3 (No. 4):408, No month '74; McKelvie P: Can J Otolaryngol 3 (No. 4):473, No month '74

932. The T classification in TNM of laryngeal carcinoma in a vocal cord tumor extending to the subglottic region or to the supraglottic region with normal or impaired (but not fixed) mobility and without fixation of the epiglottis is:
A. T_{1s}
B. T_1
C. T_{1a}
D. T_{1b}
E. T_2
F. T_3
G. T_4
REF. Nostrand AWP: Can J Otolaryngol 3 (No. 4):408, No month '74; Shepperd HWH: Can J Otolaryngol 3 (No. 4):480, No month '74

933. The assumption that cord fixation is invariably a bad prognostic sign in laryngeal cancer can be dangerous since it may occur in:
A. exophytic tumor in the anterior commissure
B. edema of the cord
C. arthritis of the crico-arytenoid joint
D. middle of radiotherapy
E. after a course of radiotherapy without apparent detriment to the patient
F. fixation of the crico-arytenoid joint due to edema
REF. Shaheen OH: Can J Otolaryngol 3 (No. 4):486, No month '74

934. There is a significantly decreased three-year survival rate in patients with laryngeal cancer with a clinically positive lymph node greater in size in cm than:
A. 1
B. 2
C. 3
D. 4
E. 5
REF. Sessions DG, Ogura JH: Can J Otolaryngol 3 (No. 4):489, No month '74

935. Wegener's granulomatosis is a disease characterized by:
A. necrotizing granulomas and vasculitis of the upper and lower respiratory tract
B. focal necrotizing glomerulonephritis with or without A
C. nasal symptoms of obstruction alone or in combination with A and/or B
D. C with or without subglottic stenosis
E. unilateral proptosis being the initial symptom
REF. Djalilian M, McDonald TJ, Devine KD, Weiland LH: Ann Otol Rhinol Laryngol 84:757, Nov '75

936. The treatment of choice in Wegener's granulomatosis is:
A. steroids alone
B. streptomycin
C. tetracycline
D. chloromycetin
E. steroids with cyclophosphamide
REF. Djalilian M, McDonald TJ, Devine KD, Weiland LH: Ann Otol Rhinol Laryngol 84:757, Nov '75

937. A nonneoplastic, nontraumatic subglottic stenosis may be a manifestation of a systemic disorder and examination should consist of:
A. chest and tracheal roentgenograms
B. complete blood count
C. erythrocyte sedimentation rate (ESR)
D. serologic studies
E. serum creatinine concentration
F. urinalysis
G. endoscopic examination of the larynx and trachea with biopsy
REF. Djalilian M, McDonald TJ, Devine KD, Weiland LH: Ann Otol Rhinol Laryngol 84:757, Nov '75

938. Which of the following significant tissue damage to vocal cords can be caused by intubation in adults?
A. ulceration of the medial surface of the arytenoid vocal process
B. granulomas of the interarytenoid region
C. webs
D. glottic strictures
E. subglottic strictures
REF. Hengerer AS, Strome M, Jaffe BF: Ann Otol Rhinol Laryngol 84:764, Nov '75

939. The usual practice in adults is conversion from intubation to a tracheotomy for continued airway assistance after the following time in days:
A. one
B. two
C. three
D. seven
E. fourteen
REF. Hengerer AS, Strome M, Jaffe BF: Ann Otol Rhinol Laryngol 84:764, Nov '75

940. The neonatal larynx responds differently to the effects of intubation as compared to the adult larynx and:
A. the duration of neonatal intubation can be extended
B. A cannot be extended
C. no definite length of time of the onset of laryngeal injuries with persistent hoarseness has been determined, as in adults
D. patients who remain hoarse after one year have significant laryngeal changes resulting from the neonatal period
E. D not always true
REF. Hengerer AS, Strome M, Jaffe BF: Ann Otol Rhinol Laryngol 84:764, Nov '75

941. Which of the following conditions can cause nontraumatic subglottic stenosis?
A. relapsing polychondritis
B. amyloidosis
C. sarcoidosis
D. Wegener's granulomatosis
E. neoplastic disease
REF. Djalilian M, McDonald TJ, Devine KD, Weiland LH: Ann Otol Rhinol Laryngol 84:757, Nov '75

942. Reactions to iodinated intravenous contrast media appear inconsistent with an allergic mechanism mediated by antibodies because:
A. incidence of reactions does not increase in patients previously exposed to the media
B. following a reaction some patients tolerate subsequent administration
C. fewer reactions follow intra-arterial administration
D. C but with intravenous administration
E. intradermal testing has no value in predicting a possible reaction
REF. Graf MW: Modern Med 43:133, Mar '75; Patterson R: Allergy Diseases, I Ed., J.B. Lippincott Co., Phila., pp. 476-478, 1972

943. Inhalation of 95 percent oxygen and five percent CO_2 instead of air can be very useful in which of the following conditions?
A. bacterial fermentation or putrefaction with release of H_2 in the intestinal tract
B. A with release of CH_4
C. A with release of H_2S, or volatile amines
D. pulmonary embolism due to air
E. subcutaneous or mediastinal emphysema
REF. Fine J: Med World News 16:17, June '75

944. A six-year-old female with a bilaterial midline vocal cord paralysis present since birth following a successful tracheo-esophageal operation should have:
A. re-implantation procedure utilizing the ansa hypoglossal nerve and strap muscle
B. transoral intra-laryngeal arytenoidectomy (Thornell procedure)
C. Woodman arytenoidectomy
D. recurrent laryngeal nerve decompression
E. do nothing until full development of the larynx
REF. Alonso WA, Novack AJ, Wallenborn WM, Wine CJ, Winborn CD, Thornell WC, Titche LL, Sydnor A, Tobin HA, Pratt LW: Coll Ltrs Int Corr Soc Oph-Otolaryngol 20:73, May '75

945. The etiologic agent of infectious mononucleosis is:
A. adenovirus
B. coxsackie virus A
C. rhinovirus
D. respiratory syncytial virus
E. Epstein-Barr virus
REF. Klein JO: Ann Otol Rhinol Laryngol 84 (Suppl. 19):30, Mar '75

946. Patients with advanced diffuse histiocytic lymphoma (reticulum-cell sarcoma) have been cured with:
A. nitrogen mustard (or cyclophosphamide)
B. procarbazine
C. vincristine
D. prednisolone
E. combination chemotherapy with A, B, C, D
REF. De Vita Jr. VT: Lancet 1:248, Feb '75

947. Arterial gas changes in animals with laryngeal obstruction shows:
A. elevated PCO_2
B. decreased PCO_2
C. decreased PO_2
D. elevated PO_2
E. increased laryngeal obstruction is associated with an increase in pulmonary resistance
REF. Ogura JH: Ann Otol Rhinol Laryngol 84 (Suppl. 19):49, Mar '75

948. Which of the following lesions of the thyroid are considered benign?
A. Hashimoto's
B. follicular adenoma
C. colloid nodules
D. Hürthle-cell adenoma
E. fetal adenoma
REF. Refetoff S, Harrison J, Karanfilski BT, Kaplan EL, DeGroot LJ, Bekerman C: N Eng J Med 292:171, Jan '75

949. Thyroid carcinoma or abnormalities occur after irradiation to which of the following areas of the neck in infancy and childhood?
A. skin (acne)
B. adenoids
C. tonsils
D. B + C
E. thymus
REF. Refetoff S, Harrison J, Karanfilski BT, Kaplan EL, DeGroot LJ, Bekerman C: N Eng J Med 292:171, Jan '75

950. In nodular irradiated thyroids removed at operation, the occurrence of carcinoma is often in the percent range of:
A. 1-5
B. 10-15
C. 20-25
D. 30-35
E. 40-50
REF. Refetoff S, Harrison J, Karanfilski BT, Kaplan EL, DeGroot LJ, Bekerman C: N Eng J Med 292:171, June '75

951. The psychotherapeutic potential of lithium carbonate is known but of all of the following side effects which occur which one should otolaryngolotists be especially aware of?
A. thyroid dysfunction
B. congenital anomalies
C. cardiac arrhythmias
D. manic psychoses
E. slurred speech
REF. Wolber PGH, King SJ: Notes and Tips, Harper & Row Pub., Inc. 5:132, Mar '75

952. Improvement of high dose methotrexate therapy in the treatment of head and neck cancer has been accomplished by the use of which one of the following drugs administered 6 to 18 hours later:
A. bleomycin
B. cyclophosphamide
C. adriamycin
D. streptozotocin
E. leucovorin
REF. Bertino JR: The Laryngoscope 85:491, Mar '75

953. Accumulated evidence clearly indicates which of the following groups of viruses are causative agents for many neoplastic diseases in animals?
A. poxvirus
B. herpesvirus
C. adenovirus
D. papova
E. leukovirus types B, C
REF. Sheinin R: The Laryngoscope 85:468, Mar '75

954. Combination chemotherapy programs with improved therapeutic results and possibly cure occur with:
A. epidermoid carcinoma
B. acute lymphatic leukemia
C. Hodgkin's disease
D. histocystic lymphoma
E. embryonal testicular tumors
REF. Bertino JR: The Laryngoscope 85:491, Mar '75

955. In the treatment of Burkitt's Lymphoma, the drug of choice is:
A. busulfan
B. chlorambucil
C. cyclophosphamide
D. phenylalanine mustard
E. nitrogen mustard
REF. Bertino JR: The Laryngoscope 85:491, Mar '75

956. Single agent therapy cures which two of the following human neoplasms?
A. epidermoid carcinoma
B. Burkitt's lymphoma
C. adenocarcinoma
D. lymphoepithelioma
E. choriocarcinoma
REF. Bertino JR: The Laryngoscope 85:491, Mar '75

957. Cultivation of cells from at least one squamous cell carcinoma of the larynx has been accomplished. These cells are susceptible to infection by herpes virus type I (HSV-1) and type 2 (HSV-2). Some cells transformed by oncogenic herpes virus make virus-coded proteins which may be available to the immune system with production of antibodies. Of 38 patients with laryngeal cancer, what percent gave evidence for serum antibodies to HSV-determined proteins?
A. 5
B. 20
C. 25
D. 80
E. 95
REF. Sheinin R: The Laryngoscope 85:468, Mar '75

958. Which of the following appears true in warts and papillomata of the larynx?
A. human warts are caused by the human papilloma virus
B. human papilloma virus unequivocally causes laryngeal papillomata
C. biopsied papillomata show electron microscopic evidence of nuclear inclusions of particles characteristic of the human papilloma virus
D. biopsied papillomata show electron microscopic evidence of intranuclear depositions of filamentous virus structures
E. human papilloma virus appears to be transmitted from genital warts in pregnant women to newborn infants
REF. Sheinin R: The Laryngoscope 85:468, Mar '75

959. In infectious mononucleosis which of the following antibiotics is indicated?
A. ampicillin
B. erythromycin
C. sulfacetamide
D. tetracycline
E. none
REF. ACA Course: Allergy News Bull 4:6 (Month=none) Issue 9, '75

960. Any wound of the face or neck more than five hours old should:
A. be considered potentially contaminated
B. have vigorous debridement
C. have immediate wound closure
D. have delayed wound closure in three to five days
E. probably have culture with sensitivity tests and antibiotic therapy
REF. Robson MC, et al.: J Surg Res 14:426, May '73

961. Disadvantages of taking a skin graft from the buttock, hip or lower abdomen are:
A. split-thickness skin grafts from these areas can assume a yellowish or light-brown hue in the recipient sites
B. donor sites require prolonged healing
C. A but lightens with time
D. A but blush response
E. A discoloration increases on exposure to sunlight or ultraviolet light
REF. Ponten B: Acta Chir Scand (Suppl.) 257:1-78, Apr '60

962. The advantages of taking a skin graft from the buttocks, hip, or lower abdomen are:
A. healed donor site, often lighter than the surrounding tissue color, is hidden by clothing
B. donor sites heal as quickly as any other body sites
C. dermis is much thicker than the epidermis making these sites ideal for cutting multiple split-thickness skin grafts
D. graft does not change color with time
E. graft color does not change on exposure to sunlight or ultraviolet light
REF. Ponten B: Acta Chir Scand (Suppl.) 257:1-78, Apr '60

963. In the treatment of seromas (accumulated serosanguineous fluid) under isograft (autograft) split-thickness skin graft on the second day after application, which of the following statements are true?
A. incision of the graft over a seroma to remove accumulated serum does not disturb the remainder of the graft
B. A does disturb as early as the second day
C. removal of the whole graft causes bleeding and probable hematoma under the reapplied graft
D. systemic antibiotics increases the percent of graft "take"
E. skin graft placed on an open wound decreases the bacterial count below a wound infection level
REF. Grabb WC, Smith JW: Plastic Surgery: A Concise Guide to Clinical Practice, Little, Brown & Co., Boston, p. 33, 1973

964. Seromas (accumulated fluid) under isograft (autograft) split-thickness skin graft on the second day after application should be treated by:
A. systemic antibiotics
B. removal of the graft and not replaced since rejection is developing
C. incision of the graft over the seromas with removal of accumulated fluid
D. removal of the whole graft and reapplied under a pressure dressing
E. removal of the whole graft, antibiotic dressing applied and regrafted in two to three days
REF. Grabb WC, Smith JW: Plastic Surgery: A Concise Guide to Clinical Practice, Little, Brown & Co., Boston, p. 33, 1973

965. Patients with cerebellar syndromes (ataxia, gait disturbances, speech disorders, vertigo) secondary to infectious mononucleosis should:
A. have thorough neuroradiologic studies
B. be treated with high doses of steroids
C. B is of unproved value regardless of dose level
D. not be treated since most patients return to completely normal function
E. have a cisternal myelogram to rule out a posterior fossa tumor
REF. Schraeder PL, Messert B, Henke TK, Peters HA: Wis Med J 74:S-25, Feb '75

966. Subnormal peripheral blood levels of T cells (spontaneous lymphocyte rosette assay) are found in:
A. melanomas
B. sarcomas
C. squamous cell carcinomas
D. inoperable malignancies
E. recurrent malignancies
REF. Potvin C, et al.: Clin Immunol Immunopath 3:476, Mar '75

967. Normal peripheral blood levels of T cells (spontaneous lymphocyte rosette assay) are found in patients clinically cured of:
A. adenocarcinomas
B. melanomas
C. sarcomas
E. squamous carcinomas
REF. Potvin C, et al.: Clin Immunol Immunopath 3:476, Mar '75

968. Which one of the following characteristics of infectious mononucleosis is not generally recognized?
A. inflammatory swelling of the lymph nodes, especially of the cervical region
B. moderate leukocytes due mostly to abnormal mononuclear cells
C. sometimes severe faucial lesions
D. sudden onset with fever and malaise
E. multiple discrete granulomas (granulomatous inflammation) in the bone marrow
REF. Rothwell DJ, Arch Path 99:508, Sept '75

969. T-cells from a Burkitt Lymphoma biopsy have which of the following important features?
A. have actually been isolated from Burkitt Lymphoma (BL) biopsy
B. can kill the autologous tumor cells (biopsy)
C. patients with infectious mononucleosis (IM) develop killer T cells which recognize BL tumor cells
D. patients with BL may benefit from transfer of immunity from patients with IM
E. D same with patients with nasopharyngeal carcinoma
REF. Jondal M, et al.: Nature 255:405, May '75

970. Following acute trauma to the neck, the most commonly found laryngeal fracture is:
A. secondary lateral arch
B. vertical midline
C. paramedial thyroid alar fracture
D. A plus B
E. A plus C
REF. Travis LW, Olson NR, Melvin JW, Snyder RG: Trans Am Acad Ophthalmol Otolaryngol 80:ORL-382, July '75

971. Following acute trauma to the neck, immediate tracheotomy is indicated in:
A. airway distress
B. laryngoscopic findings of severe edema
C. B of hematoma
D. B extensive mucosal lacerations with false passages
E. crepitation of cartilage fragments
F. hemoptysis
G. dysphonia
REF. Travis LW, Olson NR, Melvin JW, Snyder RG, Trans Am Acad Ophthalmol Otolaryngol 80: ORL-382, July '75

972. The boundaries of the supraglottic larynx consists of all of the following structures, except:
A. hyo-epiglottic ligament
B. thyrohyoid membrane
C. body of the hyoid
D. mucosa of the lingual surface of the epiglottic tip
E. mucosa of the vallecula
REF. Nostrand AWP V: Can J Otolaryngol 3 (No. 4):408, No month '74; Maguire A, Dayal VS: Can J Otolaryngol 3 (No. 4):432, No month '74

973. Which of the following statements are accurate when considering treatment of T_1 and T_2 glottic carcinomas?
A. highly curable in its early stages (irradiation)
B. tumors involving the anterior commissure show a tendency to spread inferiorly into the anterior subglottic region
C. stripping of the vocal cord for in situ cancer extending to the anterior commissure may be inadequate treatment
D. invasive cancer in the anterior commissure should be excised by an entire anterior glottic wedge
E. cancer persisting within mucous glands is a cause of radiation failure
REF. Bridger GP: Can J Otolaryngol 3 (No. 4):507, No month '74

974. Experience with 230 patients with tetanus showed:
A. male predominance
B. A female
C. survival rate greater than 84 percent
D. C less than 27 percent
E. tetanus antitoxin, 10,000 units, appears sufficient for treatment
F. diazepam provides adequate relaxation and sedation
G. tracheostomy and gastrostomy are important
REF. Garnier MJ: Am J Surg 129:459, Apr '75

975. Classic hypersensitivity - induced reactions which are bizarre and potentially serious from the use of phenytoin (diphenylhydantoin (dilantin)) - are:
A. pseudolymphoma, lymphadenopathy simulating malignant lymphoma
B. true lymphoma
C. Hodgkin's disease
D. unifocal lymphadenopathy
E. lymphadenopathy with lymph node hyperplasia (without pseudolymphoma)
REF. Archer JD: Arch Otolaryngol 101:461, Aug '75

976. The glottic and subglottic structures of the larynx are embryologically largely derived from which of the following arches?
A. I
B. II
C. III
D. IV
E. V
F. VI
REF. Nostrand AWP V: Can J Otolaryngol 3 (No. 4):408, No month '74; Hast MH: Can J Otolaryngol 3 (No. 4):412, No month '74

977. A patient with laryngeal cancer with a T_4 N_O M_O lesion is in stage:
A. I
B. II
C. III
D. IV
REF. Sessions DG, Ogura JH: Can J Otolaryngol 3 (No. 4):489, No month '74

978. What percent of T_1 and T_2 laryngeal carcinomas failed to be cured by irradiation because of clinical failure to recognize submucous extension, especially via the mucous glands?
A. 3
B. 5
C. 10
D. 15
E. 20
REF. Atkinson L, Bridger GP: Can J Otolaryngol 3 (No. 4):496, No month '74

979. Radiation failures in laryngeal carcinomas should be suspected when which of the following occur?
A. failure of symptoms to improve in T_1 and T_2 lesions
B. failure of larynx to return to a normal appearance
C. patients persist in smoking and drinking
D. crico-arytenoid joint fixation
E. extension of glottic tumors T_1 or T_2 to the subglottic region (especially epiglottic)
REF. Atkinson L, Bridger GP: Can J Otolaryngol 3 (No. 4):496, No month '74

980. Although all of the following carcinomas in situ of the larynx occur, which one type is most common?
A. bowenoid
B. verrucous
C. adenocarcinoma
D. squamous carcinoma grade I
E. squamous carcinoma grade II or III
REF. Fisher HR: Can J Otolaryngol 3 (No. 4):522, No month '74

981. The absence of histologically identifiable residual cancer in hemilaryngectomy specimens indicates that endoscopic removal of "all" of the tumor occurs in the following percent of patients:
A. 2
B. 5
C. 7
D. 11
E. 20
REF. McGavran MH, Stutsman AC, Ogura JH: Can J Otolaryngol 3 (No. 4): 526, No month '74

982. Cancer of the true vocal cord in properly selected patients can probably be successfully managed by endoscopic removal alone in the following percent of patients:
A. 1-2
B. 3-4
C. 5-10
D. 11-14
E. 15-20
REF. McGavran MH, Stutsman AC, Ogura JH: Can J Otolaryngol 3 (No. 4): 526, No month '74

983. Which of the following statements must be assumed in considering precancerous lesions of the larynx?
A. it is not certain that every carcinoma in situ becomes an invasive cancer
B. A it is certain
C. carinoma in situ may be multicentric in origin and found isolated by intervening healthy epithelium from invasive or preinvasive lesions
E. malignant change may occur in a pre-existing benign papilloma
E. D never occurs
REF. Friedmann I: Can J Otolaryngol 3 (No. 4):528, No month '74

984. Keratosis and keratosis with atypia are reactive epithelial changes and are part of the histologic picture in a variety of conditions including:
A. reactions to laryngeal deformities
B. radiation injury
C. "chronic laryngitis"
D. healing biopsy sites
E. "contact ulcers"
F. histoplasmosis
G. tuberculosis
H. vocal nodules
I. granular cell tumors
J. reaction to the presence of cancer
REF. Bauer WC: Can J Otolaryngol 3 (No. 4):533, No month '74

985. The overall frequency of carcinoma in situ associated with all invasive laryngeal carcinomas is quite high but the most common site is:
A. supraglottic
B. transglottic
C. infraglottic
D. glottic
REF. Bauer WC: Can J Otolaryngol 3 (No. 4):533, No month '74

986. Nonkeratinizing squamous carcinomas originate from endodermal or foregut derivatives and are common in the:
A. pharynx
B. oral cavity
C. larynx
D. paranasal sinuses
E. part of the nasal fossa
REF. Bauer WC: Can J Otolaryngol 3 (No. 4):533, No month '74

987. Keratinizing squamous carcinomas are ectodermally derived and are found most common in the:
A. buccal mucosa
B. floor of the mouth
C. anterior tongue
D. retromolar trigone
E. larynx
REF. Bauer WC: Can J Otolaryngol 3 (No. 4):533, No month '74

988. In the following question, each lettered item is to be matched with one or more numbered items. Each numbered choice may be used more than once:
A. microsurgical intervention
B. conservative intervention such as chordectomy
C. partial resection of the larynx with reconstruction
D. radical operation such as total laryngectomy

1. infiltrative cancer
2. invasive, infiltrative carcinoma
3. carcinoma in situ with micro-invasion
4. hyperplasia
5. hyperplasia with epithelial dysplasia
6. carcinoma in situ
REF. Padovan IF: Can J Otolaryngol 3 (No. 4):543, No month '74

989. Carcinoma in situ is:
A. precancerous disease
B. early cancer
C. best treated by radiation therapy
D. can be treated by excisional surgery
E. cancer which may recur after radiation treatment
REF. Holinger PH, Schild JA: Can J Otolaryngol 3 (No. 4):549, No month '74

990. Which of the following rules must be observed in adequate treatment of premalignant lesions of the vocal cord?
A. keratosis, keratosis with atypia and carcinoma in situ are treated in the same manner
B. stripping of the true cord, as a definitive curative procedure, is the therapy of choice in a unilateral involved cord
C. B in bilateral lesions a staged procedures is advisable
D. possibility of a subglottic cancer in the anterior commissure must be verified or excluded
E. cessation of smoking may produce a cure
REF. Som ML: Can J Otolaryngol 3 (No. 4):551, No month '74

991. Which of the following statements may be considered true in the management of keratosis and/or keratosis with atypia of the vocal cord?
A. surgical stripping of the cords is usually successful
B. radiation is the treatment of choice in recurrence following stripping
C. radiation is unwarranted and may change these lesions into true malignancy
D. cryosurgery is always successful
E. D results in occasional failure
REF. Miller D: Can J Otolaryngol 3 (No. 4):557, No month '74

992. A closed cryoprobe with a 20 sq mm surface should be used in the treatment of a T_{1S} vocal cord cancer with 30 seconds application with petrolatum strip protection to non-treated areas and with liquid nitrogen spray at a C temperature of:
A. 0
B. -5
C. -10
D. -15
E. -20
REF. Miller D: Can J Otolaryngol 3 (No. 4):557, No month '74

993. Keratosis with and without atypia and carcinoma in situ are confined to the epithelium of the vocal cord and are separated from the vocalis muscle by Reinke's space of loose areolar tissue. CO_2 surgical laser appears to be an optimal method of biopsy-excision provided there is:
A. wide exposure with binocular vision and space for bimanual manipulation
B. a time interval between excision of lesions extending across the anterior commissure to avoid web formation
C. blue-black staining of carcinoma in situ with a nuclear stain (two percent Toluidine blue or Azure blue)
D. C where areas of keratosis stand out in contrast as white areas
E. C where areas of respiratory epithelium in the ventricle and lower subglottic will not stain
REF. Strong MS: Can J Otolaryngol 3 (No. 4):560, No month '74

994. Which of the following facts must be considered in the treatment of carcinoma in situ of the vocal cord?
A. the pathologist cannot always determine the presence of multicentric areas of carcinoma in situ (or early micro-invasion) near the biopsy site
B. the laryngologist can always recognize carcinoma in situ or early invasion by the use of Toluidine blue staining and the use of microlaryngoscopy
C. carcinoma in situ should be first treated with 6000 to 6500 rads with 95 percent cure rate and preservation of voice
D. recurrences after radiation therapy should be treated with partial laryngectomy
E. D with total laryngectomy
REF. Miller D: Can J Otolaryngol 3 (No. 4):557, No month '74

995. Adequate irradiation treatment of vocal carcinoma in situ consists of a tumor dose of 6000 rads given over a five week period using a 4 Mv Linear accelerator. Reactions are not usually any problem, except with:
A. patients with sensitive skin resulting in severe dermatitis and ulceration
B. dysphagia with inability to swallow even liquids
C. persistent smokers
D. alcoholics
E. chronic bronchitis
REF. Dalby JE: Can J Otolaryngol 3 (No. 4):564, No month '74

996. There is the possibility of a long term carcinogenic radiation effect in which of the following vocal cord lesions treated with radiotherapy?
A. keratosis
B. hyperkeratosis
C. leukoplakia
D. carcinoma in situ
E. carcinoma, invasive
REF. Dalby JE. Can J Otolaryngol 3 (No. 4):564, No month '74

997. Failures after irradiation for carcinoma in situ of the vocal cord are:
A. insidious
B. manifested frequently by limited motion
C. manifested by fixation of an arytenoid
D. manifested always by mucous membrane changes
E. followed by invasive carcinoma in many more instances than when the initial treatment is stripping alone or laryngofissure
REF. Miller AH: Can J Otolaryngol 3 (No. 4):567, No month '74

998. Pathologists and clinicians agree that which one of the following terms should no longer be used for laryngeal lesions:
A. keratosis
B. keratosis with atypia
C. leukoplakia
D. carcinoma in situ
E. carcinoma in situ with microinvasion
REF. Miller AH: Can J Otolaryngol 3 (No. 4):573, No month '74

999. The most common cause of subglottic stenosis is:
A. external trauma to the larynx
B. use of cuffed tracheotomy tubes
C. high tracheotomy incision
D. congenital stenosis
E. neoplastic disease, primary or secondary
REF. Djalilian M, McDonald TJ, Devine KD, Weiland LH: Ann Otol Rhinol Laryngol 84:757, Nov '75

1000. Which of the following is necessary in the management of radiotherapy of premalignant laryngeal vocal cord lesions?
A. histological accuracy
B. clinical acumen
C. radiotherapy indicated where there is real histological uncertainty
D. C where there is a suggestion of carcinoma in situ
E. C where clinical features strongly suggest malignancy
REF. Dalby JE: Can J Otolaryngol 3 (No. 4):564, No month '74

1001. The usual sites of involvement in relapsing polychondritis are:
A. external ear
B. nasal septal cartilages
C. larynx
D. tracheal bronchial tree
E. ribs
REF. Djalilian M, McDonald TJ, Devine KD, Weiland LH: Ann Otol Rhinol Laryngol 84:757, Nov '75

1002. Audiovestibular manifestations of relapsing polychondritis are:
A. conductive hearing loss
B. sensorineural hearing loss
C. tinnitus
D. vertigo
E. may simulate endolymphatic hydrops of Ménière's disease
F. may simulate Coagan's syndrome
REF. Djalilian M, McDonald TJ, Devine KD, Weiland LH: Ann Otol Rhinol Laryngol 84:757, Nov '75

1003. The clinical picture in the acute phase of relapsing polychondritis is characterized by:
A. pain, swelling, redness and tenderness of the external ear
B. A of the nose
C. narrowing of the trachea and/or tracheobronchial tree with possible death
D. ocular manifestations of inflammation

E. fragmentation of cartilage with necrosis and chondrolysis
F. cartilage replacement by fibrous connective tissue
REF. Djalilian M, McDonald TJ, Devine KD, Weiland LH: Ann Otol Rhinol Laryngol 84:757, Nov '75

1004. The treatment of relapsing polychondritis is:
A. corticosteroids
B. antibiotics
C. A plus B
D. surgical resection of the stenosed area of the trachea and lining with skin
E. simple tracheal dilation
F. valved speaking tracheotomy tube
REF. Djalialian M, McDonald TJ, Devine KD, Weiland LH: Ann Otol Rhinol Laryngol 84:757, Nov '75

1005. The most common part of the body to be affected by localized amyloidosis (starchlike and turns blue-black when treated with iodine and sulfuric acid) is:
A. heart
B. larynx
C. tongue
D. skin
E. lung
REF. Djalilian M, McDonald TJ, Devine KD, Weiland LH: Ann Otol Rhinol Laryngol 84:757, Nov '75

1006. The most common sites of amyloidosis in the larynx in order of frequency are:
A. false cords
B. subglottic area
C. ventricles
E. aryepiglottic fold
REF. Djalilian M, McDonald TJ, Devine KD, Weiland, LH: Ann Otol Rhinol Laryngol 84:757, Nov '75

1007. The treatment of amyloidosis of the larynx consists of:
A. treatment with systemic iodine
B. A with local dilute sulphuric acid
C. A plus B
D. removal if obstruction occurs
E. excision regardless of size
REF. Djalilian M, McDonald TJ, Devine KD, Weiland LH: Ann Otol Rhinol Laryngol 84:757, Nov '75

1008. Localized amyloidosis in the larynx or other organs may be associated with
A. fibrosarcoma
B. adenocarcinoma
C. sqaumous cell carcinoma
D. multiple myeloma
E. solitary myeloma
REF. Djalilian M, McDonald TJ, Devine KD, Weiland LH: Ann Otol Rhinol Laryngol 84:757, Nov '75

1009. Subglottic stenosis of the larynx due to sarcoidosis is most effectively treated with:
A. streptomycin
B. thyrotomy and excision
C. thyrotomy with excision and skin grafting
D. direction suspension laryngoscopy with stripping of the involved subglottic area
E. injection of cortisone acetate into the involved subglottic area
REF. Djalilian M, McDonald TJ, Devine KD, Weiland LH: Ann Otol Rhinol Laryngol 84:757, Nov '75

1010. The chief presenting symptoms of a cleft larynx limited to the cricoid lamina are:
A. severe choking with solid feedings
B. cyanosis with thickened feedings
C. inspiratory stridor
D. choking with liquids in the neonate
E. airway obstruction and severe pneumonias in the neonate
REF. Cohen SR: Ann Otol Rhinol Laryngol 84:757, Nov '75

1011. A definitive diagnosis of cleft larynx with or without laryngotracheosophageal septal cleft can only be diagnosed by:
A. cine-esophagram by swallowing
B. A by injection of an opaque substance through an indwelling catheter
C. routine x-rays of the larynx
D. tomograms
E. endoscopic examination
REF. Cohen SR: Ann Otol Rhinol Laryngol 84:757, Nov '75

1012. A cleft larynx with limited cricoid lamina defect is treated:
A. medically
B. surgically
C. by gastrostomy feedings
D. by tracheotomy
E. by D only when oral secretions are aspirated into the tracheobronchial tree
REF. Cohen SR: Ann Otol Rhinol Laryngol 84:757, Nov '75

1013. An extensive laryngotracheoesophageal cleft requires:
A. medical treatment
B. surgical repair through a lateral pharyngotomy approach
C. B may require a thoracic approach
D. tracheotomy in most instances
E. D never necessary
REF. Cohen SR: Ann Otol Rhinol Laryngol 84:757, Nov '75

1014. The problem of aspiration in posterior cleft larynx is due to:
A. lateral displacement of the arytenoids
B. posterior displacement of the arytenoids
C. A plus B
D. absence or deficiency of the interarytenoid muscle
E. unopposed posticus muscle
REF. Cohen SR: Ann Otol Rhinol Laryngol 84:757, Nov '75

1015. Aspiration problems in the neonate may be caused by:
A. cricopharyngeus, spasm of
B. patulous cricopharyngeal sphincter
C. nonsphincteric spasm of the esophagus
D. cardiospasm
E. strictures
REF. Cohen SR: Ann Otol Rhinol Laryngol 84:747, Nov '75

1016. Aspiration problems in the neonate may be associated with:
A. central nervous system lesions due to prematurity, abnormal development, hypoxia, birth trauma
B. anatomic defects of the nose, nasopharynx, larynx, esophagus, trachea
C. laryngeal paralysis
D. diseases of the esophagus
E. myasthenia gravis
F. amyotonia congenita
G. autonomic dysfunction of Riley-Day
REF. Cohen SR: Ann Otol Rhinol Laryngol 84:747, Nov '75

1017. The muscles of the larynx depend for their differentiation on the development and growth of the cartilages. The first muscle to develop into a recognizable form and which arises from the sixth arch at the 9 mm stage is:
A. interarytenoid
B. cricoarytenoid
C. posticus
D. thyroarytenoid
E. cricothyroid
REF. Cohen SR: Ann Otol Rhinol Laryngol 84:747, Nov '75

1018. The ability of ionizing radiation to produce malignant neoplasms is a well-established phenomenon in all of the following sites but is rare in the:
A. skin
B. thyroid gland
C. blood
D. bone
E. lung
F. mucosa
REF. Lawson W, Som M: Ann Otol Rhinol Laryngol 84:771, Nov '75

1019. Which of the following malignant tumors of the larynx, hypopharynx, or esophagus occur following radiation to the neck for benign conditions?
A. squamous cell carcinoma
B. adenocarcinoma
C. lymphosarcoma
D. reticulum cell sarcoma
E. fibrosarcoma
REF. Lawson W, Som M: Ann Otol Rhinol Laryngol 84:771, Nov '75

1020. The oncogenetic effect of ionizing radiation has been shown by the ability of radiation to transform which of the following into malignant tumors?
A. juvenile laryngeal papillomatosis
B. goitre
C. thyrotoxicosis
D. tuberculosis cervical adenitis
E. skin
REF. Lawson W, Som M: Ann Otol Rhinol Laryngol 84:771, Nov '75

1021. The latent period of radiation-induced neoplasms is generally regarded to be in years:
A. 1-5
B. 6-10
C. 11-14
D. 15-30
E. over 30
REF. Lawson W, Som M: Ann Otol Rhinol Laryngol 84:771, Nov '75

1022. Which of the following facts appear true in the development of radiation-induced carcinomas of the larynx and laryngopharynx following therapeutic irradiation of the larynx for malignant disease?
A. cancer occurring in the postcricoid area in males, an uncommon site of primary or multicentric malignancies in this sex but within the zone of radiation
B. in A, delayed recurrence of the initial tumor after a five year disease-free interval with squamous cell carcinoma T_1 lesions does not seem logical
C. a causal relationship has been established
D. supervoltage therapy appears to enhance the radiobiologic effect of ionizing radiation when directed to laryngeal mucosa over orthovoltage therapy by lowering the latent period for the development of laryngeal or hypopharyngeal cancer from 12 to 15 years to seven years
E. radiation should probably be withheld in individuals under 50 years of age
REF. Lawson W, Som M: Ann Otol Rhinol Larngol 84:771, Nov '75

1023. Following tracheostomy, sites of tracheal stenosis occur at the site of the stoma or tracheal incision and areas of the tracheostomy cuff and tip. In preservation of the tracheal lumen and healing of the stoma, the best functional advantage occurs with the incision that is:

A. vertical
B. inverted U flap
C. oval
D. transverse
E. inverted V

REF. Lulenski GC, Batsakis JG: Ann Otol Rhinol Laryngol 84:781, Nov '75

1024. An immunosurveillance system for early evidence that a malignancy is present might be useful as a screening method for cancer and increase the accuracy of post-therapeutic detection of residual cancer. To date, immunology in carcinoma indicates:

A. humoral antitumor antibodies demonstrable in cancer patients
B. A cellular-fixed
C. tumor specific antigens (TSA) present on the cell membranes of cancer cells which are different from antigens present on normal cells and isolated from a variety of tumors in man and animals
D. lymphocytes from patients with various types of cancer destroy not only their own cancer but also cells from cancers of the same histologic type found in other patients (cross-reactivity)
E. lymphocytes from epidermoid carcinoma of the head and neck patients destroy cells in culture from carcinoma of the larynx whereas non-sensitized lymphocytes from control patients do not

REF. Krause CJ, Nysather J, McCabe BF: Ann Otol Rhinol Laryngol 84:787, Nov '75

1025. Antibody response to tumor antigens is extremely complex but which of the following appear to be facts:

A. response of the host T-lymphocyte system appears to be of paramount significance in tumor destruction
B. sensitized lymphocytes which destroy specific tumor cells remain in the peripheral circulation for about 24 months after tumor removal and then disappear unless a recurrence of the tumor develops
C. humoral antibodies against tumor antigens are associated with B-lymphocytes
D. high antibody titers directed against the Epstein-Barr virus have been found in patients with nasopharyngeal carcinoma as well as with some other head and neck carcinomas
E. elevated Epstein-Barr antibody titers fall rapidly to normal in patients who are free of tumor after treatment

REF. Krause CJ, Nysather J, McCabe BF: Ann Otol Rhinol Laryngol 84:787, Nov '75

1026. Antibodies in cancer patients:

A. are associated with B-lymphocytes
B. show high antibody titers directed against the Epstein-Barr virus and are found in patients with nasopharyngeal carcinoma as well as some other head and neck carcinomas
C. elevated antibody titers show a rapid decline to normal in those patients free of tumor after treatment
D. demonstrate elevated antibody titers against herpes simplex virus non-virion antigens in patients with head and neck cancer
E. is at present poorly understood in the rejection of tumors
F. antigen-antibody complexes may actually impair or block the action of sensitized lymphocytes against the tumor cells

REF. Krause CJ, Nysather J, McCabe BF: Ann Otol Rhinol Laryngol 84:787, Nov '75

1027. In the treatment of pyriform sinus cancer, which of the following criteria should be considered?
A. preoperative irradiation appears to have no destructive action on the laryngeal framework
B. the thyroid lobe on the involved side may be invaded and should be removed even if the cancer has not eroded through the thyroid cartilage
C. preoperative irradiation disqualifies a pyriform sinus cancer for conservation surgery
D. small growths on the medial wall of the pyriform sinus do not appear to respond well to irradiation
E. surface presentation rarely reflects the exact extent of invasion even before irradiation
F. conservation surgery must not be done when there is involvement of the apex of the pyriform sinus or of the thyroid cartilage
REF. Kirchner JA: Ann Otol Rhinol Laryngol 84:793, Nov '75

1028. In recurrent cancer after radiation therapy failure:
A. delay in diagnosis is common
B. salvage surgery is often required
C. radiation failure T_1 and T_2 laryngeal lesions can be treated by partial laryngectomy with voice preservation
D. C must be treated by total laryngectomy
E. supraglottic cancer is more apt to develop metastases than glottic cancer
REF. Skolnik EM, Martin L, Yee KF, Wheatley MA: Ann Otol Rhinol Laryngol 84:804, Nov '75

1029. In the treatment of cancer of the larynx, most otolaryngologists and radiotherapists agree that:
A. the first opportunity is the best opportunity for cure
B. the microscopic characteristics of a tumor from a biopsy specimen offer no prediction as to the response of the tumor to radiotherapy
C. T_3 and T_4 lesions are best treated by surgery initially and not by radiotherapy for cure
D. the initial treatment is radiation therapy for cure in the majority of T_1N_0 glottic patients
E. elderly patients seem to do better with surgery as a primary therapy for laryngeal cancer
REF. Skolnik EM, Martin L, Yee KF, Wheatley MA: Ann Otol Rhinol Laryngol 84:804, Nov '75

1030. The effects of radiation therapy may mask early recurrence and make diagnosis both difficult and delayed. All of the following are post-radiation complications but the most common factor responsible for the delay in diagnosis of recurrence is:
A. protracted laryngeal edema
B. perichondritis
C. cartilage necrosis
E. changes in irradiated skin
REF. Skolnik EM, Martin L, Yee KF, Wheatley MA: Ann Otol Rhinol Laryngol 84:804, Nov '75

1031. When recurrence or persistence of cancer is suspected, the diagnosis is confirmed by:
A. repeated biopsies at six to eight week intervals
B. deep biopsies since tumor cell nests may be present in the submucosal tissue
C. multiple biopsies because the recurrence may be present in tiny nests of cells
D. C contraindicated when evaluation for possible conservation surgery because the tumor margin may become indistinct
E. microlaryngoscopy, at times, with supravital staining with Toluidine blue under general anesthesia and thyrotomy
REF. Skolnik EM, Martin L, Yee KF, Wheatley MA: Ann Otol Rhinol Laryngol 84:804, Nov '75

1032. After the classical radical neck dissection with excision of the sterncleidomastoid muscle and division of the spinal accessory nerve supplying the trapezius muscle, there is weakness and deformity and often pain in the shoulder. Participating muscles which compensate for loss of the trapezius are the:
A. deltoid
B. latissimus dorsi
C. levator scapulae
D. serratus anterior
E. rhomboids
REF. Saunders WH, Johnson EW: Ann Otol Rhinol Laryngol 84:812, Nov '75

1033. The major antagonist of the trapezius muscle may be considered to be the:
A. deltoid
B. latissimus dorsi
C. levator scapulae
D. serratus anterior
E. rhomboids
REF. Saunders WH, Johnson EW: Ann Otol Rhinol Laryngol 84:812, Nov '75

1034. Which of the following procedures has been advocated for preservation of the trapezius muscle function during a radical neck dissection?
A. direct suturing of the cut ends of the spinal accessory nerve
B. grafting between the cut ends of the spinal accessory nerve using the greater auricular nerve
C. modification of the neck dissection in which both the sternocleidomastoid muscle and nerve supply (spinal accessory) are spared
D. removal of only the fascial compartments around muscles, vessels and nerves (Bocca)
E. radical neck dissection with trapezius paralysis but minimization of the associated problems by a set of exercises
REF. Saunders WH, Johnson EW: Ann Otol Rhinol Laryngol 84:812, Nov '75

1035. Pain following radical neck dissection with removal of the sternocleidomastoid muscle and division of the spinal accessory nerve with trapezius paralysis is caused by:
A. stretching of the rhomboideus minor
B. stretching of the rhomboideus major
C. stretching of the levator scapulae
D. pull of the serratus anterior
E. periarthritis of the scapulohumeral joint
F. osteoarthritis of the sternoclavicular joint on the paralyzed side
REF. Saunders WH, Johnson EW: Ann Otol Rhinol Laryngol 84:812, Nov '75

1036. There is controversy regarding the dose of irradiation which significantly impairs wound healing and increases the incidence of pharyngocutaneous fistulas complicating head and neck cancer surgery. It is generally agreed that pharyngeal dehiscence is most likely to occur with rads of:
A. 1000
B. 2000
C. 3000
D. 4500-8000
REF. Dedo DD, Alonso WA, Ogura JH: Ann Otol Rhinol Laryngol 84:833, Nov '75

1037. The common factors which predispose the majority of patients to pharyngocutaneous fistulas complicating head and neck cancer surgery are:
A. type of cancer
B. size of the lesion
C. dosage of irradiation
D. presence of systemic disease
E. failure of prior treatment modalities (surgery or irradiation)
REF. Dedo DD, Alonso WA, Ogura JH: Ann Otol Rhinol Laryngol 84:833, Nov '75

1038. To prevent pharyngocutaneous fistulas complicating head and neck cancer surgery in high risk patients and patients with abnormal wound healing (e.g., cellulitis, edema, fluid accumulation), decannulation, peroral feeding and high dose IV antibiotics are continued for the following number of weeks:

A. 1
B. 2
C. 3
D. 4
E. 5

REF. Dedo DD, Alonso WA, Ogura JH: Ann Otol Rhinol Laryngol 84:833, Nov '75

1039. Pharyngocutaneous fistulas complicating head and neck cancer surgery occur most often:

A. through carcinoma
B. adjacent to the tracheostoma
C. after radiation and surgical failures
D. in cancer involving the lateral and posterior pharyngeal walls
E. in patients with serious systemic disease
F. in patients having conservation laryngeal surgery
G. after total laryngectomies

REF. Dedo DD, Alonso WA, Ogura JH: Ann Otol Rhinol Laryngol 84:833, Nov '75

1040. Which of the following diseases produce severe obstructive conditions in the trachea, bronchi, and alveoli leading to respiratory difficulty?

A. alveolar proteinosis
B. pneumonia
C. asthma
D. bronchiectasis
E. cystic fibrosis

REF. Passy V, Ermshar C, Brothers M: Arch Otolaryngol 102:193, Apr '76

1041. Therapy for obstructive pulmonary lung diseases ranges from medical therapy to inhalation therapy to direct bronchoscopy and irrigation but the most effective method appears to be:

A. expectorants
B. liquifiers
C. coughing
D. postural drainage
E. bronchoscopy with washings
F. massive bronchopulmonary lavage

REF. Passy V, Ermshar C, Brothers M: Arch Otolaryngol 102:193, Apr '76

1042. The spread of cancer in the larynx depends on many concurrent factors among which are:

A. microscopic structure of the tumor and its type of growth
B. specific anatomical features of the larynx
C. site of the primary lesion
D. well differentiated exophytic cancers are obstructed to growth by the thyroid cartilage
E. anaplastic carcinomas infiltrate and destroy cartilages

REF. Olszewski E: Arch Otolaryngol 102:200, Apr '76

1043. Laryngeal cartilages are damaged by cancer in:

A. ossified sites
B. nonossified cartilages
C. vascularized sites
D. avascular cartilages
E. a vascular system in the presence of a tumor angiogenic factor (TAF) which plays an important role in the complex process of the spread of cancer in the larynx and its passage beyond the limits of the organ

REF. Olszewski E: Arch Otolaryngol 102:200, Apr '76

1044. Reconstruction after mandibulectomy for cancer presents a major problem in head and neck surgery and this applies in particular when the continuity of the anterior arch is lost. Procedure of choice for reconstruction appears to be:
A. immediate bone grafting
B. metallic implants
C. synthetic implants
D. stainless steel wire mesh and a fourfold stainless steel wire
E. planned staged reconstruction with (1) maintenance of preoperative occlusion relationship at time of resection with vitallium splints or monobloc acrylic appliances, (2) bone grafting of the mandible three months after resection, and (3) formation of lower buccal and lingual sulcus by skin inlay grafts about six months after the first procedure
REF. Snow GB, Kruisbrink JJ, Slooten EA Van: Arch Otolaryngol 102:207, Apr '76

1045. A lethal freeze can reach the inner perichondrium (full thickness of the vocal cord) in about two minutes after the probe tip (45-sq mm surface area) reaches -196 C. Which of the following factors determine tissue depth and degree of freeze?
A. vascular supply to the target including the size of nearby vessels
B. compression of the target tissue under the probe
C. duration of contact
D. repetition of the freeze in the same location, usually two freeze-thaw cycles
E. slow freeze and rapid thaw gives the best cryolesion
F. E rapid freeze and slow thaw
REF. Mulvaney TJ, Miller D: Arch Otolaryngol 102:226, Apr '76

1046. Problems observed in using peroral endolaryngeal crysurgery are:
A. difficulty in creating a large cryolesion safely without obstructing the laryngeal view of the target
B. immediate severe bleeding
C. slough of the necrotic cord leaving a deep ulcer with severe hemorrhage
D. slough of necrotic thyroid cartilage
E. edema
F. tracheostomy
REF. Mulvaney TJ, Miller D: Arch Otolaryngol 102:226, Apr '76

1047. Pachyonchia congenita (Jadassohn-Lewandowsky syndrome) is a genetic syndrome of epithelial dysplasia inherited as an autosomal dominant trait and consists of:
A. painful fissuring at the angles of the mouth
B. dysphonia with thickening of the posterior commissure of the larynx
C. lesions of the oral cavity, similar to the white sponge nevus, that show tendency to develop malignant changes
D. C no malignant changes
E. multiple epithelial cysts of the face, neck, and upper part of the trunk
F. abnormally coarse hair
G. hyperhidrosis and painful hyperkeratosis and blistering of the soles
REF. Cohn AM, McFarlane JR, Knox J: Arch Otolaryngol 102:233, Apr '76

1048. The microscopic appearance of laryngeal lesions in Pachyonychia Congenita (Jadassohn-Lewandowsky syndrome) consists of:
A. thickening of the epithelium with acanthosis and parakeratosis
B. intracellular vacuolization extending throughout the epithelium
C. a vascular stroma
D. a mild inflammatory infiltrate consisting mostly of mature lymphocytes in the subjacent connective tissue
E. tendency to T_1 or T_2 squamous cell carcinoma
REF. Cohn AM, McFarlane JR, Knox J: Arch Otolaryngol 102:233, Apr '76

1049. Which of the following measures have produced permanent solutions to the morbidity of Pachyonchia Congenita (Jadassohn-Lewandowsky syndrome)?
A. vitamin A (high doses)
B. vitamin E (high doses)
C. x-ray therapy
D. salicylic acid plasters
E. nail removal
F. excision and skin graft
G. at times some of these
H. none of these
REF. Cohn AM, McFarlane JR, Knox J: Arch Otolaryngol 102:233, Apr '76

1050. Most endoscopists are aware of the difficulties in removing large, hard, spherical foreign bodies from the esophagus but this can be accomplished best by:
A. urologic balloon catheters with low risk
B. A without general anesthesia
C. A without endoscopy
D. direct esophagoscopy with special Jackson forceps
E. esophagoscopy with the use of a Dormia basket
REF. Schiratski H: Arch Otolaryngol 102:238, Apr '76

1051. Closed tracheal rings occupying the entire length of the trachea are:
A. rare
B. usually the cause of death by respiratory infections in early infancy
C. difficult to diagnose during life
D. diagnosed by radiographic and endoscopic examinations
E. associated with intermittent respiratory obstruction
REF. Greene DA: Arch Otolaryngol 102:241, Apr '76

1052. The differential diagnosis in complete (closed) tracheal rings occupying the entire length of the trachea consists of:
A. laryngomalacia
B. tracheoesophageal fistula
C. tracheal webs
D. tracheomalacia
E. foreign bodies
F. extrinsic tracheal compression syndromes (such as vascular rings)
G. various infectious processes
REF. Greene DA: Arch Otolaryngol 102:241, Apr '76

1053. Malignant melanoma of the head and neck in children are:
A. congenital
B. prepubertal associated with metastases
C. those developing in a nevus pigmentosus giganticus
D. relatively benign
E. not different biologically in any substantial way from their adult counterpart
REF. Shanon E, Samuel Y, Adler A, Rapoport Y, Redianu C: Arch Otolaryngol 1012:244, Apr '76

1054. Treatment of malignant melanoma of the head and neck in children consists of:
A. early surgical extirpation with or without neck dissection as indicated
B. preoperative irradiation
C. postoperative irradiation
D. radiotherapy for cure
E. immunotherapy as a possible therapeutic adjunct
REF. Shanon E, Samuel Y, Adler A, Rapoport Y, Redianu C: Arch Otolaryngol 102:244, Apr '76

1055. Which of the following should be considered in the immunological therapy of malignant melanoma of the head and neck in children?
A. determination of delayed hypersensitivity skin reaction to 2 and 5 international units of purified protein derivative of tuberculin (PPD)
B. immunization to dinitrochlorobenzene (DNCB) after sensitization by 1000 μg applied to the skin
C. tumor tissue-specific immunization
D. nonspecific adjuvant immunotherapy with BCG vaccine in sites selected to coincide with possible eventual further sites of tumor extension to stimulate the underlying lymph nodes to adequate immunological interaction with occult tumor deposits (skin of the neck, supraclavicular, infraclavicular, scapular areas) using multiple inoculi of percutaneous BCG vaccine with the multipuncture apparatus (given three weeks later and again at nine months)
E. BCG vaccine in single punctures every six weeks
REF. Shanon E, Samuel Y, Adler A, Rapoport Y, Redianu C: Arch Otolaryngol 102:244, Apr '76

1056. Immunotherapy in malignant melanoma of the head and neck in children can be monitored by:
A. skin reaction to PPD (purified protein derivative of tuberculin)
B. skin reaction to DNCB (dinitrochlorobenzene)
C. absolute lymphocyte number per cubic millimeter of peripheral blood
D. lymphocyte stimulation by PHA (phytohemagglutinin)
E. D to PPD (purified protein derivative of tuberculin)
F. percent of E-rosette-forming cells
REF. Shanon E, Samuel Y, Adler A, Rapoport Y, Redianu C: Arch Otolaryngol 102:244, Apr '76

1057. Cysticercosis infestation from the consumption of viable cysticeri in uncooked pork is manifested by:
A. local soft, nontender mass in the tongue, buccal mucosa, neck and brain
B. x-ray visible calcifications in the soft tissues and muscles
C. biopsy of cysts
D. alterations of the sella turcica indicative of intracranial hypertension
E. complement fixation test on the cerebrospinal fluid
REF. Kinnman J, Chi CH, Park JH: Arch Otolaryngol 102:144, Mar '76

1058. The treatment for cysticercosis in otolaryngology is:
A. surgical removal in some cases
B. preventive, including the thorough cooking of pork
C. quinacrine hydrochloride
D. extract of aspidium
E. no specific treatment
REF. Kinnman J, Chi CH, Park JH: Arch Otolaryngol 102:144, Mar '76

1059. Laryngeal injury may be recognized by:
A. subtle changes in the quality of voice
B. expiratory noise
C. inspiratory noise
D. palpation revealing a displaced fracture of the thyroid cartilage or loss of cricoid prominence
E. subcutaneous crepitation
F. air passing through an open wound
G. compromise of airway
REF. Cohn AM, Larson DL: Arch Otolaryngol 102:166, Mar '76

1060. The diagnosis of laryngeal injury is made by:
A. conventional anteroposterior and lateral roentgenograms
B. xerograms
C. polytomography
D. esophagram using a water soluble solution
E. indirect laryngoscopy
F. direct laryngoscopy
REF. Cohn AM, Larson DL: Arch Otolaryngol 102:166, Mar '76

1061. Blunt trauma to the larynx more often than penetrating wounds results in subsequent formation of granulation tissue and stenosis which appears to be best prevented or treated by:
A. meticulous primary closure of mucosal lacerations
B. open reduction of cartilaginous fractures
C. use of soft stents with a tissue graft when mucosal loss cannot be approximated
D. depot steroids
E. low doses of irradiation
F. endoscopic removal
REF. Cohn AM, Larson DL: Arch Otolaryngol 102:166, Mar '76

1062. Extensive subglottic stenosis due to laryngeal injury has been successfully managed by:
A. dilation
B. excision of the connective tissue
C. tissue grafting around a stent
D. sleeve resection with utilization of skin-lined tubes, various alloplastic materials and advancement of neck flaps
E. end-to-end anastomosis with or without laryngeal release
REF. Cohn AM, Larson DL: Arch Otolaryngol 102:166, Mar '76

1063. Laryngeal injury with stenosis limited to the anterior segment of the circoid ring has been treated successfully with:
A. dilation
B. excision of the connective tissue
C. tissue grafting around a stent
D. excision of the cricoid ring with end-to-end anastomosis with or without laryngeal release
E. transposition of the midhyoid as a graft
REF. Cohn AM, Larson DL: Arch Otolaryngol 102:166, Mar '76

1064. Laryngeal injury with severe glottic stenosis has been treated successfully by:
A. dilation
B. excision of the connective tissue
C. lysis of the glottic web with insertion of a keel
D. laryngo-fissure with free tissue graft
E. D with advancement flap
F. Ogura's rehabilitation of the displaced vocal cord
REF. Cohn AM, Larson DL: Arch Otolaryngol 102:166, Mar '76

1065. Laryngeal injury with neural involvement with resultant vocal cord paralysis is frustrating and is usually approached by:
A. immediate neurorrhaphy
B. transposition of a nerve-muscle unit during the acute repair
C. anastomosis of vagal or recurrent nerve fibers or both
D. arytenoidectomy
E. intracordal implantation of polytetrafluoroethylene in an abducted paralyzed cord
REF. Cohn AM, Larson DL: Arch Otolaryngol 102:166, Mar '76

1066. Laryngeal injury with supraglottic stenosis has responded well to:
A. excision of the connective tissue
B. tissue graft around a stent
C. dilation
D. laryngo-fissure with free tissue graft
E. horizontal supraglottic laryngectomy
REF. Cohn AM, Larson DL: Arch Otolaryngol 102:166, Mar '76

1067. Laryngeal injury with comminuted fractures of the cricoid is treated by:
A. suturing of the multiple pieces of devitalized cartilage and overyling tissues
B. discarding the pieces of devitalized cartilage and suturing the overyling soft tissues
C. transposition of the midhyoid as a graft
D. resection and primary thyrotracheal anastomosis
E. resection with utilization of a skin-lined tube
REF. Cohn AM, Larson DL: Arch Otolaryngol 102:166, Mar '76

1068. In laryngeal injuries, the proper choice of tissue to use as grafting material in free grafts or tissue grafts around stents is debatable but which one of the following tissues being readily available, resistant to infection and contracts only slightly appears to be most appropriate?
A. split-thickness skin
B. sinus mucosa
C. buccal mucosa
D. full thickness skin
E. dermis (corium)
REF. Cohn AM, Larson DL: Arch Otolaryngol 102:166, Mar '76

1069. Granular cell myoblastomas:
A. are relatively uncommon tumors of unknown origin
B. are prevalent in the larynx and bronchus in the respiratory tract but may be found in any organ or site but are most common in the head and neck area
C. may occur with dyspnea, pain and dysphonia
D. tend to occur in the posterior third of the true cord
E. are featured by the presence of numerous eosinophilic granules in the cytoplasm of the myoblastomas but an overlying layer of pseudoepitheliomatous hyperplasia may dangerously resemble squamous cell carcinoma
REF. Canalis RF, Dodson TA, Turkell SB, Maenza RM: Arch Otolaryngol 102:176, Mar '76

1070. Intermittent short lasting attacks of glottic closure are not uncommon in:
A. pseudomyotonia
B. myotonia
C. tabes dorsalis
D. hysterical dysphonia
E. multiple sclerosis
REF. Levinson S, Canalis, RF, Kaplan HJ: Arch Otolaryngol 102:185, Mar '76

1071. Pseudomyotonia is a syndrome characterized by:
A. progressive muscle stiffness, weakness, myokymia, hyperhydrosis, and wasting of muscle
B. being more common in young men
C. EMG showing a state of constant rapid dysrhythmic discharge of independent muscle fibers present at rest and increased by initial muscle activity
D. C by electrical activity ceasing with the onset of relaxation
E. glottic spasm as a direct result of the continuous firing of the adductor muscles of the larynx
REF. Levinson S, Canalis RF, Kaplan HJ: Arch Otolaryngol 102:185, Mar '76

1072. Laryngeal spasm complicating pseudomyotonia can usually be controlled with therapeutic doses of:

A. phenytoin sodium
B. atropine sulfate
C. quinine
D. cortisone
E. trihexyphenidyl hydrochloride
F. adenosine triphosphate
G. triamine diphosphate
H. diazepam
I. procainamide hydrochloride
J. carbamazepine

REF. Levinson S, Canalis RF, Kaplan HJ: Arch Otolaryngol 102:185, Mar '76

1073. The identification and destruction of tumor cells is associated with:

A. the cellular immune system
B. bone-marrow-derived precursor cells which function as immuno-competent thymus-dependent lymphocytes (T-cells or T-lymphocytes) programed by the thymus
C. T-lymphocytes responsible for cell-mediated reactions such as graft rejection, defense against intracellular organisms and identification and destruction of tumor cells
D. circulating T-lymphocytes which are statistically lower in patients with advanced or recurrent squamous cell carcinoma
E. circulating lymphocytes which are not diminished in localized or nodal squamous cell carcinoma

REF. Eastham III RJ, Mason JM, Jennings BR, Belew PW, Maguda TA: Arch Otolaryngol 102:171, Mar '76

1074. The humoral immunological system:

A. is responsible for the identification and destruction of tumor cells
B. mediates the production of antibodies against foreign antigens
C. interacts with the cellular immune system and with other cells of the reticuloendothelial system under normal antigenic stimulation
D. is responsible for graft rejection and identification and destruction of tumor cells
E. consists of bursa-equivalent lymphocytes in contradistinction to T-lymphocytes

REF. Eastham III RJ, Mason JM, Jennings BR, Belew PW, Maguda TA: Arch Otolaryngol 102:171, Mar '76

1075. Depressed cell-mediated immunity in head and neck neoplasms has been demonstrated by:

A. delayed hypersensitivity reactions to common skin antigens
B. A to de novo antigens such as DNCB (dinitrochlorobenzene)
C. impairment of blastogenic transformation of lymphocytes with phytohemagglutinin
D. a depressed T-cell rosette response which measures the total peripheral circulating T-lymphocytes
E. substantial depression of the circulating T-lymphocytes in patients with advanced or recurrent squamous cell carcinoma

REF. Eastham III RJ, Mason JM, Jennings BR, Belew PW, Maguda TA: Arch Otolaryngol 102:171, Mar '76

1076. Thymus-dependent T-lymphocytes:

A. are responsible for the identification and destruction of tumor cells
B. are separated from but interact with the humoral antibody system and the reticuloendothelial system under normal antigenic stimulation
C. are responsible for graft rejection
D. defend against intracellular organisms
E. are substantially depressed in patients with advanced squamous cell carcinoma
F. are depressed in patients with localized or nodal squamous cell cancer

REF. Eastham III RJ, Mason JM, Jennings BR, Belew PW, Maguda TA: Arch Otolaryngol 102:171, Mar '76

1077. Thymus-dependent T-lymphocytes usually:
A. concentrate in the interfollicular areas within lymph nodes
B. infiltrate heavily around localized skin carcinomas in patients with normal T-cell waves
C. infiltrate very slightly around very aggressive skin cancers
D. are enhanced by BCG vaccine
E. are dramatically increased in the circulation by treatment with cryosurgery
REF. Eastham III RJ, Mason JM, Jennings BR, Belew PW, Maguda TA: Arch Otolaryngol 102:170, Mar '76

1078. The effects of drugs on thymus-dependent T-lymphocyte counts indicate:
A. no decrease of the T-cell count following treatment by methotrexate
B. no decrease with high dose of methotrexate followed by leucovorin
C. improvement with BCG vaccine
D. improvement with cryosurgery
E. improvement with BCG vaccine despite treatment of the patient with known immunosuppressive effects of radiation and chemotherapy
REF. Eastham III RJ, Mason JM, Jennings BR, Belew PW, Maguda TA: Arch Otolaryngol 102:171, Mar '76

1079. Patients with which of the following lesions may be selected for laryngeal reconstructive surgery?
A. endolaryngeal lesions of the true cords
B. A of the false cords
C. A of the ventricle
D. infiltration of the laryngeal cartilage
E. vestibular-epiglottic carcinoma not permitting an amplified horizontal supraglottic procedure
REF. Vega MF: The Laryngoscope 85:866, May '76

1080. Contraindications to laryngeal reconstructive surgery are:
A. patients with lymph nodes N-2 and N-3
B. infiltration of the laryngeal cartilage
C. lesion in the prelaryngeal muscles
D. invasion of the thyroid gland
E. extension of thyroid cancer to the larynx
F. exteriorization of tumor to the skin
G. invasion of cancer to the hypopharynx, valleculas or base of tongue
H. extension of cancer to the hyoid bone
REF. Vega MF: The Laryngoscope 85:866, May '75

1081. Mycosis fungoides is a disorder of the reticulo-endothelial system occurring in an eczematous or psoriatic stage, progressing to an infiltrated plaque stage and finally to a tumorous stage (d'emblee type). Mycosis fungoides features are:
A. involvement of the skin
B. culmination into a malignant lymphoma-reticulum cell sarcoma, lymphosarcoma or Hodgkin's disease
C. presence of mycosis cells which are large mononuclear cells with clear cytoplasm having a single "infolded cerebriform" nucleus which ultrastructurally have features of reticulum cells
D. the formation of Pautrier's microabscesses involving the epidermis which are regarded as pathognomonic
E. possible occurrence of facial nerve palsy
F. E with medial bulging of the tonsil
G. possible extension into the superior mediastinum causing pressure on the trachea and esophagus
H. that it never terminates fatally in the tumorous stage
REF. Gupta IM, Gupta OP, Samant HC, Bhatia PL, Ankaiah S: The Laryngoscope 85:898, May '75

1082. Leiomyosarcoma of the head and neck:
A. is a malignant tumor of smooth muscle origin mainly (in the head and neck region) in blood vessel walls and the erector pili musculature of the skin
B. is usually not circumscribed but irregular and soft
C. tend to be larger than leiomyomas and most likely malignant if over 2.5 cm in size
D. is most effectively treated by wide surgical resection for both primary and recurrent tumors
E. requires a unilateral or bilateral radical neck dissection for adequate control
REF. Mindell RS, Calcaterra, TC, Ward PH: The Laryngoscope 85:904, May '75

1083. Surgical speech rehabilitation in the laryngectomized patient:
A. has the disadvantage of multiple stage procedure of relatively considerable extent in the Asai operation
B. has the disadvantage of saliva and foods passing into the respiratory tract in the Asai and other procedures
C. A and B can be controlled partly by placing the pharyngostomy at the lingual base in the Asai operation
D. has the disadvatage that the patient must acquire some motor skill to block the cricostomy without a simultaneous occlusion of the vocal cord
E, has been limited mainly to the supracricoid laryngectomy with preservation of structures of the posterior part of vestibulum laryngis
F. can be effected at times by an arytenoid vocal shunt in patients with supracricoid laryngectomy with preservation of one or two arytenoids or the interarytenoid fold alone but the anterior phyaryngeal wall must lie in the plane of the arytenoids or somewhat posteriorly
REF. Mozolewski ES, Zietek E, Wysocki R, Jach K, Jassem W: The Laryngoscope 85:853, May '75

1084. The cricopharyngeus muscle:
A. is part of the inferior constrictor muscle
B. can be classified as in independent sphincter
C. arises bilaterally from the lateral arches of the cricoid and runs transversely around the posterior wall of the esophagus
D. possesses a median raphe like the inferior pharyngeal constrictor
E. inferiorly, blends with the transverse and circular fibers of the cervical esophagus
REF. Calcaterra TC, Kadell BM, Ward PH: Arch Otolaryngol 101:726, Dec '75

1085. The most effective chemotherapeutic agent available to treat malignant melanoma with a 20-30 percent response rate is:
A. Daunorubicin-adriamycin
B. Nitrosoureas
C. Streptozotocin
D. Dimethyltriazeno imidazole carboxamide (DTIC)
E. Adriamycin + cyclophosphamide
REF. Bertino JR: The Laryngoscope 85:491, Mar '75

1086. The innervation of the cricopharyngeus muscle is:
A. believed to be supplied by the vagopharyngeal plexus
B. by the recurrent nerves that innervate the cervical esophagus
C. affected only when the vagus nerve is sectioned above the ganglion nodosum
D. by sympathetic nerve impulses which contract the cricopharyngeus muscle
E. by parasympathetic nerve impulses which result in relaxation
REF. Calcaterra TC, Kadell BM, Ward PH: Arch Otolaryngol 101:726, Dec '75

1087. Which of the following conditions produces cricopharyngeal achalasia with dysphagia?
A. myasthenia gravis
B. thyrotoxicosis
C. muscular dystrophy
D. bulbar polio
E. stroke
F. Parkinson disease
G. basilar arterial thrombosis with brain stem damage usually involving the nucleus ambiguus
H. partial pharyngectomy
I. supraglottic laryngectomy
J. high unilateral vagal injuries
K. Zenker diverticulum
L. idiopathic, usually in the elderly
REF. Calcaterra TC, Kadell, BM, Ward PH: Arch Otolaryngol 101:726, Dec '75

1088. The treatment of choice in intractable dysphagia secondary to cricopharyngel muscle dysfunction or achalasia is:
A. gastrostomy
B. skeletal muscle relaxants such as chlorzoxazone
C. ataractics with relief of skeletal muscle spasm such as diazepam
D. prolonged nasogastric tube feeding
E. cricopharyngeal myotomy
REF. Calcaterra TC, Kadell BM, Ward PH: Arch Otolaryngol 101:726, Dec '75

1089. Chylous fistula following radical neck dissection is an unusual and serious complication resulting from accidental sectioning of the thoracic duct on the left or right lymphatic duct. A chylous fistula leak:
A. should be stopped during surgery by ligation of the injured lymphatic duct
B. shows no sequelae when the thoracic duct or right lymphatic duct is ligated
C. is always accompanied by sequelae handled medically
D. may result in chylothorax with symptoms of sudden onset of dyspnea followed by respiratory embarrassment, shock, and death
E. will rapidly deplete the body stores of fluid, proteins and electrolytes with shock and death
REF. Myers EN, Dinerman WS: The Laryngoscope 85:835, May '75

FIGURE FOR SECTION IV

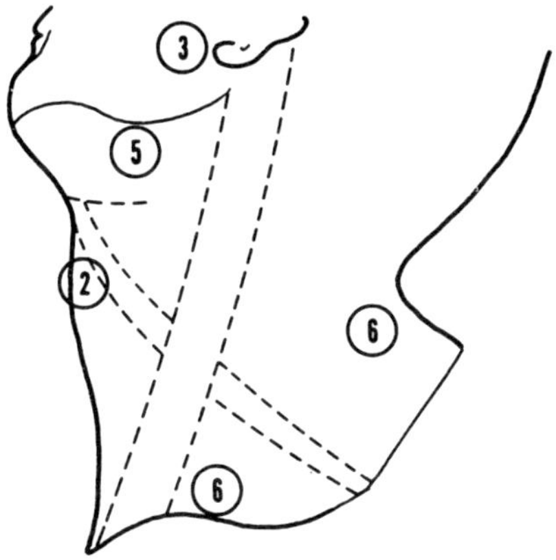

Fig. 23. Tuberculous cervical adenitis. Location of cervical tuberculous lymphadenitis. Number of cases located in parotid, submandibular, anterior cervical, posterum cervical, and supraclavicular areas. The incidence of cases has increased during the past three years. Below is the incidence by year:

1962	2	1968	2
1963	1	1969	1
1964	1	1970	3
1965	1	1971	4
1966	1	1972	3
1967	3		

(Courtesy of Ord, R.J., Matz, G.J.: Arch Otolaryng, 99:327, May '74)

1090. Which of the following is a contraindication to the external approach to rhinoplasty?
A. congenital deformities of the nose
B. major nasal septal deformities
C. large hump nose with cartilaginous deformities
D. major augmentation procedures accompanied by cartilaginous deformities
E. transverse columellar incision through severe scarring
REF. Goodman WS: Canadian J Otolaryngol, 2:3, 207,'73

1091. Which of the following is the only contraindication for not performing the external approach to rhinoplasty?
A. bifid tip correction difficulty
B. excessive subcutaneous scar tissue development
C. re-operation necessary with major deformity
D. reluctance to make a transverse incision through the columella and inexperience of the surgeon in this technique
E. inability to excise large dermoid cysts
REF. Goodman WS: Canadian J Otolaryngol, 2:3, 207,'73

1092. The septum and lower lateral cartilages assume their definite shape and proportions at the age of:
A. six months
B. five years
C. puberty
D. eighteen years
E. twenty-one years
REF. Briant TDR, Paradisgarten A, Jansen V: Canadian J Otolaryngol, 2:3, 217,'73

1093. The lower lateral cartilages develop from the cartilaginous nasal capsule and are well advanced as cartilaginous structures by the following month of embryonic life:
A. one
B. two
C. three
D. four
E. six
REF. Briant TDR, Paradisgarten A, Jansen V: Canadian J Otolaryngol, 2:3, 217,'73

1094. Ossification centers appear in the embryo which form the bony fragment of the nose at the month of:
A. one
B. two
C. three
D. four
E. six
REF. Briant TDR, Paradisgarten A, Jansen V: Canadian J Otolaryngol, 2:3, 217,'73

1095. The projection of the nasal tip where the basal width exceeds the height may be increased by:
A. Weir type procedure
B. Goldman procedure
C. Lippsett procedure
D. basal implants
E. interposed baton or button at the nasal tip
REF. Briant TDR, Paradisgarten A, Jansen V: Canadian J Otolaryngol, 2:3, 217,'73

1096. The projection of the nasal tip may be decreased by shortening the medial crura by:
A. Weir type procedure
B. Goldman procedure
C. Lippsett procedure
D. narrowing of cleft tip
E. separation upper lateral cartilages from the septum
REF. Briant TDR, Paradisgarten A, Jansen V: Canadian J Otolaryngol, 2:3, 217,'73

1097. A procedure which has fallen into disfavor because of tendency to slip or extrude in nasal tip surgery to increase projection is:
A. Weir type procedure
B. Goldman procedure
C. Lippsett procedure
D. basal implants
E. buttons in the nasal tip
REF. Briant TDR, Paradisgarten A, Jansen V: Canadian J Otolaryngol, 2:3, 217,'73

1098. The aging mechanism is obviously unknown. Of the following possible etiological factors which one shows definite histological signs of aging in the skin?
A. hormonal withdrawal
B. heat
C. sunlight
D. excessive massage
E. catabolic disease states
REF. Ellis DAF: Canadian J Otolaryngol, 2:3, 231,'73

1099. Which one of the following groups age at a lesser rate?
A. negroes
B. Irish
C. Scotch
D. Swedish
E. Danish
REF. Ellis DAF: Canadian J Otolaryngol, 2:3, 231,'73

IN THE FOLLOWING QUESTION MATCH EACH LETTERED ITEM WITH ONE NUMBERED ITEM. EACH CHOICE MAY BE USED ONLY ONCE.

1100. Surgical techniques and their indications in the aging face are:
A. chemical skin peeling
B. dermabrasion
C. rhytidectomy (face lift)
D. brow lift
E. blepharoplasty
F. shortening the nose

1. acne pitted face
2. sagging brow
3. youthful appearance
4. fine circumoral wrinkling
5. baggy eyelids and narrow palpebral fissure
6. jowl and submental sagging

REF. Ellis DAF: Canadian J Otolaryngol, 2:3, 231,'73

1101. Although mentoplasty is considered a safe and simple operation, which of the following complications do occur?
A. hematoma
B. infection
C. shift of the prosthesis
D. early or late rejection of the foreign body
E. bone resorption
REF. Newton RA: Canadian J Otolaryngol, 2:3, 235,'73

IN THE FOLLOWING QUESTIONS, MATCH EACH LETTERED ITEM WITH ONE NUMBERED ITEM. EACH CHOICE MAY BE USED MORE THAN ONCE.

1102. The patient with an underdeveloped chin may have:
A. micrognathia
B. microgenia

1. entire mandible is underdeveloped
2. angle class 2 malocclusion
3. pronounced overjet of maxillary teeth
4. lower first molar posterior to the maxillary first molar
5. cephalometric x-ray examination shows the SNP (Sellae-Nasion-Pogonion) angle significantly less than the 80 degrees considered normal
6. normal occlusion but chin alone is underdeveloped either absolutely or relatively to the prominence of the nose

REF. Newton RA: Canadian J Otolaryngol, 2:3, 235,'73

IN THE FOLLOWING QUESTION MATCH EACH LETTERED ITEM WITH ONE NUMBERED ITEM. EACH CHOICE MAY BE USED ONLY ONCE.

1103. The treatment of an underdeveloped chin is:
A. mandibular advancement or maxillary recession
B. augmentation mentoplasty

1. microgenia
2. micrognathia

REF. Newton RA: Canadian J Otolaryngol, 2:3, 235,'73

1104. In augmentation mentoplasty which one of the following autogenous and homogenous tissues or alloplastic material appears to be a safe, curable and inert substance?
A. silicone
B. cartilage
C. fat
D. dermal fat (buttock)
E. bone

REF. Newton RA: Canadian J Otolaryngol, 2:3, 235,'73

1105. The port wine stain or naevus flammeus is a localized or extensive, dull red, non-raised, non-palpable foci consisting histologically of dilatation and increased numbers of capillaries in the subdermal, dermal and subepidermal layers of the skin. The most effective treatment is:
A. carbon dioxide snow
B. dermabrasion
C. electrolysis
D. surgical tattooing
E. boiling water injection

REF. Newton RA: Canadian J Otolaryngol, 2:3, 251,'73

IN THE FOLLOWING QUESTION MATCH EACH LETTERED ITEM WITH ONE NUMBERED ITEM. EACH CHOICE MAY BE USED MORE THAN ONCE.

1106. The pigment used in surgical tattooing for port wine stain is:
A. titanium oxide
B. iron oxide
C. mercuric sulfide
D. cobalt blue
E. hydrated chrome oxide

1. green
2. black
3. blue
4. red
5. yellow
6. white

REF. Newton RA: Canadian J Otolaryngol, 2:3, 251,'73

1107. In maxillofacial injuries which one of the following fractures is most common?
A. zygoma
B. nose
C. maxilla
D. orbit
E. frontal

REF. Forget G, Belanger C: Canadian J Otolaryngol, 2:3, 254,'73

1108. The facial nerve anastomoses in the human (and throughout the order of mammals) with many nerves in the face but the strongest and most constant of all is between the facial and which one of the following nerves?
A. supraorbital
B. infraorbital
C. cervical cutaneous
D. glossopharyngeal
E. auriculotemporal

REF. Baumel JJ: Arch Otolaryngol, 99:34, Jan'74

1109. Partial paralysis of facial muscles due to disturbances of muscle sense can occur after destruction of:
A. trigeminal nerve
B. cervical plexus
C. auriculotemporal nerve
D. glossopharyngeal nerve
E. complete destruction of facial nerve

REF. Baumel JJ: Arch Otolaryngol, 99:34, Jan'74

1110. The greatest number of sensory nerve endings occur in which of the following muscles?
A. frontalis
B. orbicularis oculi
C. muscles of lips and angle of mouth
D. masseter
E. platysma
REF. Baumel JJ: Arch Otolaryngol, 99:34, Jan'74

1111. An unexpected result of direct electrical stimulation of the trigeminal root or ganglion in man and cat is:
A. contracture of facial musculature
B. numbness of the face
C. pain in the face
D. tingling sensation in the face
E. no sensation
REF. Baumel JJ: Arch Otolaryngol, 99:34, Jan'74

1112. Those investigators who consider the facial nerve as the sole motor supply of the facial muscles believe facial paralysis results during surgery of the trigeminal ganglion from:
A. elevation of the dura creating tension on the underlying greater petrosal branch of the facial
B. tension on the geniculate ganglion causing actual trauma
C. tension on the geniculate ganglion with secondary inflammation
D. trauma to motor fibers of the facial nerve in the facial canal
REF. Baumel JJ: Arch Otolaryngol, 99:34, Jan'74

1113. Facial nerve anastomoses (under favorable conditions: clean cut, matching of fasciculi, minimal scarring) regeneration in regard to substantial return of function is best described as:
A. excellent with 100 percent recovery
B. superior 80-90 percent recovery
C. moderate 50 percent recovery
D. around 25 percent recovery
E. usually disappointing
REF. Baumel JJ: Arch Otolaryngol, 99:34, Jan'74

1114. In surgery on the bony nasal vault which of the following anatomic facts pertinent to cosmetic rhinoplasty must be observed?
A. in performing a controlled curved lateral osteotomy, it is quite futile to carry a lateral osteotomy close to the frontal bone since the nasal bones cannot physically be compressed at this level and narrowing at this level is not really desirable
B. in attempting to narrow the nose after hump removal, bends in the ethmoidal plate of the septum may interfere with medial approximation of the lateral bony components after lateral osteotomy
C. the curved lateral osteotomy cuts through the frontal process of the maxilla starting at a level corresponding to the infraorbital rim but ascends forward and upward to the nasion
D. a routine medial osteotomy is always done
E. as the curved lateral osteotome is driven up towards the nasion, the long axis of the osteotome is twisted medially so as to push the bony wall inward and create an oblique fracture 2 to 3 mm short of the midline
REF. Bernstein L: Arch Otolaryngol, 99:67, Jan'74. (See Fig. 24)

1115. The following description of the anatomy of the lateral cartilages is accurate except for:
A. two lateral or upper lateral cartilages together with the quadrilateral cartilage of the septum form a single uninterrupted unit being enclosed in a common perichondrial sheath
B. upper borders of lateral cartilages always articulate over the nasal bones to a greater or lesser extent
C. lateral crura of the tip cartilages overlap the caudal edges of the lateral cartilages

D. inferiorly, the caudal edge of the lateral cartilage tends to recurve sharply outward and upward, forming a scroll
E. laterally, the lateral cartilage is short of the pyriform edge of the maxilla
REF. Bernstein L: Arch Otolaryngol, 99:67, Jan'74

1116. The following description of the anatomy of the tip cartilages is accurate except for:
A. each lower lateral, or tip, cartilage is usually made up of a single piece of cartilage consisting of a medial and a lateral crus
B. medial crus lies immediately under the very thin skin of the columella
C. lateral crus is usually rounded along its upper part
D. cephalic edge of the lateral crus overlaps the caudal part of the lateral cartilage
E. scrolls of the lateral and tip cartilages abut each other and curve in the same direction. Thus, the lateral crus can pivot and slide up and down along its scroll
REF. Bernstein L: Arch Otolaryngol, 99:67, Jan'74

1117. The following description of the anatomy of the columella is accurate except for:
A. columella consists of two medial crura without any intervening tissue
B. two medial crura are covered by extremely thin skin with very little underlying subcutaneous tissue
C. anteriorly, the crura flare to a greater or lesser extent as they contribute the framework for the width of the tip
D. posteriorly, the free curved ends of the medial crura flare to accommodate the posterior part of the caudal edge of the quadrilateral cartilage of the septum
E. D and frequently also the anterior nasal spine
REF. Bernstein L: Arch Otolaryngol, 99:67, Jan'74

1118. The following description of the anatomy of the septum is accurate except for:
A. the rhinion is the bony-cartilaginous junction of the dorsum of the septum
B. dorsal component plays an important part in the shape of the cartilaginous profile above the lobule
C. caudal part has a direct bearing on the position of the columella
D. junction of the dorsal and caudal margins of the quadrilateral cartilage is referred to as the "anterior septal angle" and is a fairly sharp curve rather than an angle and is situated just above the level of the domes of the tip cartilages
E. bony septum plays a major role in cosmetic rhinoplasty but after surgery it never grows forward postoperatively even in hump removal at an early age
REF. Bernstein L: Arch Otolaryngol, 99:67, Jan'74

1119. The following description of the anatomy of the investing soft tissues of the nose is accurate except for:
A. the disparity between the external skin profile and that of the underlying bony-cartilaginous pyramid is usually greatest in noses with large dorsal humps
B. the nasofrontal region is filled quite markedly with the procerus muscle and its investing areolar tissue
C. the skin reaches its thickest dimension over the rhinion
D. the rhinion usually corresponds to the greatest prominence of the dorsal convexity of the nasal pyramid
E. from the rhinion to the intercrural space, the skin progressively becomes thin
REF. Bernstein L: Arch Otolaryngol, 99:67, Jan'74. (See Fig. 25)

1120. Patients with unilateral exophthalmos in addition to the usual x-rays of the sinuses and skull should have a careful head and neck examination supplemented by which of the following refined studies?
A. tomography
B. arteriography with subtraction
C. orbital venography
D. contrast orbitography
E. ultrasonography
REF. Calcaterra TC, Hepler RS, Hanafee WN: The Laryngoscope, 84:231, Feb'74

1121. Which of the following conditions may give a misleading appearance of unilateral exophthalmos?
A. tumors arising within the muscle cone
B. unilateral enophthalmos
C. lid retraction
D. unilateral myopia
E. weakness extraocular muscles
REF. Calcaterra TC, Hepler RS, Hanafee WN: The Laryngoscope, 84:231, Feb'74

1122. Pure axial displacement of unilateral exophthalmos is most likely due to which one of the following conditions?
A. tumors within the nuscle cone, such as optic nerve glioma
B. acute inflammation of the frontal sinuses
C. acute ethmoiditis
D. tumors of the lacrimal gland
E. tumors of the temporal fossa
REF. Calcaterra TC, Hepler RS, Hanafee WN: The Laryngoscope, 84:231, Feb'74

1123. Unilateral exophthalmos with the eye displaced downward and/or laterally usually arises from:
A. acute frontal sinusitis
B. acute ethmoiditis
C. chronic mucopyoceles of the frontal sinus
D. chronic mucopyoceles of the ethmoid sinuses
E. tumors of the lacrimal gland
REF. Calcaterra TC, Hepler RS, Hanafee WN: The Laryngoscope, 84:231, Feb'74

1124. Unilateral exophthalmos with the eye displace medially is usually due to:
A. tumors of the lacrimal gland
B. tumors of the maxillary sinus
C. acute frontal sinusitis
D. acute ethmoiditis
E. tumors of the temporal fossa
REF. Calcaterra TC, Hepler RS, Hanafee WN: The Laryngoscope, 84:231, Feb'74

1125. Unilateral exophthalmos with the eye pushed upward is most often due to:
A. tumors of the lacrimal gland
B. tumors of the maxillary sinus
C. acute ethmoiditis
D. acute frontal sinusitis
E. tumors of the temporal fossa
REF. Calcaterra TC, Hepler RS, Hanafee WN: The Laryngoscope, 84:231, Feb'74

1126. Absolute measurements of exophthalmos may be obtained with the Hertel exophthalmometer. Normal values range from 14 to 20 mm. Relative exophthalmos exist when a forward displacement of one globe is greater than the other in mm of:
A. 1
B. 2
C. 3
D. 4
E. 5
REF. Calcaterra TC, Hepler RS, Hanafee WN: The Laryngoscope, 84:231, Feb'74

1127. Unilateral exophthalmos pulsations without bruit of the globe indicate:
A. arterial-venous vascular malformations
B. endocrine exophthalmos
C. intracranial pulsations due to loss of bony partition between the frontal lobe and orbital contents
D. intracranial pulsations due to loss of bony partition between the temporal lobe and orbital contents
E. cystic lesion
REF. Calcaterra TC, Hepler RS, Hanafee WN: The Laryngoscope, 84:231, Feb'74

1128. In unilateral exophthalmos, bruits (auscultation) suggest:
A. arterio-venous vascular malformations
B. endocrine exophthalmos
C. intracranial pulsations due to loss of bony partition between the frontal lobe and orbital contents
D. intracranial pulsations due to loss of bony partition between the temporal lobe and orbital contents
E. cystic lesion
REF. Calcaterra TC, Hepler RS, Hanafee WN: The Laryngoscope, 84:231, Feb'74

1129. In unilateral exophthalmos, transillumination may reveal:
A. arterio-venous vascular malformations
B. endocrine exophthalmos
C. intracranial pulsations due to loss of bony partition between the frontal lobe and orbital contents
D. intracranial pulsations due to loss of bony partition between the temporal lobe and orbital contents
E. cystic lesion
REF. Calcaterra TC, Hepler RS, Hanafee WN: The Laryngoscope, 84:231, Feb'74

1130. In unilateral exophthalmos, lid retraction, lid lag on upward gaze, restriction on elevation of the globe, and injection of the blood vessels over the rectus muscles all implicate:
A. inflammatory lesion
B. orbital varix
C. arterio-venous vascular malformations
D. endocrine exophthalmos
E. cystic lesion
REF. Calcaterra TC, Hepler RS, Hanafee WN: The Laryngoscope, 84:231, Feb'74

1131. In unilateral exophthalmos, chemosis, cellulitis and fluctuance of the eyelid suggest:
A. inflammatory lesion
B. orbital varix
C. arterio-venous vascular malformations
D. endocrine exophthalmos
E. cystic lesion
REF. Calcaterra TC, Hepler RS, Hanafee WN: The Laryngoscope, 84:231, Feb'74

1132. Increasing unilateral exophthalmos with congestion of the conjunctival vessels occurring during coughing or valsalva maneuver may be seen with:
A. inflammatory lesions
B. orbital varix
C. arterio-venous vascular malformations
D. endocrine exophthalmos
E. cystic lesion
REF. Calcaterra TC, Hepler RS, Hanafee WN: The Laryngoscope, 84:231, Feb'74

1133. Although all of the following may occur, the earliest sign of corneal damage in exophthalmos is:
A. circumcorneal congestion
B. loss of normal corneal brightness
C. generalized ocular infection
D. corneal ulceration (demonstrated by fluorescein stain)
E. blindness
REF. Calcaterra TC, Hepler RS, Hanafee WN: The Laryngoscope,84:231, Feb'74

1134. In unilateral exophthalmos where the lesion is not well established on clinical grounds or localizable by radiographic studies, the treatment is:
A. surgical exploration by anterior orbitotomy
B. surgical exploration through an infraorbital rim or lower lid sub-ciliary incision
C. Caldwell-Luc incision
D. periodic re-examination rather than surgical exploration
E. trial of systemic corticosteroids to rule out a pseudotumor
REF. Calcaterra TC, Hepler RS, Hanafee WN: The Laryngoscope, 84:231, Feb'74

1135. In unilateral exophthalmos with lesions lying in the anterior and middle third of the orbit, the best surgical approach is:
A. anterior orbitotomy through the eyebrow and supraorbital periosteum
B. an infraorbital rim or lower lid sub-ciliary incision
C. Caldwell-Luc
D. Kronlein operation with removal of the lateral orbital bone
E. transfrontal craniotomy
REF. Calcaterra TC, Hepler RS, Hanafee WN: The Laryngoscope, 84:231, Feb'74

1136. In unilateral exophthalmos with lesions lying in the floor of the orbit, the best surgical procedures are:
A. anterior orbitotomy through the eyebrow and supraorbital periosteum
B. an infraorbital rim or lower lid sub-ciliary incision
C. Caldwell-Luc
D. Kronlein operation with removal of the lateral orbital bone
E. transfrontal craniotomy
REF. Calcaterra TC, Hepler RS, Hanafee WN: The Laryngoscope, 84:231, Feb'74

1137. In unilateral exophthalmos with lesions near the apex, either within the extraocular muscles or outside the muscle cone, the best surgical procedures are:
A. anterior orbitotomy through the eyebrow and supraorbital periosteum
B. an infraorbital rim or lower lid sub-ciliary incision
C. Caldwell-Luc
D. Kronlein operation with removal of the lateral orbital bone
E. transfrontal craniotomy
REF. Calcaterra TC, Hepler RS, Hanafee WN: The Laryngoscope, 84:231, Feb'74

1138. In unilateral exophthalmos with erosion of the optic foramen, superior orbital fissure, or foramen rotundum, the operative procedure of choice is:
A. anterior orbitotomy through the eyebrow and supraorbital periosteum
B. an infraorbital rim or lower lid sub-ciliary incision
C. Caldwell-Luc
D. Kronlein operation with removal of the lateral orbital bone
E. transfrontal craniotomy
REF. Calcaterra TC, Hepler RS, Hanafee WN: The Laryngoscope, 84:231, Feb'74

1139. Which of the following terms have been used to describe abnormally protruding ears?
A. lop
B. flop
C. butterfly
D. protruding
E. prominent
REF. Gay EC: The Laryngoscope, 84:468, Mar'74

1140. It is generally accepted that the abnormally protruding ear is due to:
A. increased angle between the concha and the mastoid process
B. excessive constriction of the superior auricular muscle
C. excessive constriction of the posterior auricular muscle
D. shortening of the posterior ligament (lig. auriculare posterius)
E. absence of a normal antihelix
REF. Gay EC: The Laryngoscope, 84:468, Mar'74

1141. Which of the following is the most important structure in providing support for the auricle?
A. posterior muscle (m. auricularis posterior)
B. superior muscle (m. auricularis superior)
C. posterior ligament (lig. auriculare posterius)
D. superior ligament (lig. auriculare superius)
E. anterior ligament (lig. auriculare anterius)
REF. Gay EC: The Laryngoscope, 84:468, Mar'74

IN THE FOLLOWING QUESTION MATCH EACH LETTERED ITEM WITH ONE NUMBERED ITEM. EACH CHOICE MAY BE USED ONLY ONCE.

1142. In the anatomy of the external ear, the ligaments and their attachments to the skull are:
A. posterior ligament (lig. auriculare posterius)
B. superior ligament (lig. auriculare superius)
C. anterior ligament (lig. auriculare anterius)

1. from spine of the helix to the bony external acoustic meatus on its superior margin
2. from the eminence of the concha to the mastoid process
3. from helix and tragus to the zygoma and completing the front of the external meatus

REF. Gay EC: The Laryngoscope, 84:468, Mar'74

1143. The arterial supply to the auricle consists of:
A. internal carotid
B. posterior auricular
C. vertebral
D. ascending pharyngeal
E. superficial temporal
REF. Gay EC: The Laryngoscope, 84:468, Mar'74

1144. Which of the following sensory nerves give off branches to the auricle?
A. greater auricular (C2 and 3)
B. small occipital (C2 and 3)
C. auriculotemporal (CN V)
D. vagus (nerve of Arnold) (CN X)
E. facial (CN VII)
REF. Gay EC: The Laryngoscope, 84:468, Mar'74

1145. The most common postoperative complication following otoplasty surgery is:
A. infection without perichondritis
B. hematoma
C. suture extrusion
D. skin incision separation
E. unsatisfactory cosmetic result
REF. Gay EC: The Laryngoscope, 84:468, Mar'74

1146. Serious complications of otoplasty surgery such as perichondritis and hematoma with cauliflowering of the pinna probably occur because:
A. elastic cartilage of the external ear is devoid of blood vessels
B. all nutrition to the cartilage must be supplied by the vessels in the perichondrium
C. perichondrium must not be separated from the cartilage to ensure life in the cartilage
D. inadequate suturing
E. secondary infection
REF. Gay EC: The Laryngoscope, 84:468, Mar'74

IN THE FOLLOWING QUESTION MATCH EACH LETTERED ITEM WITH ONE NUMBERED ITEM. EACH CHOICE MAY BE USED ONLY ONCE.

1147. In the external ear, the muscles and their attachments to the skull are:
A. posterior muscle (m. auriculares posterior)
B. superior muscle (m. auricularis superior)
C. anterior muscle (m. auricularis anterior)

1. origin upon tendon of the sternocleidomastoideus muscle and its insertion on the conchal eminence
2. origin on the galea aponeurotica and insertion on the eminentia fossae triangularis
3. origin from galea oponeurotica and insertion in the spine of the helix
REF. Gay EC: The Laryngoscope, 84:468, Mar'74

1148. Recidivism is defined as the incidence of return to prison or return to criminal behavior. The effects of plastic surgery on the recidivistic rate of inmates with facial disfigurements indicate which of the following to be realistic?
A. severe psychotics may be helped
B. an individual who attributes all of his problems to his physical deformity and uses it as a crutch on which to rest his sense of failure can throw away his crutch
C. "burned out" addict well motivated is helped
D. prisoner becomes grateful for an unusual favor and feels obligated to the surgeon and society
E. interpreted by prisoner as a completely disinterested social act by a representative of society and results in a relationship of communication and understanding
REF. Lewison E: Canadian J Otolaryngol, 3:1, 42,'74

1149. Following excisional surgery of a circular skin lesion on the face, the resultant defect can be treated successfully by:
A. elliptical excision with direct closure
B. local flap
C. distant flap
D. split-thickness skin graft
E. full thickness skin graft
REF. Cotton RT: Canadian J Otolaryngol, 3:1, 51, '74

1150. The use of the rhomboid flap following excisional surgery on the face has which of the following advantages?
A. geometrically simple to understand and design
B. safe from point of view of blood supply
C. may be used on irradiated skin
D. produces an irregular closure line with good cosmetic result
E. there is never any secondary defect which must be closed
REF. Cotton RT: Canadian J Otolaryngol, 3:1, 51, '74

1151. The main types of external ear deformities which encompasses almost all the abnormalities encountered in clinical practice are:
A. microtia
B. lop ear
C. cup ear
D. protruding ear
E. total absence
REF. Mallen RW: Canadian J Otolaryngol, 3:1, 74, '74. (See Fig. 26)

1152. Microtia has which of the following features?
A. malformed and underdeveloped
B. arrest of ear development at the sixth to eighth week
C. associated with other abnormalities in the development of first branchial arch
D. associated with other abnormalities in the development of the first and second branchial arches
E. occurs frequently in Treacher-Collins syndrome
REF. Mallen RW: Canadian J Otolaryngol, 3:1, 74, '74.

1153. The lop ear has which of the following features?
A. characteristic severe downward folding of the upper pole of the ear
B. deficient rigidity of the helix
C. deficient rigidity of scapha
D. cartilage does not lack resiliency
E. usually associated with a deficient antihelix
REF. Mallen RW: Canadian J Otolaryngol, 3:1, 74, '74

1154. The cup ear has which of the following features?
A. excessively deep and concave concha
B. shortened helix
C. lobule never cupped forward
D. usually the ear is smaller than normal
E. cartilage is much thicker and more resilient, making surgical correction difficult to maintain
REF. Mallen RW: Canadian J Otolaryngol, 3:1, 74, '74

1155. The protruding ear has which of the following features?
A. does not resemble the normal ear in shape
B. unfurling of the body of the antihelix and/or the superior crus
C. excessive conchal cartilage
D. excess size or protrusion of the lobule
E. inadequate folding of the helical rim producing the "shell" ear
REF. Mallen RW: Canadian J Otolaryngol, 3:1, 74, '74

1156. The most rapid growth period of the human face occurs during which of the following week period of embryonic life?
A. 1 - 2
B. 3 - 4
C. 4 - 8
D. 8 - 12
E. 12 - 16
REF. Mallen RW: Canadian J Otolaryngol, 3:1, 74, '74

1157. The primitive external ear does not appear until the end of which of the following weeks?
A. 1
B. 2
C. 3
D. 4
E. 5
REF. Mallen RW: Canadian J Otolaryngol, 3:1, 74, '74

1158. The primitive external ear is represented by the appearance of six hillocks, three mandibular and three hyoid around the first branchial cleft. These hillocks fuse and the antihelix develops at about which week?
A. 1
B. 2
C. 3
D. 6
E. 8
REF. Mallen RW: Canadian J Otolaryngol, 3:1, 74, '74

1159. In the fully developed ear which of the following anatomical parts are of mandibular origin?
A. superior crus
B. anterior crus of helical margin
C. concha
D. scapha
E. tragus
REF. Mallen RW: Canadian J Otolaryngol, 3:1, 74, '74

1160. In the fully developed ear which of the following anatomical parts are derived from the hyoid arch?
A. superior crus
B. anterior crus of helical margin
C. concha
D. scapha
E. tragus
REF. Mallen RW: Canadian J Otolaryngol, 3:1, 74, '74

1161. The adult normal ear has which of the following characteristics?
A. the lobule is on a lower plane than the scapha
B. adult size ear measures 6 cm in height
C. adult size ear is reached by the sixth to seventh year
D. cephaloconchal angle should be less than 45 degrees
E. the conchoscaphal angle dependent on the antihelix should approximate 90 degrees
REF. Mallen RW: Canadian J Otolaryngol, 3:1, 74, '74

1162. Many surgical procedures have been devised for the correction of protruberant ears, the most important aim being to:
A. diminish size of ear
B. "pin" the ear back against the mastoid
C. increase protrusion of lower portions of the ear
D. eliminate the post-auricular sulcus
E. produce a smoothly rounded antihelix and superior crus
REF. Mallen RW: Canadian J Otolaryngol, 3:1, 74, '74

1163. There is a high incidence of poor results following otoplasty including most commonly:
A. upper pole of ear continues to protrude due to failure to develop a superior crus
B. helix is hidden due to excess prominence of the antihelix
C. ear protrudes at top and bottom "telephone ear" due to excessive conchal reduction or skin removal
D. protruberant lobule due to failure to surgically correct the cauda helicis
E. antihelix is much too sharp due to inappropriate incision of cartilage along the line of the antihelix
REF. Mallen RW: Canadian J Otolaryngol, 3:1, 74, '74

1164. To avoid pitfalls in correcting protruding ears the surgeon must attempt to accomplish which of the following?
A. correction of the protrusion of the upper one-third of the ear without protrusion of the lower portions
B. antihelix and superior crus must be smoothly rounded and curved forward in a continuous C-shaped fashion
C. helix must be visible in front at least down to the middle third and preferably all the way
D. post-auricular sulcus need not be maintained
E. both ears must be a symmetrical distance from the head making surgery on both ears almost mandatory
REF. Mallen RW: Canadian J Otolaryngol, 3:1, 74, '74

1165. Pseudocysts of the auricle appear to have which of the following features?
A. rare
B. etiology unknown
C. no epithelial lining to the cyst wall
D. similar to subperichondrial effusions or hematomas where fluid or blood collects between the perichondrium and cartilage
E. best treatment appears to be incision and drainage with application of 1% iodine into the cyst cavity and the application of contour pressure dressings for six days
REF. Santos VB, Polisar IA, Ruffy ML: Ann Otol, 83:9, Jan-Feb'74

1166. The most common site in frontal sinus fractures is:
A. anterior wall
B. posterior wall
C. medial wall
D. inferior wall
E. nasofrontal duct
REF. Newman MH, Travis LW: The Laryngoscope, 83:1281, Aug'73

1167. The three most common sites in frontal sinus fractures are:
A. anterior wall
B. posterior wall
C. medial wall
D. inferior wall
E. nasofrontal duct
REF. Newman MH, Travis LW: The Laryngoscope, 83:1281, Aug'73

1168. In frontal sinus fractures cerebrospinal fluid rhinorrhea suggests dural tears through which of the following walls?
A. anterior
B. medial
C. floor
D. lateral
E. posterior
REF. Newman MH, Travis LW: The Laryngoscope, 83:1281, Aug'73

1169. In a frontal sinus fracture with severe injury to the nasofrontal duct, the preferred method of treatment appears to be:
A. removal intersinus septum
B. A plus reconstructing the damaged nasofrontal duct
C. thorough removal sinus mucous membrane
D. occlusion of the nasofrontal duct
E. obliteration of the sinus cavity (osteoplastic frontal sinusotomy) with fat obliteration - exception: involvement posterior table
REF. Newman MH, Travis LW: The Laryngoscope, 83:1281, Aug'73

1170. Nondisplaced fractures of the posterior table of the frontal sinus demonstrated by lateral laminagraphs are best treated by:
A. exploration, as soon as the patient's general condition permits
B. no exploration unless symptoms develop
C. exploration if there is a persistent cerebrospinal fluid leak after three-week period to allow for any spontaneous closure

D. C with antibiotic coverage
E. exploration if nasofrontal duct is damaged - development of sinus clouding by Caldwell frontal radiograph
REF. Newman MH, Travis LW: The Laryngoscope, 83:1281, Aug'73

1171. The most common pathologic condition affecting the frontal sinuses is:
A. mucocele
B. benign tumors such as osteoma
C. infectious diseases
D. Malignancies
E. trauma
REF. Newman MH, Travis LW: The Laryngoscope, 83:1281, Aug'73
Discussion: Dickinson J

1172. When facial nerve anastomoses is unsuccessful, it is usually due to which of the following causes?
A. Schwann tubules fail to align themselves properly across the anastomosis
B. secondary to poor stabilization of the nerve endings with tortion and movement preventing proper alignment
C. excessive ingrowth of granulation tissue between nerve endings
D. formation of fibroblasts between nerve endings
E. C and D resulting in a classic disorganized pattern of a neuroma
REF. Miglets AW, Thomas JR: The Laryngoscope, 83:1027, July'73

1173. Experimentally, the functional return of severed facial nerves appeared best under which of the following conditions?
A. careful neurolemmal anastomosis (nerve sheath)
B. neurorrhaphy protected by a section of vein (intimal surface next to the sheath) after neurorrhaphy
C. segment of vein slipped over proximal segment of cut nerve prior to neurorrhaphy, then after repair of the sheath, the vein is positioned over the anastomosis
D. Millipore filters placed around nerve anastomosis
E. silastic as a protection of nerve anastomosis
REF. Miglets AW, Thomas JR: The Laryngoscope, 83:1027, July'73

1174. In patients with short columellas, cleft lip deformities or with inadequate anterior septal support due to previous trauma or radical submucous resection can be most successfully treated with:
A. Bone implants
B. cartilage implants (bank)
C. septal cartilage
D. V-Y columellar advancement procedure
E. injectable teflon - polytef
REF. Goode RL, Ross J: The Laryngoscope, 83:1123, July'73

1175. Which of the following statements are true about malignant fibrous histiocytoma of the maxilla?
A. rare
B. mesenchymal soft tissue tumor usually composed of tissue histiocytes, fibroblasts, foam cells, and bizarre or multinucleated giant cells
C. at times difficult to classify as benign or malignant
D. mitotic figures by themselves are not reliable criteria for malignancy
E. irradiation does not appear to be effective
REF. Spector GJ, Ogura JH: Arch Otolaryngol, 99:385, May'74

1176. Some excellent uses of dermal grafts in head and neck operations include all of the following, except:
A. bone coverage inside the mouth
B. carotid artery coverage after radiotherapy or extensive head and neck surgery or both
C. to fill in facial contour defects (this includes dermal-fat grafts)
D. pharyngeal suture line coverage
E. replacement of mucous membrane in the mouth, pharynx and hypopharynx
F. soft tissue grafts to the nasal dorsum
G. myringoplasty
REF. Cairns JR, AB: Tr Am Acad Ophth Otol 80:ORL-510, Nov '75

1177. Using an electric dermatone, a strip of split thickness skin 0.03 cm (0.012 inch) is elevated and left attached at one end. With the cutting width narrowed slightly, a second pass with the dermatone is made over the same area removing a dermal graft that measures in cm in thickness:
A. 0.01-0.02
B. 0.03-0.05
C. 0.07-0.09
D. 0.10-0.15
E. 0.20-0.25
REF. Cairns JR, AB: Tr Am Acad Ophth Otol 80:ORL-510, Nov '75

1178. Muscle grafts used for carotid coverage are:
A. often only large enough to cover the carotid bulb
B. never long enough to cover both the carotid and the suture line
C. always adequate to cover both the carotid and the suture line
D. often destroyed when blood and nefve supply to the muscle are not transferred intact
E. unsatisfactory since the use of the levator scapula muscles make the already disabled shoulders worse (e.g., sacrifice of the spinal accessory nerves with subsequent trapezium muscle paralysis)
REF. Cairns JR, AB: Tr Am Acad Ophth Otol 80:ORL-510, Nov '75

1179. The advantages of dermal grafts are numerous and include:
A. early vascularization (three to five days)
B. derivation of its blood supply from both sides of the graft
C. capacity to survive in face of infection, dessication, and salivary leak
D. no postoperative absorption
E. being strong and pliable (can be layered if needed)
REF. Cairns JR, AB: Tr Am Acad Ophth Otol 80:ORL-510, Nov '75

1180. In secondary nasal revisions after rhinoplasties:
A. standard preoperative photographs are mandatory
B. palpation of the nose reveals better than simple inspection the condition of the nasal bones and cartilages
C. observation of the nose during quiet and forceful breathing shows the existence of nasal alar collapse
D. protrusion of upper lateral cartilages into the nasal vestibulum may be an important factor for the impairment of breathing after rhinoplasties
E. anterior nasal spine and caudal tip of the septum must be evaluated prior to any surgical intervention
F. septal cartilage and ear cartilage with adherent perichondrium are adequate for reconstruction
REF. Walter CD: Tr Am Acad Ophth Otol 80:ORL-519, Nov '75

1181. Chemexfoliation:
A. is contraindicated in patients with renal disease
B. A is not contraindicated
C. is contraindicated in patients with hepatic disease
D. C is not contraindicated
E. is more successful in fair-skined patients with fine to moderate skin wrinkling than those individuals with a dark complexion
REF. Ariagno RP, Briggs DR: Tr Am Acad Ophth Otol 80:ORL-536, Nov '75

1182. Complications of extensive undermining and redraping of the skin in rhinoplasty include:
A. increased edema
B. increased ecchymosis
C. furuncle formation
D. transient seborrheic type of dermatitis
E. skin necrosis
F. skin atrophy
REF. Feit LJ: Tr Am Acad Ophth Otol 80:ORL-540, Nov '75

1183. Defects usually associated with saddle nose deformity include:
A. lack of tip projection and support
B. retracted columella
C. bulbosity of the lobule
D. widened alar base
E. flattening and widening of the nasal bones
REF. Beekhuis GJ: Tr Am Acad Ophth Otol 80:ORL-596, Nov '75

1184. There are a variety of methods described to treat depressed, comminuted anterior frontal sinus wall fractures including all of the following but the procedures of choice appear to be:
A. no treatment unless there are signs of intracranial complications
B. exploration of all fractures since sophisticated radiographic techniques (necessary for legal purposes) do not accurately show the extent of injury
C. elevation of the anterior wall by stripping the sinus mucosa and filling the cavity with fat
D. wiring of the bony fragments to a stable portion of the skull
E. elevation of the bony fragments and utilizing a Foley catheter to splint the fragments and drain the sinus
REF. Oppenheimer RP: Tr Am Acad Ophth Otol 80:ORL-507, Nov '75

1185. Polyamide mesh as filler material in saddle nose deformity has given outstanding good results but which of the following complications have occurred:
A. postsurgical swelling
B. transient redness and swelling
C. overcorrection with slight convexity of the nasal dorsum or supratip fullness
D. accumulation of fluid
E. spontaneous extrusion
REF. Beekhuis GJ: Tr Am Acad Ophth Otol 80:ORL-596, Nov '75

1186. Osteogenic sarcoma of the mandible:
A. is a rare tumor
B. is the most common primary malignant tumor of the mandible
C. is most commonly located in the body of the mandible
D. appears initially as a mass increasing in size followed by pain, loose teeth and paresthesias
E. is best treated by wide local excision or disarticulation of the mandible on the involved side depending on the tumor site with free margins and curettings from the marrow space confirmed by frozen section
REF. Pease GL, Maisel RH, Cantrell RW: Arch Otolaryngol 101:761, Dec '75

1187. Desmoplastic fibroma of the mandible must be differentiated from:
A. fibrous dysplasia
B. chondromyxoid fibroma
C. non-ossifying fibroma
D. unicameral and aneurysmal bone cysts
E. metastatic carcinoma of thyroid origin
F. E of renal origin
G. musculo-aponeurotic fibromatosis
H. fibrosarcomas
REF. Badger GA, Syed AA, Malby FC: Can J Otolaryngol 3 (No. 4):605, '74

1188. The indications for the decortication operation in functional rhinosurgery are:
A. long hump nose
B. rhinokyphosis combined with pathology of the shape of the nasal septum especially its ventocaudal angle
C. deformities of the nasal pyramid
D. C combined with congenital abnormalities of the lip, upper jaw and palate
E. post-traumatic deformities of the nasal pyramid
REF. Padovan IF: CanJ Otolaryngol 4 (No. 3):522, No month '75

1189. Osteotomy and resection rather than composite resection is indicated in:
A. T_1 cancer of the tonsil region and tongue base
B. T_2 cancer of the tonsil region and tongue base
C. periosteum of mandible involved with cancer
D. poor-risk patients
E. glandular tumors
REF. De Santo LW, Whicker JH, Devine KD: Arch Otolaryngol 101:652, Nov '75

1190. The principal characteristics of the nevoid basal cell carcinoma syndrome are:
A. cysts (keratocysts) of the jaws
B. multiple, early-appearing, basal cell carcinomas of the skin
C. developmental anomalies of the skeleton
D. peculiar dyskeratotic pitting of the hands and feet
E. ectopic soft tissue calcifications
REF. McClatchey K, Batsakis JG, Hybels R, Wieren CR Van: Arch Otolaryngol 101:613, Oct '75

1191. Odontogenic keratocysts in patients with the nevoid basal cell carcinoma syndrome commonly appear:
A. multiple, bilateral and with continuous development resulting in persistence after incomplete enucleation
B. in the cuspid-to-first molar region
C. in the maxillary second molar region with extension into the maxillary sinus and symptoms of chronic sinusitis
D. microscopic to several centimeters in diameter
E. associated occasionally with ameloblastoma
REF. McClatchey K, Batsakis JG, Hybels R, Wieren CR Van: Arch Otolaryngol 101:613, Oct '75

1192. Nevoid basal cell carcinoma syndrome with odontogenic keratocysts should be suspected when:
A. multiple (may be thousands) of basal cell carcinomas occur often between the ages of seven and 14 years but below 30 years
B. the carcinomas are always pigmented
C. carcinomas have a predilection for the skin around the eyes, nose, mouth, and ears
D. recognizable osteoid tissue is present within the neoplasm
E. jaw cysts precede the cutaneous lesions by several or more years
REF. McClatchey K, Batsakis JG, Hybels R, Wieren CR Van: Arch Otolaryngol 101:613, Oct '75

1193. Silicone injections are most useful in which of the following facial defects?
A. vertical glabellar lines
B. horizontal forehead lines
C. "crow's feet"
D. small pits and holes, the so-called ice pick variety of acne scarring
E. small folds running down from the corners of the mouth
REF. Berger RA: Arch Otolaryngol 101:525, Sept '75

1194. Osteoradionecrosis of the mandible is a dreaded late complication of irradiation for cancer of the oral cavity and is characterized by:
A. pain
B. trismus
C. fistula and cicatrix formation
D. abnormal fractures
E. loss of soft and osseous tissue
REF. Mainous EG, Hart GB: Arch Otolaryngol 101:173, Mar '75

1195. Osteoradionecrosis of the mandible following irradiation for cancer of the oral cavity has been treated effectively by:
A. excision of the affected part of the mandible through an intraoral approach
B. external incision through irradiated skin with resection of the mandibular necrotic area
C. drilling holes from the irradiated necrotic bone into viable bone to allow growth of healing granulation tissue into the necrotic bone
D. hemimandibulectomy
E. use of hyperbaric oxygen
REF. Mainous EG, Hart GB: Arch Otolaryngol 101:173, Mar '75

1196. The forehead flap has been utilized in:
A. the management of gingival and buccal mucosal defects
B. internal cheek reconstruction because of viability, accessibility and nonhair bearing quality
C. rehabilitation of the tongue
D. rehabilitation of the palate
E. rehabilitation of the mouth
REF. Hamaker RC, Conley J: Arch Otolaryngol 101:189, Mar '75

1197. The forehead flap:
A. was staged initially when first used
B. does not have to be delayed because its vascularity is based on the superficial temporal artery
C. offers 100 to 120 cm of available surfacing area
D. must not include the posterior auricular artery
E. may be used when the external carotid arterial system has been ligated by basing the forehead flap laterally on the scalp with nourishment from the opposite external carotid artery
REF. Hamaker RC, Conley J: Arch Otolaryngol 101:189, Mar '75

1198. The adipose tissue graft is obtained from the abdominal wall or from the thigh together with the deep fascia which serves to give the graft special orientation and to obliterate defects or to fix the grafts to the weakest part of the wall. Free-fat tissue grafts are useful in otology in:
A. postauricular defects with adhesion of the skin to the bone with or without displacement of the auricle
B. postauricular fistulae after mastoidectomy
C. adhesions of skin or scar tissue to the sigmoid sinus
D. mastoid cavity defects at the time of surgery
E. after acoustic neurinoma removal by the transmastoid-labyrinthine approach in order to obliterate the dead space and as a treatment for subarachnoid postoperative fistulae
REF. Tato JM: Arch Otolaryngol 100:467, Dec '74

1199. Adipose tissue grafts are useful in sinus surgery in:
A. chronic frontal sinusitis or pyocele
B. frontal sinus trauma with displacement of the anterior wall
C. cerebrospinal rhinorrhea after trauma of the frontal and ethmoid sinuses
D. spontaneous cerebrospinal rhinorrhea
E. intracranial pneumocele following frontal sinus injury
REF. Tato JM: Arch Otolaryngol 100:467, Dec '74

1200. Adenoid cystic carcinoma is also known as:
A. squamous cell carcinoma
B. adenocarcinoma
C. mixed tumor
D. adenocystic carcinoma
E. cylindroma
REF. Horrée WA: Arch Otolaryngol 100:469, Dec '74

1201. The most common site of occurrence of adenoid cystic carcinoma which develops in the minor salivary glands is the:
A. hard palate
B. maxilla
C. oral cavity
D. upper respiratory tract
E. mandible
REF. Horrée WA: Arch Otolaryngol 100:469, Dec '74

1202. Which of the following two neoplasms occur most often in the maxilla naming them in their order of frequency?
A. squamous cell carcinoma
B. adenocarcinoma
C. fibrosarcoma
D. chrondrosarcoma
E. adenoid cystic carcinoma
REF. Horrée WA: Arch Otolaryngol 100:469, Dec '74

1203. Which of the following clinical or radiological signs indicate inoperability in cancer of the maxilla?
A. destruction of the bony posterior wall of the maxillary sinus
B. destruction of the upper part of the pterygopalatine process
C. invasion in the base of the skull
D. invasion in the posterior part of the ethmoid bone
E. invasion of the hard palate
REF. Horrée WA: Arch Otolaryngol 100:469, Dec '74

1204. Maxillary sinus sarcomas:
A. are less frequently encountered than carcinomas
B. A more frequently encountered
C. etiology remains obscure
D. etiology has been proven to be due to a virus
E. lymphosarcomas and reticulum cell sarcomas are treated by irradiation being very radiosensitive
F. are most often treated by preoperative radiotherapy followed by total maxillectomy and orbital exenteration
REF. Prasanna NM: Mendelsohn M: Can J Otolaryngol 4 (No. 4):704, No month '75

1205. Which of the following lesions must be considered in the differential diagnosis of parosteal osteogenic sarcoma of the mandible?
A. adenocarcinoma
B. myositis ossificans
C. osteochondroma
D. squamous cell carcinoma
E. intramedullary osteogenic sarcoma
REF. Solomon MP, Biernack J, Slippen M, Rosen Y: Arch Otolaryngol 101: 754, Dec '75

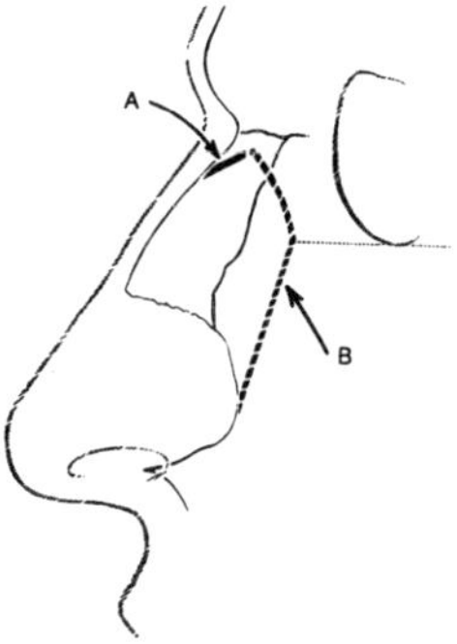

Fig. 24A. Controlled curved lateral osteotomy. Heavy broken line (B) has vertical and curved components. Horizontal dotted line indicates level at which curved part of osteotomy is begun. (A) oblique green-stick fracture near dorsum.

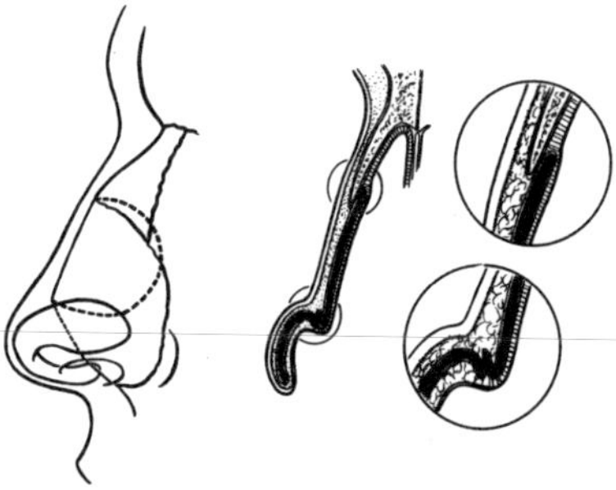

Fig. 24B. External nasal pyramid. Left, relationships of upper and lower cartilages to each other, to nasal bones, and to pyriform edge. Right, relationships demonstrated in coronal section. Insets show details of relationships.

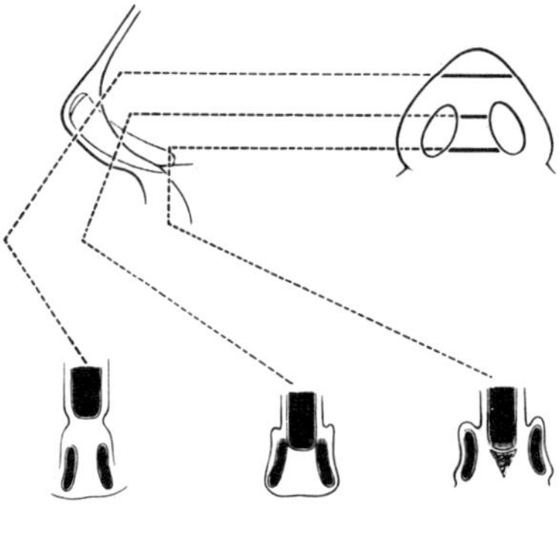

Fig. 24C Relationships between medial crura, membranous septum, and caudal edge of quadrilateral cartilage. (All figures courtesy of Bernstein, L.: Arch Otolaryng, 99:67, Jan'74)

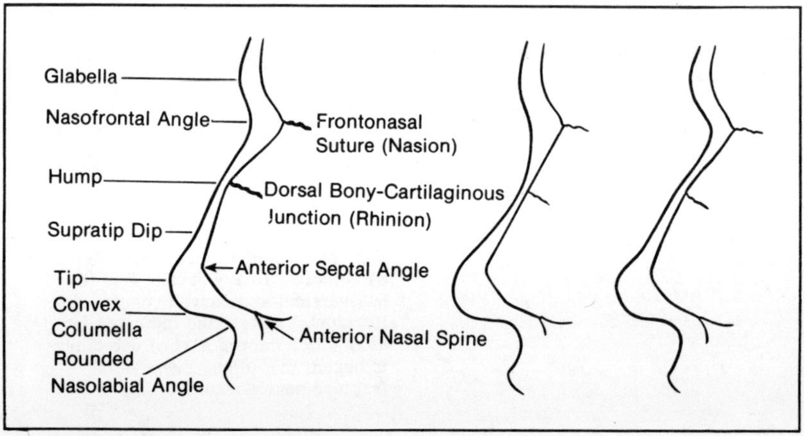

Fig. 25. Left, sagittal section showing corresponding thicknesses of soft tissues in respect to underlying skeletal outline. Center, predicted profile if skeletal dorsum is reduced to straight line. Profile reduction should be designed to accomodate uneven thickness of overlying soft tissues (right). (All figures courtesy of Bernstein, L.: Arch Otolaryngol, 99:67, Jan'74)

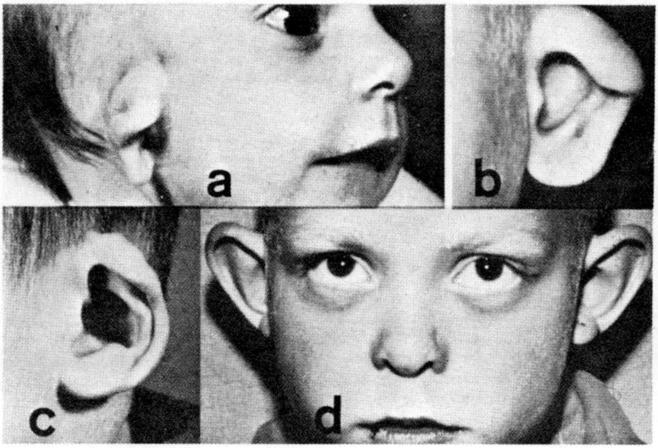

Fig. 26. Types of external ear deformity: a) lop ear; b) cup ear; c) lesser degree of cup ear; d) typical protruberant ear. (Courtesy of Mallen, R. W.: Canadian J Otolaryngol, 3:1, 74, '74)

1206. Local immunotherapy by nose drops or aerosol of aqueous pollen extracts of blue grass or western ragweed pollens induce significantly higher titers of nasal secretory specimen antibodies of:
A. IgA
B. IgD
C. IgE
D. IgG
E. IgM
REF. Tse KE: Allergy News Bulletin, III, No. 4:7, '74

1207. Parental immunotherapy by injection of aqueous pollen extracts of blue grass or western ragweed pollens induce significantly higher titers of serum blocking antibodies of:
A. IgA
B. IgD
C. IgE
D. IgG
E. IgM
REF. Tse KS: Allergy News Bulletin, III, No. 4:7, '74

1208. There appears to be no difference in the localization of which of the following immunoglobulins in nasal mucosal specimens of allergic and nonallergic individuals?
A. IgA
B. IgG
C. IgE
D. IgD
E. IgM
REF. Bass RM, Potter EV, Barney PL: Arch Otolaryngol, 99:446, June'74

1209. Reaginic antibodies comprise which one of the following distinct class of immunoglobulins?
A. IgA
B. IgM
C. IgD
D. IgE
E. IgG
REF. Bass RM, Potter EV, Barney PL: Arch Otolaryngol, 99:446, June'74

1210. Routine light microscopy observations of nasal polyps and of biopsy specimens of nasal mucosa from the middle or inferior turbinates demonstrate which of the following?
A. inflammatory cells are more numerous in the nasal polyps than in the nasal mucosa of allergic patients
B. nasal polyps vary markedly in their content of eosinophils
C. nasal polyps vary markedly in their content of plasma cells
D. relatively few eosinophils and plasma cells are observed in allergic nasal mucosa in most cases
E. no consistent difference is found in the number or distribution of eosinophils and plasma cells between individuals with and without allergic history
REF. Bass RM, Potter EV, Barney PL: Arch Otolaryngol, 99:446, June'74

1211. The origin of nasal polyps is a subject of controversy. Which of the following have been implicated in the pathogenesis of nasal polyps?
A. bacteria
B. viruses
C. allergy
D. hormonal imbalance
E. depolymerization of mucopolysaccharides
REF. Bass RM, Potter EV, Barney PL: Arch Otolaryngol, 99:446, June'74

1212. The specific role of immunoglobulins in the production of nasal polyps appears to be:
A. based on the production and localization of IgE
B. A but with IgG
C. A but with IgA
D. A but with IgM
E. no evidence of any specific role
REF. Bass RM, Potter EV, Barney PL: Arch Otolaryngol, 99:446, June'74

1213. The immunological function of the tonsil is a fundamental problem associated with the question of value or harmful effects of tonsillectomy. Which of the following facts appear true?
A. central lymphatic organs such as thymus or bursa fabricius are capable of recognizing antigen but do not produce antibodies
B. A but produces antibodies
C. IgM-antibody producing cells are found in palatine tonsils, spleens, lymph-nodes of all cases in both young and adult groups
D. ^{3}H - labeled thymocytes are found in tonsils
E. IgG antibody producing cells are not always found in tonsils and lymph nodes
REF. Suzuki M, Imai A, Kojima K, Kitami O: Jap Jour Otol, 76:1045, Jul-Dec'73

1214. Malignant granulomatous reticulosis has which of the following features?
A. nodular lesions with ulcers
B. electrophoresis of immunoglobulins (IgG, IgA, IgM) may show an increase
C. a complex of anticancer agents VEMP (vincristin, endoxan, 6-mercaptopurine, predonin) is curable
D. CO teletherapy may give temporary regression
E. antibiotics combined with steroids are curable
REF. Shigeka K, Kimura M, Nagai K: Jap Jour Otol, 76:1440, Jul-Dec'73

1215. In recent studies on nasal allergy, which of the following conclusions were made:
A. nasal provocative tests by placing house dust or mite and ragweed pollen extract discs on inferior turbinates might be worthy from a diagnostic point of view when it is compared with the skin test only
B. antigenic coincidence between house dust and mite (dermatophagoides farinae) extract was confirmed by means of skin tests, nasal provocation and P-K tests in patients with nasal allergy
C. hyposensitization therapy by mite extract is successful in treating patients allergic to house dust and mite
D. effects of hyposensitization can be determined by means of periodic skin tests and nasal provocation tests
E. effects of hyposensitization can be determined by means of P-K test and measurement of blocking antibody titer (bis-diazotized benzidine) hemagglutination test
REF. Shimada T, Ishikawa T, Miyashita H, Fujita Y: Jap Jour Otol, 76:1360, 1368, 1405, Jul-Dec'73

1216. The most sensitive in vitro technique for the demonstration of specific antibody is:
A. microimmunodiffusion
B. hemagglutination
C. complement-fixation
D. immunofluorescence
E. neutralization
REF. Kniker WT: Allergy News Bulletin (Ann Meeting AAIA), 2:10:6, '73

1217. Deficiency in surface immunity often is heralded by a relative increase in secretory:
A. IgM
B. IgG
C. IgA
D. IgD
E. IgE
REF. Kniker WT: Allergy News Bulletin, (Ann Meeting AAIA), 2:10:6, '73

1218. Phytohemagglutinin induces changes in sensitized lymphocytes similar to those induced by:
A. specific antibodies
B. transfer factor
C. migration inhibitory factor
D. antigen
E. corticosteroids
REF. Kniker WT: Allergy News Bulletin (Ann Meeting AAIA), 2:10:6, '73

1219. In agar double diffusion adjoining precipitate lines that cross each other signify that antigens are:
A. identical
B. partially identical (cross-reactive)
C. not related
D. none of these
E. cannot tell by this approach
REF. Kniker WT: Allergy News Bulletin (Ann Meeting AAIA), 2:10:7, '73

1220. When DNCB is used to assay cellular immunity in vivo:
A. 10 percent sensitization does precedes the 0.1 percent challenge dose
B. 10 percent challenge dose follows the 0.1 percent sensitizing dose
C. no challenge dose is necessary following sensitization
D. 0.1 percent challenge dose precedes the 0.1 percent sensitizing dose
E. challenge should follow sensitization within one week
REF. Kniker WT: Allergy News Bulletin (Ann Meeting AAIA), 2:10:7, '73

1221. Functional capacities of blood lymphocytes isolated by Ficoll-hypaque gradient sedimentation can be measured. Human T-lymphocytes are commonly detected by:
A. histologic demonstration of thymic chromatin
B. enumerating lymphocytes forming rosettes with sheep erythrocytes
C. counting lymphocytes forming rosettes with antigen-antibody-complement coated erythrocytes
D. demonstration of secretory villi by electron scanning
E. secretion of anti-theta antibodies
REF. Kniker WT: Allergy News Bulletin (Ann Meeting AAIA), 2:10:7, '73

1222. B-lymphocytes can easily be identified by their:
A. pyroninophilic staining
B. sparse endoplasmic reticulum
C. surface immunoglobulins demonstrated by fluorescence
D. rosette formation with sheep erythrocytes
E. spontaneous clumping in hypertonic saline
REF. Kniker WT: Allergy News Bulletin (Ann Meeting AAIA), 2:10:7, '73

1223. Normally the total of both T and B lymphocytes as compared to all blood lymphocytes should be in what percent?
A. 100
B. 90
C. 70
D. 50
E. 30
REF. Kniker WT: Allergy News Bulletin (Ann Meeting AAIA), 2:10:7, '73

IN THE FOLLOWING QUESTION, EACH LETTERED ITEM IS TO BE MATCHED WITH ONE NUMBERED ITEM. EACH CHOICE MAY BE USED ONLY ONCE.

1224. The in vitro phenomenon matching the in vivo hypersensitivity state is:
A. linear immunofluorescent staining of basement membranes
B. complement fixation
C. double diffusion in agar
D. Schulz-Dale reaction
E. cryoprecipitates

1. bronchial asthma
2. drug induced neutropenia
3. Arthus reaction
4. Goodpasture's syndrome
5. acute glomerulonephritis
REF. Kniker WT: Allergy News Bulletin (Ann Meeting AAIA), 2:10:7, '73

1225. The efficacy of transfer factor therapy in a non-sensitized recipient can readily be assessed by:
A. positive lymphocyte blastoid transformation tests in vivo
B. delayed hypersensitivity skin tests in vivo

C. alterations in serum electrophoresis patterns
D. appearance of specific antibodies to the proper antigen
E. development of a chimeric state (two genetically dissimilar populations of lymphocytes)
REF. Kniker WT: Allergy News Bulletin (Ann Meeting AAID), 2:10:7, '73

1226. Which of the following are produced by sensitized lymphocytes?
A. immunoglobulin
B. interferon
C. transfer factor
D. migration inhibition factor
E. all of the above
F. none of the above
REF. Slavin RG: Allergy News Bulletin (Ann Meeting AAIA), 2:10:7, '73

1227. IgE has a particular affinity for:
A. lymphocytes
B. basophils
C. platelets
D. macrophages
E. all of the above
F. none of the above
REF. Slavin RG: Allergy News Bulletin (Ann Meeting AAIA), 2:10:7, '73

1228. Franklin's disease or heavy chain disease is marked by the presence in the urine of a fragment of:
A. fab
B. Fc
C. kappa chain
D. lambda chain
E. all of the above
F. none of the above
REF. Slavin RG: Allergy News Bulletin (Ann Meeting AAIA), 2:10:8, '73

1229. Which of the following types of immunosuppression acts primarily before antigen recognition by lymphocytes?
A. azathioprine
B. cortisone
C. radiation
D. exogenous antibody
E. all of the above
F. none of the above
REF. Slavin RG: Allergy News Bulletin (Ann Meeting AAIA), 2:10:8, '73

1230. Which of the following types of immunosuppression acts after release of mediators?
A. azathioprine
B. cortisone
C. radiation
D. exogenous antibody
E. all of the above
F. none of the above
REF. Slavin RG: Allergy News Bulletin (Ann Meeting AAIA), 2:10:8,'73

1231. Which of the following drugs may induce the L. E. phenomenon?
A. apresoline
B. pronestyl
C. Dilantin
D. penicillin
E. all of the above
F. none of the above
REF. Slavin RG: Allergy News Bulletin (Ann Meeting AAIA), 2:10:8, '73

1232. In the positive L. E. prep, the necessary ingredients are:
A. normal white cell, nuclear material, L. E. serum
B. L. E. white cell, nuclear material, normal serum
C. L. E. white cell, normal white cell, normal serum
D. normal white cell, L. E. serum
E. none of the above
REF. Slavin RG: Allergy News Bulletin (Ann Meeting AAIA), 2:10:8, '73

1233. Atopic persons respond normally to intradermal injections of which of the following drugs?
A. epinephrine
B. prostaglandins
C. saline
D. acetylcholine
E. kinins
F. norepinephrine
REF. Kahn G: Allergy News Bulletin (Ann Meeting AAIA), 2:10:3, '73

1234. Atopic persons respond abnormally to intradermal injections of which of the following drugs?
A. acetycholine
B. kinins
C. norepinephrine
D. all of the above
E. none of the above
REF. Kahn G: Allergy News Bulletin (Ann Meeting AAIA), 2:10:3, '73

1235. Which one of the following areas of the body is most susceptible to contact sensitization?
A. scalp
B. scrotum
C. eyelids
D. palm
E. back of hand
F. finger nail
REF. Kahn G: Allergy News Bulletin (Ann Meeting AAIA), 2:10:3, '73

1236. Patients with atopic dermatitis should not wear wool caps because in comparison to the normal population they:
A. are more allergic to wool
B. have a lowered itch threshold
C. neither of the above
D. both A and B
REF. Kahn G: Allergy News Bulletin (Ann Meeting AAIA), 2:10:3, '73

1237. In asthma, the airways causing the increase in airway resistance are:
A. small airway, less than 2 mm in diameter
B. larger airways, more than 2 mm in diameter
C. the respiratory bronchioles
D. trachea and main stem bronchi
E. all of the above
REF. Avery W: Allergy News Bulletin (Ann Meeting AAIA), 2:10:3, '73

1238. The residual volume is normally what percent of the total lung capacity in percent?
A. 50-60
B. 30-40
C. 20-25
D. 10-15
E. 5-10
REF. Avery W: Allergy News Bulletin (Ann Meeting AAIA), 2:10:3, '73

1239. In pure chronic respiratory acidosis the total CO_2 is:
A. increased
B. decreased
C. unchanged
D. compensated
E. usually increased, but may be low or normal
REF. Avery W: Allergy News Bulletin (Ann Meeting AAIA), 2:10:3, '73

IN THE FOLLOWING QUESTION, MATCH EACH LETTERED ITEM WITH ONE NUMBERED ITEM. EACH CHOICE MAY BE USED ONLY ONCE:

1240. A. type A chronic obstructive lung disease
B. type B chronic obstructive lung disease
C. "small airways disease"
D. upper airway obstruction
E. none of the above

1. normal FEV, abnormal "closing volume"
2. reduced diffusing capacity, marked increase in residual volume
3. marked increase in airway resistance, moderate increase in residual volume
4. normal distribution, normal diffusing capacity, normal lung volumes, increased airway resistance

REF. Avery W: Allergy News Bulletin (Ann Meeting (AAIA), 2:10:3, '73

1241. Total CO_2 26 mEq, p CO_2 40 mm, actual bicarbonate 20 mEq, CO_2 content 40 mEq blood gas report values indicate?
A. metabolic acidosis
B. respiratory alkalosis
C. compensated respiratory acidosis
D. incorrect data
REF. Avery W: Allergy News Bulletin (Ann Meeting AAIA), 2:10:3, '73

1242. Which of the following are true?
A. number of alpha receptors in the skin is greater than that of beta receptors
B. all agents which are contact sensitizers can be primary irritants
C. all agents which are primary irritants can be contact sensitizers
D. people with atopic dermatitis are less susceptible to delayed hypersensitivity compared to non-atopic people
REF. Kahn G: Allergy News Bulletin (Ann Meeting AAIA), 2:10:3, '73

1243. Nasal polyposis being predominantly an adult disease is so unusual in children that the physician should always rule out:
A. allergy
B. infection
C. cystic fibrosis
D. malignancy
E. A and B
REF. Neely JG, Doggett RG, Harrison GM: The Laryngoscope, 82:910, May'72

1244. Which one of the following tests appears to be the most accurate in testing for food allergy?
A. deliberate food testing
B. intradermal provocative food tests (Rinkel)
C. cytotoxic tests
D. scratch tests
E. food diary
REF. Draper WL: Arch Otolaryng, 95:169, Feb'72

1245. Substance showing the most promising immunosuppressive therapy with least side effects is:
A. radiation
B. cytotoxic chemicals such as cyclophosphamide (alkylating agent)
C. antibiotics (Actinomycin C)
D. heterologous antilymphocyte serum (ALS)
E. alpha globulin
REF. Mogi G, Harvey JE, Ohyama M, Ueda N, Ogura JH: The Laryngoscope, 82:61, Jan'72

1246. steroids are members of a related group of lipoid compounds and are secreted by:
A. gonads
B. adrenal cortex
C. placenta
D. all of the above
E. none of the above
REF. Baker DC: Trans Am Acad Ophthalmol and Otolaryngol, 76:297, Mar-Apr'72

1247. Steroid hormones should be used cautiously because their effects are:
A. estrogenic, spermatogenic and androgenic
B. progestional corticoid, renotrophic, sodium secreting
C. anesthetic, thermogenic, and antitumorigenic
D. A and B
E. all of the above
REF. Baker DC: Trans Am Acad Ophthalmol and Otolaryngol, 76:297, Mar-Apr'72

1248. Which two of the following glucocorticosteroids (sugar-active steroids) exert an anti-inflammatory and immune (anti-allergic) response 30 times as potent as cortisone?
A. dexamethasone (decadron)
B. prednisolone
C. methylprednisolone
D. triamcinolone (aristocort)
E. betamethasone (celestone)
REF. Baker DC: Trans Am Acad Ophthalmol and Otolaryngol, 76:297, Mar-Apr'72

1249. The most common technique used by otolaryngologists today to facilitate diagnosis of allergic diseases is:
A. optimal dosage therapy of Hansel
B. serial dilution titration and provocative testing of Rinkel, Williams, Lee, Brown, Willoughby, etc.
C. cytology and leukocytic cytotoxic reactions for food and chemical allergies by Bryan and Bryan
D. Randolph's development of diagnosis by ingestion after five or more days of fasting with complete environmental control (chemical allergy)
E. therapeutic trial with antihistamines, pseudoephedrine and/or glucocorticosteroids
REF. Bryan WTK, Bryan MP: The Laryngoscope, 82:1231, July'72

1250. The most recent technique of greatest interest developed for the diagnosis of obscure allergic diseases is:
A. optimal dosage technique of Hansel
B. serial dilution and provocative tests of Rinkel et al
C. cytology and leukocytic cytotoxic reactions of Bryan
D. Randolph's technique of fasting with ingestion of food with complete environmental control
E. therapeutic trial
REF. Bryan WTC, Bryan MP: The Laryngoscope, 82:1231, July'72

1251. The immunosuppressive immunoglobulin in antilymphocyte serum (ALS) or antithymocyte plasma (ATP) with profound peripheral blood lymphopenia and enhanced survival of skin allografts is:
A. IgA (gamma A globulin)
B. IgM
C. IgD
D. IgE
E. IgG
REF. Mogi G, Harvey JE, Ogura JH: The Laryngoscope, 82:998, June'72

1252. Tachyphylaxis is a rapid diminution in magnitude or duration of a response to a drug when administered frequently. Drug tolerance is a progressive diminution of susceptibility to the effect of a drug resulting from continued administration. Repeated injection (every 5 to 10 minutes) of escalating doses tends to induce tachyphylaxis most rapidly. The drug well known for tachyphylactic tendencies is:
A. ephedrine isomers
B. alcohol
C. narcotics
D. hypnotics
E. anticholinergics
REF. Dempsey JE, Jackson RT: Arch Otolaryngol, 96:216, Sept'72

1253. The role of histamine release is unknown but it is released from the following cell:
A. mast
B. eosinophile
C. small lymphocyte
D. large lymphocyte
E. polymorphonuclear leukocyte
REF. Calcaterra TC: Arch Otolaryng, 96:341, Oct'72

1254. The complement system (basis of immune function) behaves so that the activation of one complement leads to the activation of the next. C'1 esterase is the first of the nine components of the complement system and its inhibitor, when low, engenders hereditary angioneurotic edema. The first component of complement may be fixed on:

A. aggregated Y-globulin
B. cryoglobulins
C. cold agglutinins
D. all of the above
E. none of the above

REF. Calcaterra TC: Arch Otolaryngol, 96:341, Oct'72

1255. The basis of immune function is the complement system and includes:

A. histamine release
B. phagocytosis
C. anaphylatoxin generation
D. binding of immune complexes to the basement membrane
E. all of the above

REF. Calcaterra TC: Arch Otolaryngol, 96:341, Oct'72

1256. Allergy can cause Ménière's disease (tinnitus, sensorineural hearing loss and episodic vertigo) and appears to be the most common etiologic factor (14 percent). Which of the following groups of allergens are most commonly involved in Ménière's disease?

A. foods
B. trees, grasses, weed pollens
C. molds
D. dust
E. all of the above

REF. Pulec JL: The Laryngoscope, 82:1703, Sept'72

1257. Craving for a certain food, postprandial bloating, and fatigue indicate allergy most likely to:

A. foods
B. trees, grasses, weeds, pollens
C. molds
D. dust
E. all of the above

REF. Pulec JL: The Laryngoscope, 82:1703, Sept'72

1258. Investigation of allergic causes of symptoms is complicated, time consuming, and difficult. Which of the following are most important?

A. history
B. conventional scratch, intradermal and provocative skin tests
C. nasal smears for eosinophiles and the more complicated cytotoxic food tests
D. challenge feeding tests, etc.
E. all of the above

REF. Pulec JL: The Laryngoscope, 82:1703, Sept'72

1259. Hypersensitivity to one or more foods should be considered with which of the following groups of symptoms?

A. abdominal flatulence and distention and fluid retention of undetermined origin
B. nuchal myalgia
C. early morning insomnia and post-prandial fatigue
D. periodic mental depression or amnesia and specific food cravings or food intolerance
E. all of the above

REF. Wilson WH: The Laryngoscope, 83:1726, Sept'72

1260. Challenge feeding test requires complete elimination of the selected food and its products from the diet for the following number of days with reintroduction on the next day. Provocation of symptoms constitute a positive test response:

A. one day with reintroduction second day
B. two days with food third day
C. three days with food fourth day

D. four days with food fifth day
E. five days with food sixth day
REF. Wilson WH: The Laryngoscope, 82:1726, Sept'72

1261. In the presence of nasal allergy, surgery should not be performed without which of the following effective and intensive measures?
A. corticosteroids
B. antihistamines, allergy tests with desensitization
C. decongestants
D. antibiotics
E. all of the above
REF. Eichel BS: The Laryngoscope, 82:1806, Oct'72

1262. In obstructive nasal polyposis, the operative procedure of choice is:
A. external
B. transantral
C. intranasal with removal of middle turbinate
D. intranasal with preservation of middle turbinate
E. polypectomy alone
REF. Eichel BS: The Laryngoscope, 82:1806, Oct'72

1263. The basic immunoglobulins are:
A. IgG
B. IgM
C. IgA
D. IgD
E. IgE
REF. Davison RC: Canadian J Otolaryngol, 1:107, No. 2, '72

1264. Which of the following immunopathological diseases are not due to circulating antibodies combining with human antigens?
A. cytotoxic or cytolytic
B. atopic or anaphylactic
C. granulomatous
D. toxic complex of Arthus
E. neutralization or inactivation
REF. Davison RC: Canadian J Otolaryngol, 1:107, No. 2, '72

1265. Many patients react to all of the following allergens but the most common allergen is:
A. dust
B. hormodendrum
C. alternaria
D. T.O.E. (trichophyton, oidiomycin, epidermophyton)
E. cephalosporium
REF. Davison RC: Canadial J Otolaryngol, 1:107, No. 2, '72

1266. All of the following factors must be considered in evaluating chronic nasal obstruction in which allergy treatment has failed but which one of the following conditions is probably most important in most instances?
A. nasopharyngeal growths such as adenoids and neoplasms
B. emotional disturbances such as stress, exhaustion, depression
C. infections in the nasal passages, nasopharynx and/or sinuses
D. environmental problems - dust or chemical fumes at work or home
E. anatomic dysfunction and deformities such as septal deviations and the broad flat nose
REF. Hinderer K: Trans Am Soc Ophthalmol and Otolaryngol Allergy, 12:59, Sept'71

1267. Sinus surgery is contraindicated in the allergic patient in which of the following conditions?
A. during the patient's allergy season even though the allergy is under desensitization control
B. during acute infections
C. after sudden withdrawal of steroids in patients taking large doses

D. in severe obstructive lung disease
E. all of the above
REF. Williams RI: (Discussion: Farrior RT, Wilson W, Sanders SH) Trans Amer Laryng Assoc, 93:85, Apr'72

1268. The glucocorticosteroids have an important role in allergy. Which of the following is true?
A. their effect in allergy is attributed to alleviation of the inflammation caused by the antigen-antibody reactions
B. affect the immune response with an immediate breakdown of lymphoid tissue adding to the pool of plasma gamma globulin and the substrate for the formation of new antibodies
REF. Baker DC: Trans Am Acad Ophthalmol and Otolaryngol, 76:297, Mar-Apr'72

1269. The corticosteroids sustain life and affect metabolism and are divided into two groups. Which of the following is true?
A. glucocorticoids facilitate the formation of carbohydrates from non-carbohydrate sources and are anti-inflammatory with a breakdown in connective tissue. Examples are cortisone and corticosterone
B. mineral corticoids affect water and electrolyte metabolism with the retention of sodium and excretion of potassium and are inflammatory provoking. Examples are deoxycorticosterone and aldosterone
REF. Baker DC: Trans Am Acad Ophthalmol and Otolaryngol, 76:297, Mar-Apr'72

IN THE FOLLOWING QUESTIONS MATCH EACH LETTERED ITEM WITH ONE NUMBERED ITEM. EACH CHOICE MAY BE USED ONLY ONCE:

1270. In food allergy, symptoms and signs suggest hypersensitivity to certain foods:
A. addiction
B. obese patient snacking on bakery products
C. gastric distress or ulcer diathesis from ice cream
D. gastric distress from popcorn or carbonated beverages
E. gastric distress from fermented alcohol and hypersensitivity to penicillin

1. wheat
2. yeast, fungal ingestants and products of fermentation
3. milk
4. corn
5. coffee
REF. Wilson WH: The Laryngoscope, 82:1726, Sept'72

1271. In food allergy the possibility of antigenic cross-reactivity requires consideration of hypersensitivity to biogenetically related foods such as:
A. beef
B. pork
C. white potato
D. chicken
E. fungal ingestants and products of fermentation

1. egg
2. tomato
3. cow's milk
4. corn
5. yeast
REF. Wilson WH: The Laryngoscope, 82:1726, Sept'72

1272. The glucocorticosteroids are best used as follows:
A. hypertrophy of the inferior turbinates due to vasomotor or allergic rhinitis
B. acute severe allergic rhinitis, such as hayfever
C. chronic vasomotor rhinitis
D. perennial rhinosinusitis

1. by mouth or I. M. injection (a quick-acting steroid) or three intranasal injections of prednisolone tertiary butylacetate. Adjunct to but not a replacement for desensitization
2. long-acting corticosteroid such as tertiary butylacetate prednisolone (hydeltra-T. B. A.), insoluble so its effect is local for as many as six months - 3 to 4 injections of 0. 3 ml in each turbinate of a solution containing 20 mg/ml - injections at weekly intervals for a total steroid dosage of 36 mg
3. adjunct only to complete allergy work-up and desensitization, glucocorticoids only - no corticoids
4. adjunct to other therapy such as one table every other day of glucocorticoids only - no mineral corticoids

REF. Baker DC: Trans Am Acad Ophthalmol and Otolaryngol, 76:297, Mar-Apr'72

1273. It is suggested that immunoglobulins may have an important role in host defense mechanism against potentially pathogenic organisms. Which one of the following statements is incorrect?

A. the electrophoretic patterns of nasal discharge and saliva are not similar to those of the corresponding sera
B. protein components of effusions (joint exudates) and external secretions (nasal discharge, saliva, bronchial fluid) are similar to each other
C. external secretions (nasal discharge, saliva) contain immunoglobulins which bathe mucous-membrane surfaces
D. immunoglobulin A (IgA) is the predominant immunoglobulin in external nasal and other secretions
E. IgA in secretions is mostly 11S in sedimentation whereas IgA in serum is 7s, and IgA (11S) differs from IgA (7s) by the possession of an additional nonimmunoglobulin glycoprotein with distinct antigenic characteristics

REF. Mogi G, Honjo S: Ann Otol, 81:99, Feb'72

1274. All of the following ephedrine isomers are pressor agents except:

A. D (-) ephedrine
B. L (+) ephedrine
C. D (-) pseudoephedrine
D. L (+) pseudoephedrine

REF. Dempsey JE, Jackson RT: Arch Otolaryngol, 96:216, Sept'72

1275. Bilateral experimental vasomotor rhinitis (parasympathicomimetic state) has all of the following features except:

A. nasal mucosa shows exaggerated reactions to external stimuli
B. usually shows eosinophiles and mast cells in the nasal secretions
C. increased pulmonary resistance in the lower respiratory tract
D. increased nasal obstruction with noisy breathing, snoring, and sneezing
E. anterior nasal mucosa appears pale and swollen

REF. Krajina Z, Harvey JE, Ogura JH: The Laryngoscope, 82:1068, June '72

1276. Histamine is associated with inflammatory reactions (including allergy). All of the following are true except:

A. histamine is associated with the initial phase of vascular permeability
B. vascular permeability is inhibited by antihistamines
C. antihistamines along with aldosterone are more effective than anti-histamines alone in the treatment of allergic problems
D. antihistamine with glucocorticoids are more effective than antihistamines alone in the treatment of allergy
E. antihistamines are helpful in allergy, but leave much to be desired and although they appear to have few side effects, they are increasing in number

REF. Baker DC: Trans Am Acad Ophthalmol and Otolaryngol, 76:297, Mar-Apr'72

1277. All of the following are effective anti-inflammatory drugs except:
A. deoxycorticosterone
B. sulfa drugs
C. antibiotics
D. antihistamines
E. glucocorticoids
REF. Baker DC: Trans Am Acad Ophthalmol and Otolaryngol, 76:297, Mar-Apr'72

1278. The most common allergic diseases are:
A. hay fever
B. asthma
C. infantile eczema
D. hives
E. gastrointestinal food reactions (atopic diseases)
REF. Wolf AF: Consultant, 55, May'74

1279. The outlook for determining the cause of hives or urticaria is dim. Hives have which of the following characteristics?
A. likely not of a generalized allergic origin
B. may be only a sign of a minor allergic reaction
C. only sign of neoplastic disease, especially lymphoma
D. all of the above
E. none of the above
REF. Wolf AF: Consultant, 55, May'74

1280. Eyelid edema and tearing is usually:
A. not allergic
B. may be due to either hyperthyroidism or hypothyroidism
C. chronic infectious blepharitis
D. tearing from blocked nasolacrimal duct or conjunctivitis
E. eye drop sensitizers in medication especially mercury
REF. Wolf AF: Consultant, 55, May'74

1281. Acute allergic rhinitis is characterized by which of the following:
A. itchiness of the nose, palate, pharynx and mouth
B. clear, watery nasal discharge
C. sneezing
D. tearing
E. purulent postnasal drip
REF. Wolf AF: Consultant, 57, May'74

1282. Which of the following must be considered in the differential diagnosis of acute allergic rhinitis?
A. pansinusitis
B. vasomotor rhinitis
C. rhinitis medicamentosa
D. patients on Rauwolfia derivatives
E. cerebrospinal rhinorrhea
REF. Wolf AF: Consultant, 57, May'74

1283. All of the following occur in vasomotor rhinitis except:
A. nasal congestion due to temperature changes
B. reddish-colored rather than pale mucous membranes
C. eosinophiles in nasal smears
D. nasal congestion due to emotional disturbances
E. associated with nonspecific vasodilators such as alcohol, sweet odors such as chocolate, odors from fabrics or dyes, and fumes such as tobacco smoke
REF. Wolf AF: Consultant, 57, May'74

1284. An increase in eosinophiles in nasal smears occurs in which of the following conditions?
A. acute allergic rhinitis due to pollen
B. rhinitis medicamentosa
C. vasomotor rhinitis
D. pansinusitis
E. foreign body reaction
REF. Wolf AF: Consultant, 57, May'74

1285. Although most of the following conditions are usually considered in a patient with a chronic cough with pneumonitis, wheezing, rhonchi, and dyspnea, the actual cause can be:
A. pneumonia
B. asthma
C. foreign body
D. bronchiectasis
E. hiatal hernia with nocturnal reflux
REF. Wolf AF: Consultant, 57, May '74

1286. In a patient with hives or urticaria, which of the following conditions may be involved?
A. drugs
B. inhalants
C. contactants
D. foods
E. physical factors
REF. Weary PE: Consultant, 151, May '74

1287. In a patient with hives or urticaria which of the following conditions are usually not thought of but have long been recognized as causes?
A. focal bacterial infections (usually low grade) of sinuses, tonsils, ears, teeth, prostate, gallbladder
B. tinea pedis in association with onychomycosis
C. candida albicans in mouth, vagina, stools
D. tinea corporis
E. fungus focal infection reinforced by outside antigenic substances from related organisms or exposure to outside sources of high fungal density such as musty basements or stored clothing
REF. Weary PE: Consultant, 151, May '74

1288. In a patient with hives or urticaria of undetermined etiology, which of the following specific therapies should be used to uncover the cause?
A. broad spectrum antibiotic, such as tetracycline, for five days in a dosage of 250 mg 4 times a day - improvement is a presumptive evidence of a focal infection
B. skin testing with bacterial antigens - may provoke a widespread flare of lesions
C. hyposensitization with autogenous vaccines (FDA regulations make many stock vaccines unavailable)
D. griseofulvin with 5 percent undecylenic acid and 20 percent zinc undecylenate ointment for topical application to feet fungal infections
E. challenged with oral Candida antigen or bakers' or brewers' yeast with worsening of hives (skin tests may be negative) - evidence hives due to candida albicans
F. nystatin - 100,000 units orally 3 times daily for 2 weeks - followed by nystatin - 500,000 units 3 times daily for 2 weeks, plus amphotericin B troches twice daily for 1 week (and in women add nystatin vaginal suppositories twice daily for 1 week) and combined with a low yeast diet - evidence candida albicans hives
G. corticosteroid therapy - evidence of hives due to antigens, perhaps bacterial or fungal when improvement occurs
REF. Weary PE: Consultant, 151, May '74

1289. A patient with hives or urticaria of undetermined etiology with no improvement in the hives after a therapeutic trial with broad-spectrum antibiotics indicates:
A. presumptive evidence of no focal infection
B. does not necessarily mean there is no infection present
C. transient improvement does not always mean infection
D. in a disorder as capricious as hives, any temporary improvement may not be significant
REF. Weary PE: Consultant, 151, May '74

1290. In a child with primary immunodeficiency, which of the following kinds of immunodeficiency need be considered?
A. antibody
B. cellular (deficient delayed hypersensitivity)
C. combined antibody and cellular
D. phagocytic (granulocytic)
E. opsonic (involving the serum complement system)
REF. Stiehm ER: Consultant, 65, May '74

1291. Immune serum globulin is the best treatment for which one of the following deficiencies?
A. antibody
B. selective IgA
C. cellular
D. phagocytic
E. opsonic
REF. Stiehm ER: Consultant, 65, May '74

1292. In caring for immunodeficient children, which of the following must be seriously considered?
A. do adenotonsillectomies only with strict indications
B. avoid all live virus vaccines (cellular immunodeficiency)
C. avoid blood or fresh plasma transfusions (cellular immunodeficiency)
D. erythrocytes for transfusions must be at least two weeks old and treated with 3,000 roentgens of irradiation - and then transfuse only if absolutely necessary
E. splenectomy contraindicated (loss of spleen's phagocytic ability)
REF. Stiehm ER: Consultant, 65, May '74

1293. In the use of immune serum globulin (gamma globulin) in the treatment of antibody deficiency, which of the following statements may be considered accurate?
A. never exceed 20 to 30 ml but dose must be more accurate than this and given intramuscularly
B. intravenous injection may result in anaphylactic reactions
C. intracutaneous injections are most effective
D. do not give to thrombocytopenic patients (danger hematoma)
E. nausea, vomiting, malaise, cyanosis and loss of consciousness may occur but it is one of the safest biologics
REF. Stiehm ER: Consultant, 65, May '74

1294. When used in children fresh frozen plasma infusions in dosages of 15 to 20 ml/kg per month are particularly valuable in which of the following?
A. thrombocytopenia
B. hypogammaglobulinemia
C. ataxia telangiectasia
D. IgA deficiency
E. IgG deficiency
REF. Stiehm ER: Consultant, 65, May '74

1295. The most common antibody deficiency in children is:
A. IgG
B. IgM
C. IgA (selective)
D. IgD
E. IgE
REF. Stiehm ER: Consultant, 65, May '74

1296. Do not use gamma globulin, blood or plasma in which one of the following conditions because severe anaphylactic reactions may occur?
A. selective IgA deficiency
B. thrombocytopenia
C. hypogammaglobulinemia
D. ataxia telangiectasia
REF. Stiehm ER: Consultant, 65, May '74

1297. Transfer factor is a nonviable extract of immune lymphocytes and when given subcutaneously induces immunity to a specific antigen in the recipient for a period in months of:
A. one to two
B. three to four
C. six to twelve
D. eighteen to twenty-four
E. life-time
REF. Stiehm ER: Consultant 65, May'74

1298. Which of the following factors may be considered true as far as the transfer factor is concerned?
A. valuable for the treatment of combined immunodeficiencies
B. useful for the therapy of some mucocutaneous candidiasis
C. useful for the treatment of Wiskott-Aldrich syndrome
D. valuable in the DiGeorge syndrome
E. involves no risk of graft-versus-host reactions and has minimal side-effects
REF. Stiehm ER: Consultant, 65, May'74

1299. Skin tests can be used to evaluate a seriously ill patient's immune status. Negative skin tests responses to all skin tests (anergy) can occur in which of the following conditions?
A. widespread cancer
B. viral or other infections
C. sarcoidosis
D. lymphatic leukemia
E. uremia
F. patients receiving immunosuppressive drugs, such as steroids
REF. Palmer DL: Consultant, 91, May'74

1300. Blastomycin skin test for suspected infection such as in the larynx is:
A. virtually worthless
B. characterized by an extensive cross-reactivity with other agents
C. results usually negative even if the patient has active blastomycosis
D. test probably should never be used
REF. Palmer DL: Consultant, 91, May'74

1301. If a patient has active tuberculosis of the sinuses or larynx, the PPD or Mantoux intradermal test (0. 5 cm of liquid stabilized PPD injected intradermally on flexor surface of the forearm) may be:
A. negative (after 48 to 72 hours
B. less than 0 to 4 mm
C. 5 to 9 mm
D. 10 to 15 mm
E. 16 mm or more
REF. Palmer DL: Consultant, 91, May'74

1302. After 48 to 72 hours the Mantoux (PPD) test should be measured in the transverse diameter by a millimeter ruler. The significant response to measure is:
A. redness
B. induration
C. B plus A
REF. Palmer DL: Consultant, 91, May'74

1303. The skin test (Mantoux) with PPD is considered significant (positive reaction) when the induration measures in a transverse diameter in millimeters of:
A. 0 to 4
B. 5 to 9
C. 10 to 15 or more
REF. Palmer DL: Consultant,91, May'74

1304. If the Mantoux test with PPD shows an area of induration of 0 to 4 mm and there is strong clinical, cultural and x-ray evidence of active tuberculosis (larynx) which of the following skin tests should be done (anergy suspected)?
A. repeat PPD test
B. test with candida
C. test with trichophyton
D. test with mumps
E. test for atypical bacteria
REF. Palmer DL: Consultant, 91, May'74

1305. If the Mantoux test with PPD shows an area of induration 5 to 9 mm and there is strong clinical, cultural and x-ray evidence of active tuberculosis (larynx), which of the following skin tests should be done (anergy suspected)?
A. repeat PPD test
B. test with candida
C. test with trichophyton
D. test with munps
E. test for atypical bacteria
REF. Palmer DL: Consultant, 91, May'74

1306. If the Mantoux test with PPD shows an area of induration of 10 to 15 mm or greater and there have been no cultural or x-ray tests, which of the following should be done in a suspected laryngeal ulceration which has been biopsied and is negative for neoplastic changes?
A. x-rays of lungs
B. acid fast smears and cultures of sputum
C. reflects active infection without further tests
D. reflects inactive infection without additional tests
E. prophylaxis or treatment probably indicated if all other findings are negative
REF. Palmer DL: Consultant, 95, May'74

1307. In a severe illness with a patient's inability to react to infection (anergy), a patient may have an active tuberculosis (larynx, lungs) with a negative PPD test. If anergy is suspected, it is confirmed by skin testing with at least two additional antigens (plus PPD) using munps, trichophyton, or candida. Which of the following results indicate true anergy?
A. all tests negative
B. 5 mm or greater induration with PPD
C. 5 mm or greater induration with any one of the tests
D. 5 mm or greater induration with all of the tests
E. 10 mm or greater with any one test
REF. Palmer DL: Consultant, 91, May'74

1308. Skin tests can give a good indication of susceptibility or lack of immunity (exposure). Lack of immunity to tuberculosis (PPD), mumps antigen, coccidioidomycosis or histoplasmosis is indicated when the induration of the skin tests measure in mm:
A. negative (no reaction)
B. 2 - 4
C. 5 - 9
D. 10 - 15
E. 16 or more
REF. Palmer DL: Consultant, 91, May'74

1309. In some parts of the U. S., particularly the southeast, induration of the Mantoux test from 5 to 10 mm reflects exposure to or infection with:
A. tuberculosis
B. histoplasmosis
C. coccidioidomycosis
D. blastomycosis
E. atypical mycobacteria (such as Battey bacillus
REF. Palmer DL: Consultant, 91, May'74

1310. A patient with a negative PPD (Mantoux) test with x-ray findings of old, calcified granulomas may have active or previous infection with histoplasmosis or coccidioidomycosis if the induration of the specific skin test is greater in mm than:
A. 1 - 2
B. 3 - 4
C. 5 - 6
D. 7 - 8
E. 10 or more
REF. Palmer DL: Consultant, 91, May '74

1311. Skin tests for fungus during the course of the disease can be:
A. usually positive
B. negative early
C. negative when infection is severe
D. negative when infection is disseminated
E. antigens can cross-react with each other (rarely false positives)
REF. Palmer DL: Consultant, 91, May '74

1312. When false-negative reactions occur in fungal skin tests, which of the following tests should be very helpful?
A. complement-fixation or precipitin test with a rising titer
B. A with a decreasing titer
C. repeat PPD with stronger antigen
D. repeat histoplasmosis with stronger antigen
E. repeat coccidioidomycosis with stronger antigen
REF. Palmer DL: Consultant, 91, May '74

1313. Which of the following precautions should be taken in skin testing with histoplasmin when a complement-fixation test is contemplated?
A. serum sample should be taken before the skin test
B. serum sample may be taken after the skin test
C. histoplasmin can elevate complement-fixation titers
D. histoplasmin does not elevate complement-fixation titers
REF. Palmer DL: Consultant, 91, May '74

1314. Antigen-antibody reaction is the beginning of an immune reaction and various effectors such as complement do the basic work of cellular or bacterial destruction. The complement system is made up of the following number of proteins:
A. 3
B. 6
C. 9
D. 11
E. 13
REF. Stroud RM: Consultant, 144, May '74

1315. Complement proteins are measured by both of the following methods but the most recent technique is:
A. radical immunodiffusion
B. hemolytic assays
REF. Stroud RM: Consultant, 144, May '74

1316. Complement proteins are numbered 1 through 9 but there are 11 in all since C1 has three subcomponents which are?
A. $C1_a$
B. $C1_p$
C. $C1_q$
D. $C1_r$
E. $C1_s$
REF. Stroud RM: Consultant, 144, May '74

1317. A deficiency of which of the following complement proteins appears to predispose to collagen diseases (lupus, polymyositis) and is an autosomal recessive trait?
A. C_2
B. C_3
C. C_6
D. C_7
E. C_8
REF. Stroud RM: Consultant, 144, May '74

IN THE FOLLOWING QUESTION, MATCH EACH LETTERED ITEM WITH ONE NUMBERED ITEM. EACH CHOICE MAY BE USED ONLY ONCE.

1318. Immunoglobulins is a group of proteins including all molecules with antibody activity and all molecules structurally related to those with antibody activity.

The following properties are characteristic of which serum immunoglobulin?

A. IgG
B. IgA
C. IgM
D. IgD
E. IgE

1. protects intravascular spaces
2. acts as an antibody within the body but its main function seems to protect the mucous membrane surfaces
3. Reagin or skin sensitizing antibody-responsible for the classic Prausnitz-Küstner passive transer of skin sensitizing antibody
4. main immunoglobulin of the body and responsible for opsonization, immobilization, agglutination, fixation of complement, etc. Individuals without this immunoglobulin must have supportive therapy with injections of this immunoglobulin or die
5. function unknown

REF. Allansmith MR: Trans Amer Soc Ophthal-Otolaryngol Allergy, 13:9, Sept'72. (See Fig. 27A, B, C and D)

1319. The oldest of the complement-associated inborn errors is hereditary angioedema in which the attacks of edema are painless if subcutaneous but very painful in the intestine. Edema of the larynx or trachea can be fatal and a tracheostomy may be life-saving. Episodes of edema are triggered by injury, menses, exertion or emotional upsets by activating the Hageman factor which converts plasminogen to plasmin which in turn activates the C_1 molecule. Which of the following proteins inherited as an autosomal dominant is responsible for hereditary angioedema?

A. C6
B. C7
C. C5
D. C1 inhibitor deficiency
E. C3 inactivator deficiency

REF. Stroud RM: Consultant, 144, May'74

IN THE FOLLOWING QUESTION, MATCH EACH LETTERED ITEM WITH ONE NUMBERED ITEM. EACH CHOICE MAY BE USED ONLY ONCE:

1320. In the following types of allergic reactions, which procedures are used for diagnosis?

A. type I - release of histamine and SRS-A, slow reacting substance of anaphylaxis from cells previously sensitized by antigen or allergens (atopic diseases)
B. type II - triggered by direct action of antigens and antibodies on cell surfaces resulting in cellular destruction (cytotoxic reactions) (transfusion reactions)
C. type III - toxic antigen - antibody complexes which are soluble and circulate generally (lupus erythematosus and serum sickness) or insoluble and deposited as precipitates in specific tissues elicitng inflammation (Farmer's Lung, glomerulonephritis)
D. type IV - delayed or cellular hypersensitivity reactions set in motion by specifically sensitized lymphocytes rather than antibodies (homograft reaction, allergic eczematous contact dermatitis)

1. primarily complex hematologic tests
2. intradermal tests (PPD), histoplasmin, patch tests, eosinophilia, hypergammaglobulinemia, hypocomplementemia
3. direct skin test, Prausnitz-Küstner reaction, (caution: hepatitis), radioallergosorbent test (Rast-experimental)
4. gel diffusion procedures for precipitating antibodies in the serum

REF. Wolf AF: Consultant, 55, May'74

1321. Autoimmune disease means:
A. normal automatic immunity reaction of the body to disease such as hay-fever
B. abnormal immunity reaction of the body to disease
REF. Stroud RM: Consultant, 144, May'74

1322. Dinitrochlorobenzene (2-4 DNCB) appears to have which of the following characteristics?
A. forms a hapten with skin protein in a covalent bond when applied to the skin
B. a delayed hypersensitivity reaction with second application to the skin is useful to measure cell-mediated immunity as a gross measure of cancer immunity
C. few people have been exposed to 2-4 DNCB
D. 2-4 DNCB-skin antigen complex reacts to produce small lymphocytes with a memory for this new foreign material
E. DNCB test is a more accurate predictor of delayed hypersensitivity than the lymphocyte count
REF. Maisel RH, Ogura JH: The Laryngoscope, 82:2012, Dec'73

1323. Immunity appears to be important in cancer because:
A. many tumor specific antigens with antibodies have been identified
B. neoplasia is more virulent in animals and humans treated with medication inhibiting reaction to antigenic material
C. carcinoma and lymphoma are more common than actuarially expected in kidney transplant recipients
D. immunologic deficiency exists in patients with lymphomas and Hodgkin's where transplant-rejection is defective
E. delayed hypersensitivity reaction is defective in patients with lymphomas
REF. Maisel RH, Ogura JH: The Laryngoscope, 83:2012, Dec'73

1324. Anergy (hyporeactive immune state) appears to be present in patients with Hodgkin's disease because:
A. abnormal lymphocyte function
B. delayed hypersensitivity
C. high incidence of skin homograft acceptance
D. greatly decreased incidence of response to PPD (Mantoux test) and other skin tests
E. leukocytosis
REF. Maisel RH, Ogura JH: The Laryngoscope, 83:2012, Dec'73

1325. The humoral limb of the immune system is the bursal system and is derived from mammalian tissue comparable to the bursa of fabricius in fowl. These B cells are mostly stationary and among them are the plasma cells which act to produce:
A. circulating antibodies
B. circulating immunoglobulins
C. initial antigen recognition
D. memory retention
E. involved in transplant rejection
REF. Maisel RH, Ogura JH: The Laryngoscope, 83:2012, Dec'73

1326. The cell mediated limb of the immune system involves the thymus derived cells (T cells) and their prime agent is the small lymphocyte which circulates in the blood and lymph. T cells (small lymphocytes)are involved in:
A. circulating antibodies or immunoglobulins
B. transplant rejection
C. delayed skin tests such as PPD and fungus
D. initial antigen recognization
E. memory retention
REF. Maisel RH, Ogura JH: The Laryngoscope, 83:2012, Dec'73

1327. B cells are found in:
A. medullary cords
B. central lymph follicles
C. peripheral cortical regions of lymph nodes
D. splenic red pulp
E. subepithelial lymphoid follicles
REF. Maisel RH, Ogura JH: The Laryngoscope, 83:2012, Dec'73

1328. T cells are found in:
A. deep cortical areas of lymph nodes
B. periarteriolar areas of the spleen
C. circulate in the blood
D. circulate in the lymph
E. thymus
REF. Maisel RH, Ogura JH: The Laryngoscope, 83:2012, Dec'73

1329. Young children with bilateral nasal polyps may have?
A. pansinusitis
B. allergy
C. foreign bodies
D. hypertrophied adenoids
E. cystic fibrosis
REF. Meyers D, Myers EN: The Laryngoscope, 84:833, May'74

1330. If both parents are allergic, the following percent of children will develop some allergic manifestations:
A. 10
B. 25
C. 50
D. 75
E. 95
REF. Meyers D, Myers EN: The Laryngoscope, 84:833, May'74

1331. The following percent of allergic patients have a family history of allergy:.
A. 10
B. 25
C. 50
D. 75
E. 95
REF. Meyers D, Myers EN: The Laryngoscope, 84:833, May'74

IN THE FOLLOWING QUESTION, MATCH EACH LETTERED ITEM WITH ONE NUMBERED ITEM. EACH CHOICE MAY BE USED ONLY ONCE:

1332. In the treatment of nasal obstruction which of the following is used?
A. acute microbial inflammation
B. neutralize allergies
C. eliminate obstructive edema

1. antihistamines
2. corticosteroids
3. antibiotics
REF. Meyers D, Myers EN: The Laryngoscope, 84:833, May'74

1333. Corticosteroids inhibit the inflammatory responses due to which of the following inciting agents?
A. chemical
B. bacterial
C. mechanical
D. immunological
REF. Meyers D, Myers EN: The Laryngoscope, 84:833, May'74

1334. Nasal polyposis may be due to:
A. allergy
B. collagen disease
C. cystic fibrosis
D. infection
E. cardiac decompensation
REF. Meyers D, Myers EN: The Laryngoscope, 84:833, May'74 Semenov H: Trans Amer Acad Ophthal and Otolaryng, P. 121, May-Apr '52

1335. Nasal surgical procedures should be avoided on allergic patients with:
A. acute allergic exacerbations such as hayfever
B. asthmatic attacks
C. acute infections
D. undetermined pulmonary function studies in asthmatics and patients with emphysema
E. cardiac decompensation
REF. Meyers D, Myers EN: The Laryngoscope, 84:833, May'74

1336. Which of the following will cause regression of nasal polyps?
A. 0.5 to 1cc of a sterile suspension of triamcinolone acetonide (Kenalog 40 R) injected into the body of the polyp with a 27-gauge three and one half inch needle and repeated each five to seven days
B. dexamethasone sodium phosphate in aerosol form (systemic absorption occurs)
C. prednisolone 40 mgm per day for five days
D. intramuscular injection of triamcinolone acetonide suspension 40-80 mgm
E. D with methyl prednisolone
REF. Meyers D, Myers EN: The Laryngoscope, 84:833, May'74

1337. Alternate day therapy (ADT) with oral corticosteroids in which twice the usual daily dose of corticoid is administered minimizes undesirable side effects by eliminating adrenocortical suppression. Serum ACTH levels rise to a resultant maximal plasma corticoid level by 8 a.m. Therefore, exogenous steroids suppress adrenocortical activity least when given at:
A. 5 a.m.
B. 8 a.m.
C. noon
D. 5 p.m.
E. bedtime
REF. Meyers D, Myers EN: The Laryngoscope, 84:833, May'74

1338. Surgery in nasal polyposis is reserved for which of the following patients?
A. allergy management (tests with desensitization, etc.) has been partly or totally unsuccessful
B. refuse allergy tests
C. over use of antihistamines, pseudoephedrine, nasal sprays or drops
D. allergy drugs contraindicated-diabetes, tuberculosis, ulcers (stomach)
E. disease too extensive for medical control
REF. Meyers D, Myers EN: The Laryngoscope, 84:833, May'74

1339. Which of the following patients should not use steroids?
A. hypertension
B. ulcer disease (peptic)
C. tuberculosis
D. psychiatric illness
E. diabetes
F. glaucoma
REF. Meyers D, Myers EN: The Laryngoscope, 84:833, May'74

1340. In patients with numerous polyps obstructing the entire nasal airway, in addition to a polypectomy which of the following procedures should be considered?
A. nasal septoplasty or submucous resection
B. outfracture the inferior and/or middle turbinates
C. injection of steroids in the inferior and/or middle turbinates
D. submucous resection of the inferior and/or middle turbinates
E. mucosal electrodessication of the inferior turbinates
REF. Meyers D, Myers EN: The Laryngoscope, 84:833, May'74

1341. Which of the following complications occur in performing an intranasal ethmoidectomy for polyps?
A. injury to the roof of the ethmoid with cerebrospinal fluid leak and rhinorrhea
B. A with meningitis
C. A with brain abscess

D. optic nerve injury with blindness
E. injury to the medial rectus muscle with diplopia
REF. Meyers D, Myers EN: The Laryngoscope, 84:833, May'74

1342. Which of the following may cause sudden sensori-neural hearing loss?
A. diabetes
B. hypercholesterolemia
C. metastatic carcinoma
D. allergy
E. multiple sclerosis
REF. Simmons FB: The Laryngoscope, 83:1221, Aug'73

1343. A preponderance of eosinophils is frequently considered diagnostic of allergy. The role of the eosinophil in the immune response, however, is not clear. Eosinophilia is associated with which of the following conditions?
A. food, drug, respiratory allergies
B. cutaneous hypersensitivity
C. infections
D. parasitic infestations
E. pernicious anemia
F. chronic myelogenous leukemia
G. Hodgkin's disease
H. myeloma
I. collagenous diseases
J. sarcoidosis
K. neoplasms
L. radiation exposure
M. Löffler's syndrome
N. Löffler's endocarditis parietalis fibroplastica
O. disseminated eosinophilic collagenosis
P. eosinophilic leukemia
Q. eosinophilic granulomas
REF. Zuker-Franklin D: Consultant, 14:No. 6: 131, June '74

1344. The eosinophils have which of the following features?
A. functionally resemble neutrophils
B. ameboid motion
C. phagocytize certain bacteria, mycoplasmas, inert particles, sensitized erythrocytes
D. inactivate histamine
E. inactivate bradykinin
F. probably inactivate serotonin
REF. Zuker-Franklin D: Consultant, 14:No. 6: 131, June '74

1345. Eosinophilia has the ability to:
A. protect guinea pigs from anaphylaxis induced by small amounts of histamine
B. protect guinea pigs from anaphylaxis induced by small amounts of carefully titrated allergens
C. ingest immune complexes
D. develop in agammaglobulinemia
E. develop in immunodeficiency syndromes
REF. Zuker-Franklin D: Consultant, 14:No. 6: 131, June '74

1346. Although all of the following are true, which features are unique with eosinophils?
A. during phagocytosis, the granules of the eosinophil coalesce with the phagocytic vacuole as is the case with neutrophils
B. granules possess all the hydrolytic enzymes found in lysosomes from other tissues and are considered therefore primary lysosomes
C. granules have a particularly high peroxidase content
D. granules have an usual ultrastructure (crystalline core)
E. crystalline core of the eosinophil granule is poorly soluble in physiologic fluids and when the eosinophil disintegrates as in the sputum of bronchial asthma, the crystalline core of the granules aggregate to form the nidus of Charcot-Leyden crystals
F. granular cores are not disrupted by chemical or osmotic lysis or by lysis by physiologic agents (trypsin, pepsin, streptolysin-o)
REF. Zuker-Franklin D: Consultant, 14:No. 6:131, June '74. (See Fig. 28)

1347. History is important in the evaluation of a patient with (or might develop) a drug reaction. Which of the following questions are significant?
A. do you have seasonal hay fever or asthma?
B. do you have reactions on exposure to any animals or insects?
C. do you have reactions on exposure to poison ivy?
D. do you have reactions on exposure to penicillin, sulfa, aspirin, local anesthetics?
E. do you have any unusual reactions during routine immunizations?
REF. Grater WC: Consultant, 14:No. 6: 119, June '74

1348. Aspirin is a frequent cause of drug allergy and the mechanism is due to:
A. aspirin (antigen) combines with circulating antibody (Reagin) giving off chemical mediator histamine producing patient's allergic symptoms
B. A but giving off serotonin causing symptoms
C. A but giving off bradykinin causing symptoms
D. A but giving off slow-reacting substance causing symptoms
E. unknown
REF. Grater WE: Consultant, 14:No. 6: 119, June'74

IN THE FOLLOWING QUESTION, MATCH EACH LETTERED ITEM WITH ONE NUMBERED ITEM. EACH CHOICE MAY BE USED ONLY ONCE:

1349. Drug sensitivity reactions fall into three major classifications:
A. protein and vegetable gums
B. crystalloid drugs
C. contact dermatitis

1. drug (antigen) combines with circulating antibody (Reagin) giving off chemical mediators (such as histamine) causing allergic symptoms
2. drug or hapten (partial antigen) combines with a body protein to form a complete antigen with the usual antigen-antibody reaction
3. cellular reaction of delayed inflammatory type with repeated exposure (local or injection) 4 to 72 hours later causing local allergic reaction (contact dermatitis)

REF. Grater WC: Consultant, 14:No. 6: 119, June'74

1350. Chemical mediators in the usual antigen-antibody (Reagin) reaction include which of the following?
A. histamine
B. serotonin
C. bradykinin
D. slow-reacting substance (material that contracts smooth muscle more slowly and for a longer time than histamine)
E. none of the above
REF. Grater WC: Consultant, 14:No. 6: 119, June'74

1351. The most practical (immediate or delayed reaction) tests for allergy to protein and vegetable gums (including some drugs) are:
A. patch
B. scratch or pressure puncture
C. intradermal
D. PK (Prausnitz-Küstner)
E. rechallenge
REF. Grater WC: Consultant, 14:No. 6: 119, June'74

1352. The most practical tests for allergy to crystalloid drugs (most drugs used today) are:
A. patch
B. scratch or pressure puncture
C. intradermal
D. PK (Prausnitz-Küstner)
E. rechallenge
REF. Grater WC: Consultant, 14:No. 6: 119, June'74

1353. The scratch or pressure puncture test is performed by placing a drop of aqueous solution of allergen on the patient's skin and a prick or scratch made through the drop (drop may be placed on the scratch). The scratch or pressure test is:
A. usually read in 20 minutes
B. less accurate but less dangerous than the intradermal test
C. should always precede the intradermal test
D. may have false negatives
E. response varies from one to four plus (wheal with pseudopods)
REF. Grater WC: Consultant, 14:No. 6: 119, June '74

1354. The intradermal test of a small amount of allergen is:
A. more sensitive than any other test available to the average allergist
B. more dangerous than the scratch or pressure test
C. should be performed when the scratch test is negative or at most weakly positive
D. may have false positives
E. can cause instant death
REF. Grater WC: Consultant, 14:No. 6: 119, June '74

1355. The Prausnitz-Küstner (PK) test is performed by injecting the allergic person's serum into the skin of a nonallergic individual and then:
A. expecting an erythematous reaction in 24 hours
B. A in 48 hours
C. A in one week
D. challenging the sensitized site with the allergen after a period of 24 to 48 hours
E. D after a period of nine days
REF. Grater WC: Consultant, 14:No. 6: 119, June '74

1356. Probably the most dangerous test to determine a suspected drug allergen is:
A. scratch or pressure
B. intradermal
C. PK (Prausnitz-Küstner)
D. patch
E. rechallenge
REF. Grater WC: Consultant, 14:No. 6: 119, June '74

1357. A patch test should not be performed until the patient has recovered from the initial bout of contact dermatitis. The patch containing the suspected allergen is placed on the patient's unbroken skin for a period in days of (depending on patient's complaints of irritation):
A. 1
B. 2
C. 3
D. 4
E. 5
REF. Grater WC: Consultant, 14:No. 6: 119, June '74

1358. Which of the following allergy tests available only in research departments appear to be probable clinical realities?
A. histamine release from leukocytes
B. lymphocyte transformation test
C. skin window test
D. immunoglobulin E test
E. lymphokine determinations
REF. Grater WC: Consultant, 14:No. 6: 119, June '74

1359. In the differential diagnosis of bilateral nasal polyps, which unusual one of the following conditions should be considered?
A. allergy
B. infection
C. cystic fibrosis
D. antro-choanal polyps
E. chromophobe adenoma of the pituitary gland
REF. Sadick MK, Nagori MA, Jafarey NA: J Laryngol & Otol, 88:379, Apr '74

1360. The most common associated disease with allergic rhinitis and nasal polyps is which one of the following:
A. maxillary sinusitis
B. frontal sinusitis
C. nasopharyngitis
D. sphenoiditis
E. bronchial asthma
REF. Yassin A, Fouad H, Abu-el-Ezz F, Issa H, Basyouni A: J Laryngol & Otol, 88:39, Apr '74

1361. Auto-immunity in nasal allergy should be considered because:
A. two types of autoantibodies against sinus tissue have been reported, one which cross-reacted with lung tissue
B. nasal infection with Staphylococcus aureus may change the proteins in the mucous membrane and become antigenic and cause intrinsic bronchial asthma
C. atrophic rhinitis may be an autoimmune disease as precipitating and agglutinating autoantibodies can be demonstrated against nasal mucosa
D. repeated bacterial or viral infections in cases of polypi and allergy change the antigenicity of nasal mucosa which then becomes "foreign" to the body
E. infecting microorganisms and nasal mucosa may share an antigenic determinant bringing about a cross-reacting antibody which reacts with both microorganisms and nasal mucosal antigens (true of rheumatic fever)
F. repeated polypectomies may release cellular proteins hidden from the immune system without early development of tolerance and these released auto-antigens induce the formation of autoantibodies such as in thyroiditis
REF. Yassin A, Fouad H, Abu-El-Ezz F, Issa H, Basyouni A: J Laryngol & Otol, 88:39, Jan'74

1362. Studies on the immunobiological position and local immunity of the tonsil in rabbits indicate:
A. the tonsil is a peripheral lymphatic organ with capacity for local immunity
B. the tonsil has no capacity for local immunity
C. IgM-antibody producing cells are recognized in tonsils in both young and adults groups
D. IgM is not found in tonsils
E. IgG is not found in all tonsils
REF. Suzuki M, Imai A, Kojima K, Kitami O: Jap Jour Otol, 76:1045, Jul-Dec'73

1363. In recent studies on nasal allergy, the immunoglobulin E (IgE) was not detected in:
A. epithelial cells or basement membrane of nasal mucosa in non-allergic patients
B. epithelial cells or basement membrane of nasal mucosa in allergic patients
C. tonsils
D. lymph nodes
E. intestinal mucosa
REF. Ishikawa T, Miyashita H, Shimada T: Jap Jour Otol, 76:1095, Jul-Dec'73

1364. Nasal polyps result from pathological changes in the nasal and sinus mucosa and the following influence the production of nasal polyps:
A. reaction to allergens
B. reaction to infection
C. reaction to systemic conditions such as cystic fibrosis
D. reaction to A and B combination
E. any or all of the above
REF. Saunders SH: Trans Amer Laryng Assoc. 93:73, Apr'72

1365. Nasal polyposis most frequently begins with:
A. pollenosis
B. infection
C. cystic fibrosis
D. A and then B
E. B and then A
REF. Saunders SH: Trans Amer Laryng Assoc, 93:73, Apr'72

1366. Allergic reaction including nasal polyposis can only be prevented from progressing by:
A. antihistamines
B. corticosteroids
C. antibiotics
D. hyposensitization
E. combination A, B and C
REF. Saunders SH: Trans Amer Laryng Assoc, 93:73, Apr'72

1367. Basic types of food allergy are:
A. fixed
B. cyclic
C. thermal
D. A and B
E. A and C
REF. Williams RI: Trans Amer Laryng Assoc, 93:85, Apr'72

1368. Undesirable surgical sequelae due to pansinus surgery for chronic sinus disease and polyps are:
A. diplopia following detachment of the trochlea from the orbital rim
B. anesthesia of the forehead if the supraorbital nerve is cut
C. enophthalmos when a large portion of the ethmo-orbital wall and floor of the frontal sinus is removed
D. pain and swelling of the eyelids and forehead with or without osteomyelitis
E. postoperative mucoceles and pyoceles
REF. Saunders SH: Trans Amer Laryng Assoc, 93:73, Apr'72

1369. The second stage of cyclic food allergy occurs when food is completely avoided for at least the following number of days, that is, the patient's reaction to food will change from a stage of masking (no, or reduced, reaction) to a stage of hyperacute reaction or an accentuated reaction, compared to the previous masked reaction:
A. one day
B. two days
C. three days
D. four days
E. five days
REF. Williams RI: Trans Amer Laryng Assoc, 93:85, Apr'72

1370. Which of the following groups of foods are most capable of producing allergic edema?
A. wheat, corn, tomato, soy, lettuce, celery, potato
B. egg, chicken
C. beef, milk
D. fruit juices
E. yeast
REF. Williams RI: Trans Amer Laryng Assoc, 93:85, Apr'72

1371. Active sensitization to food implies that the food causes symptoms every time it is eaten. Latent sensitization to foods may be very confusing to both patient and physician. In testing the patient, which of the following is important?
A. test the food and determine any immediate reaction
B. if no reaction to A, feed the food every fifth day for six feedings
C. if no reaction to B, feed the food once daily every third day
D. if no reaction to A, B, or C, masking may have occurred and the food may be tolerated
E. if reaction occurs to A, B, or C, the food should be completely avoided until food tolerance is gained later (12 days to as long as two years)
REF. Williams RI: Trans Amer Laryng Assoc, 93:85, Apr'72

1372. Mold control in shower stalls or damp basements can be controlled by:
A. skin testing with desensitization of the offending mold
B. desensitization to trichophyton alone
C. desensitization to oidiomycin alone
D. desensitization to T. O. E. (trichophyton, oidiomycin and epidermophyton)
E. 5 to 10 ccs of formaldehyde (37%) in small saucers every 50 square feet of floor space
REF. Williams RI: Trans Amer Laryng Assoc, 93:85, Apr'72

1373. Food allergy is dynamic, not static, and can be influenced by which of the following:
A. thermal changes when patient is exposed to a low temperature critical for that patient and usually resulting in fever and purulent sinus disease
B. seasonal factors such as a superimposed pollen allergic reaction
C. geographic changes
D. changes in food habits (eating same food twice in one day instead of once daily) (Hippocrates)
E. emotion
REF. Williams RI: Trans Amer Laryng Assoc, 93:85, Apr'72

1374. All of the following are accepted methods of treating food allergies but the best treatment is:
A. complete avoidance until food tolerance is gained
B. injections of the neutralizing dosage as determined by the provocative food test, once or twice weekly until tolerance is gained
C. sublingual therapy
D, information to patients outlining possible contact
E. all of the above
REF. Williams RI: Trans Amer Laryng Assoc, 93:85, Apr'72. Rinkel HJ, Randolph TG, Zeller M: Food Allergy, Springfield, Ill. Charles C. Thomas Co., 1951

1375. Sudden severe and alarming laryngeal edema can occur from:
A. foods such as ice cream, candy bars, chewing gum (chicle), beef
B. bee stings
C. antibiotic therapy such as penicillin
D. drugs such as coal tar products (aspirin)
E. inhalant factors such as animal danders, house dust, cosmetics, molds, volatile oils or emanations from plants and commonly termed terpenes, pollens of trees-grasses-weeds
REF. Williams RI: Trans Amer Laryng Assoc, 93:85, Apr'72. Frank DI: Arch Otolaryng, 32:1067, '40. Paparella MM: J. Laryng, 78:89, '64. Jacobs CC, Hansel FK; Bull Hansel Foundation, 1:61, '52. Hansel FK: Clinical Allergy, St. Louis, C. V. Mosby Co., '53. Anderson OE: Arch Otolaryng, 54:34, '51.

1376. In the treatment of allergic cochleovestibular disturbances (Ménière's disease, hydrops) which of the following methods of treatment have been successful? (See Fig. 29)
A. provocative food testing by deliberate injection of an antigen to provoke a mild systemic reaction and neutralization by the immediate injection of a usually weaker dilution of the identical antigen to relieve symptoms
B. 150 mg nicotinic acid three times daily before meals
C. dilute histamine injected subcutaneously twice weekly
D. 20 mg diazepam (valium) daily and/or 500 mg chlorothiazide (diuril) daily
E. Klockhoff's glycerin test
REF. Clemis JD: Trans Am Acad Ophthalmol-Otolaryngol, 76:1444, Nov-Dec, '72. Rinkel HJ, Lee CH, Brown DW Jr. et al: Arch Otolaryng, 79:71, '64. Klockhoff I, Lindblom U: Acta Otolaryng, Suppl 224, 449, '67.

1377. Which of the following cell types have phagocytic function?
A. neutrophils
B. macrophages
C. basophils
D. mast cells
E. lymphocytes
REF. Bellanti J: Allergy News Bulletin (Ann Meeting AAIA), 2:10:3, '73

1378. Which one of the following cell types is characteristically seen in acute inflammation?
A. macrophage
B. eosinophil
C. neutrophil
D. basophil
E. lymphocyte
REF. Bellanti J: Allergy News Bulletin (Ann Meeting AAIA), 2:10:3, '73

1379. Which of the following cells are important in antibody production?
A. T
B. B
C. A
D. C
E. D
REF. Bellanti J: Allergy News Bulletin (Ann Meeting AAIA), 2:10:3, '73

1380. The most abundant of the immunoglobulins in the serum are:
A. IgM
B. IgG
C. IgA
D. IgD
E. IgE
REF. Bellanti J: Allergy News Bulletin (Ann Meeting AAIA), 2:10:3, '73

1381. Which of the following are synthesized predominatly in the linings of the respiratory and intestinal tracts?
A. IgM
B. IgG
C. IgA
D. IgD
E. IgE
REF. Bellanti J: Allergy News Bulletin (Ann Meeting AAIA), 2:10:3, '73

1382. The IgG molecule contains:
A. two light chains and two heavy chains
B. five light chains and five heavy chains
C. a secretory piece
D. all of the above
E. none of the above
REF. Bellanti J: Allergy News Bulletin (Ann Meeting AAIA), 2:10:3, '73

1383. The activation of which complement component is affected in hereditary angioedema?
A. C3
B. C5
C. C7
D. $C1_q$
E. C8
REF. Bellanti J: Allergy News Bulletin (Ann Meeting AAIA), 2:10:3, '73

1384. All are examples of antigen-antibody interactions except:
A. precipitation
B. agglutination
C. complement-fixation
D. neutralization
E. MIF production
REF. Bellanti J: Allergy News Bulletin (Ann Meeting AAIA), 2:10:3, '73

1385. The basic difference between tolerance and immunosuppression is that:
A. tolerance is antigen specific, immunosuppressions is more generalized
B. tolerance is only seen in newborns
C. immunosuppression is antigen specific
D. all of the above
E. none of the above
REF. Bellanti J: Allergy News Bulletin (Ann Meeting AAIA), 2:10:3, '73

1386. Which of the following are seen in the DiGeorge syndrome?
A. absence of parathyroid
B. absence of thyroid
C. absence of thymus
D. all of the above
E. none of the above
REF. Bellanti J: Allergy News Bulletin (Ann Meeting AAIA), 2:10:3, '73

FIGURES FOR SECTION VI

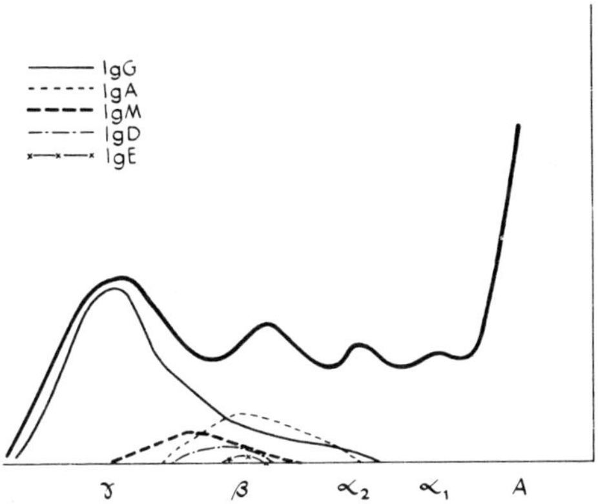

Fig. 27A. Distribution of immunoglobulin in normal human serum after electro-phoresis. Areas under respective lines indicate relative amounts and electro-phoretic distribution of IgG, IgA, IgD and IgE.

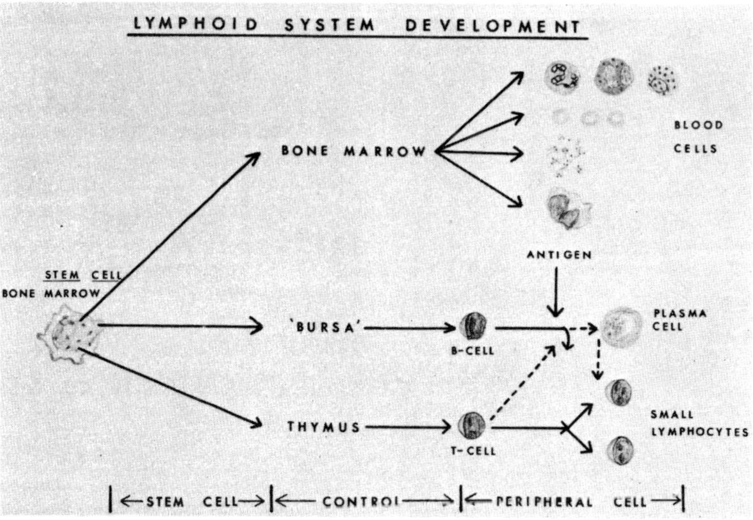

Fig. 27B. Development of lymphoid system

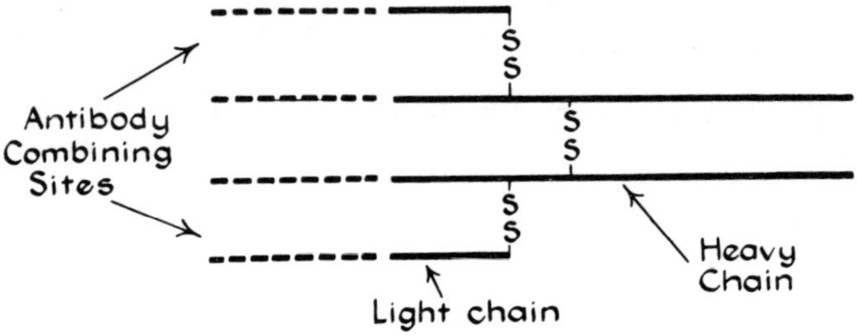

Fig. 27C. Schematic representation of the four-chain structure of IgG linked by three interchain disulfide bridges. Broken lines show variable portion of chains. (After Porter and Press, 1962, modified by Cohen and Milstein, 1967)

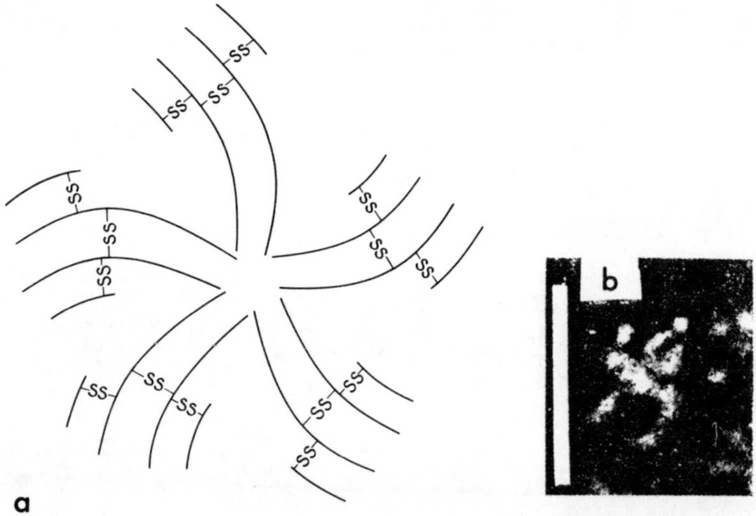

Fig. 27D. (a) One possible schematic model of IgM structure. Five 7S subunits are arranged in a spiral. (b) An electron micrograph showing a spiral five subunit structure. (From Svehag, et al., 1967). (Courtesy of Allansmith, M. R.: Trans Amer Soc Ophth-Otolaryng Allergy, 13:9, Sept '72)

Figs. 27A, B, C and D courtesy of Allansmith, M. R.: Trans Amer Soc Ophth-Otolaryng Allergy, 13:9, Sept '72

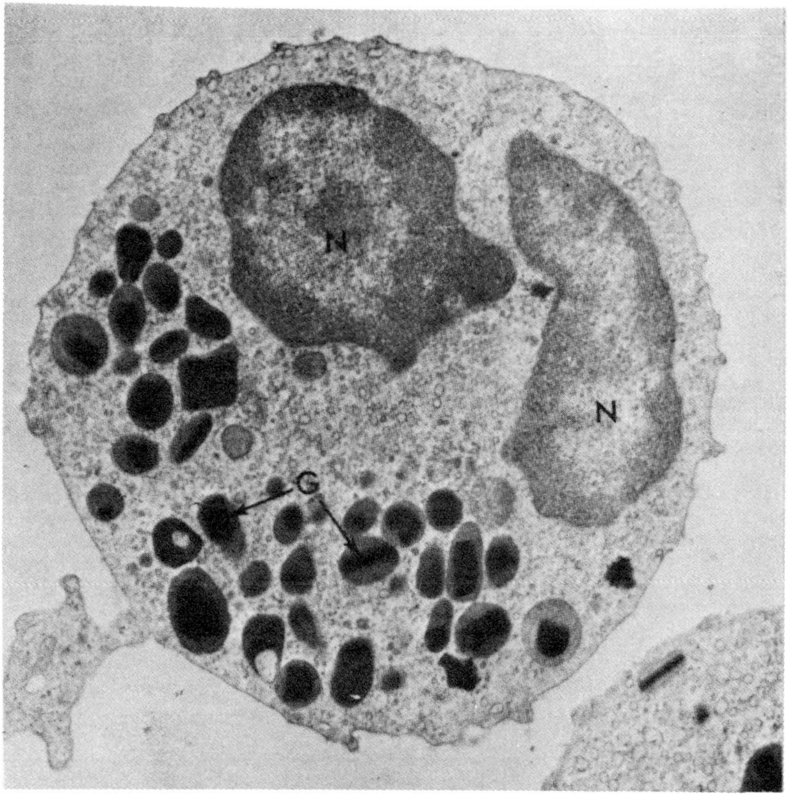

Fig. 28. Human eosinophil showing characteristic ultrastructure of the granules (G). Arrows point to cores of granules which probably form the nidus of Charcot-Leyden crystals. Nucleus (N). (Courtesy of Zucker-Franklin, D.: Consultant 14; No. 6:131, June, 1974)

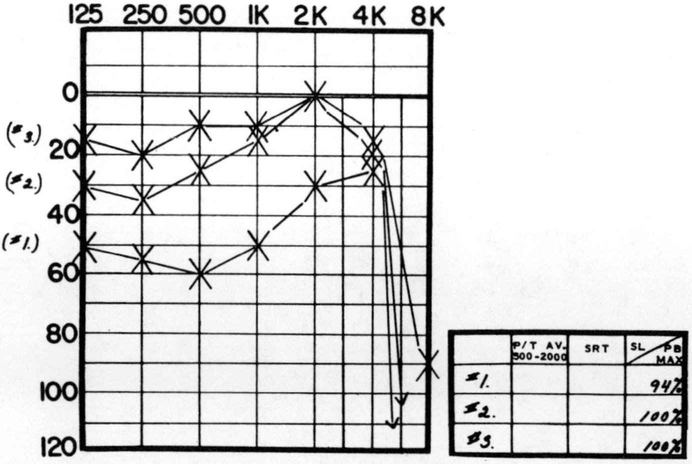

Fig. 29A. Audiogram demonstrating progressive improvement in auditory acuity and discrimination during therapeutic allergic management over three months. (Courtesy of Clemis, J. D. : Trans Amer Soc Ophthal-Otolaryng Allergy, 13:59, Sept '72)

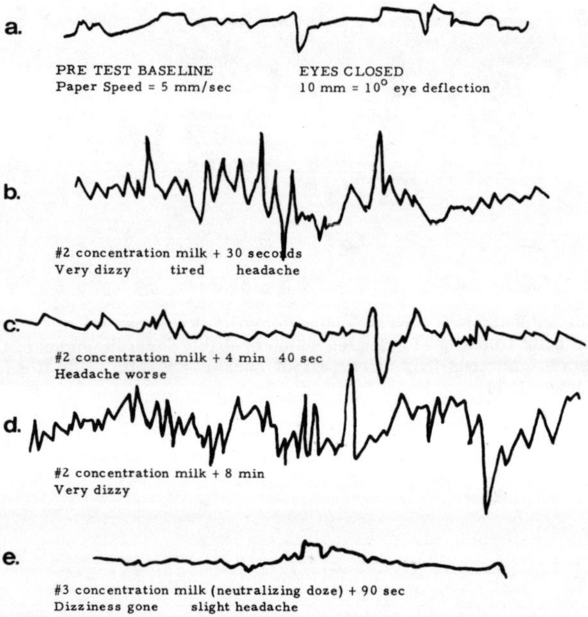

Fig. 29B. Electronystagmograph demonstrating allergic cochleovestibular disturbances. (Courtesy of Clemis, J. D. : Trans Amer Soc Ophthal-Otolaryng Allergy, 13:59, Sept '72)

1387. Acquired nasopharyngeal stenosis is an uncommon lesion and is most frequently observed as a complication of:
A. infections, acute
B. adenotonsillectomy
C. chemical burns
D. gunshot wounds
E. infections chronic, such as tuberculosis
REF. Pratt LW: The Laryngoscope, 84:707, May'74

1388. Nasopharyngeal stenosis is:
A. partial obstruction of the nasopharynx caused by scar tissue
B. complete obstruction of the nasopharynx caused by scar tissue
C. partial absence of nasopharyngeal opening caused by congenital maldevelopment
D. complete absence of nasopharyngeal opening caused by congenital maldevelopment
E. choanal atresia
REF. Pratt LW: The Laryngoscope, 84:707, May'74

1389. Nasopharyngeal atresia is:
A. partial obstruction of the nasopharynx caused by scar tissue
B. complete obstruction of the nasopharynx caused by scar tissue
C. partial absence of nasopharyngeal opening caused by congenital maldevelopment
D. complete absence of nasopharyngeal opening caused by congenital maldevelopment
E. choanal atresia
REF. Pratt LW: The Laryngoscope, 84:707, May'74

1390. The symptoms of nasopharyngeal stenosis are usually:
A. nasal obstruction
B. mouth breathing
C. alteration in tone and timbre of the voice
D. dysphagia
E. considerable nasal watery discharge
REF. Pratt LW: The Laryngoscope, 84:707, May'74

1391. Acquired nasopharyngeal stenosis is usually traumatic (iatrogenic) with an incidence rate of how many cases following 100, 000 adenotonsillectomies?
A. one
B. three
C. twenty-two
D. forty-seven
E. one hundred two
REF. Pratt LW: The Laryngoscope, 84:707, May'74

1392. In nasopharyngeal stenosis the nasal mucosa appears:
A. thickened
B. atrophic
C. more edematous than usual
D. pale
E. purplish or violaceous color
REF. Pratt LW: The Laryngoscope, 84:707, May'74

1393. Which of the following infections can cause nasopharyngeal stenosis?
A. syphilis
B. tuberculosis
C. rhinoscleroma
D. diphtheria
E. lupus
F. scarlet fever
REF. Pratt LW: The Laryngoscope, 84:707, May'74

1394. The etiology of nasopharyngeal stenosis secondary to adenotonsillectomies is usually due to:
A. adenoidectomy with a hot adenotome or extensive electrocauterization of the nasopharynx to control bleeding from the adenoid bed
B. adenotonsillectomy with resection of unusually large lateral bands
C. revisional surgery

D. keloid or cicatrizing diathesis
E. surgery (T & A) in the presence of acute pharyngitis, purulent sinusitis (and active syphilis)
REF. Pratt LW: The Laryngoscope, 84:707, May '74

1395. Which of the following can cause nasopharyngeal stenosis?
A. postnasal packing
B. repair velopalatial insufficiency
C. removal of nasopharyngeal tumors
D. ammonia chemical burn
E. sodium and potassium hydroxide burns
REF. Pratt LW: The Laryngoscope, 84:707, May '74

1396. Which one of the following chemicals when swallowed is most likely to cause nasopharyngeal stenosis?
A. ammonia
B. sodium hydroxide
C. potassium hydroxide
REF. Pratt LW: The Laryngoscope, 84:707, May '74

1397. Although all of the following have been successful, which one of the following surgical techniques appears to be the most logical procedure for repair of a nasopharyngeal stenosis?
A. simple dilatation-finger
B. obturator
C. suturing
D. seton with lead shot, or skin graft, or obturator with graft, or flap
E. atretic nasopharynx opened surgically, scar tissue resected, raw surfaces covered with viable mucosal flaps (regional-pharynx or palate; pedicle-cheek or pharynx or palate)
REF. Pratt LW: The Laryngoscope, 84:707, May '74

1398. Nasopharyngeal stenosis due to rhinoscleroma may be cured by:
A. surgical resection
B. surgical resection with graft (split-thickness)
C. self-limiting
D. antibiotics
E. radiation therapy
REF. Pratt LW: The Laryngoscope, 84:707, May '74

1399. Nasopharyngeal angiofibroma challenges the otolaryngologist in considering the extent of the tumor and treatment. Which one of the following procedures is most important in the diagnosis and assessment of an angiofibroma in the nasopharynx (grayish or red mass with epistaxis)?
A. biopsy
B. routine sinus x-rays
C. polytome x-rays
D. arteriography
E. surgical removal with frozen section
REF. Biller HF, Sessions DG, Ogura JH: The Laryngoscope, 84:695, May '74

1400. Which of the following adjuncts appear to be most successful in diminishing blood supply to nasopharyngeal angiofibromas prior to surgical removal?
A. estrogen therapy
B. cryotherapy
C. arterial occlusions with beads inserted at the initial arteriogram
D. transantral ligation of the internal maxillary artery
E. temporary occlusion of external carotid artery
REF. Biller HF, Sessions DG, Ogura JH: The Laryngoscope, 84:695, May '74

1401. The purpose of labyrinthine cryosurgery is relief of:
A. vertigo even with hearing loss
B. vertigo without hearing loss
C. tinnitus improvement
D. vertigo and tinnitus improvement
E. vertigo with hearing improvement
REF. Wolfson RJ, Ishiyama E: The Laryngoscope, 84:757, May '74

1402. In performing cryosurgery, a cryogenic application is made to the thinned bony wall of the horizontal semicircular canal for a total of six minutes (three applications of two minutes each) using a termperature of:
A. -30° C
B. -40° C
C. -70°C
D. -160° C
E. -190° C
REF. Wolfson RJ, Ishiyama E: The Laryngoscope, 84:757, May '74

1403. Vertigo following labyrinthine cryosurgery is relieved in what percent of cases?
A. 15
B. 25
C. 50
D. 75
E. 90
REF. Wolfson RJ, Ishiyama E: The Laryngoscope, 84:757, May '74

1404. Histological otosclerosis with pure sensorineural hearing loss with atrophy of the supporting sensory and neural structures:
A. does not necessarily involve the stapes
B. invariably fixes the stapes
REF. Schuknecht HF, Kirchner JC: The Laryngoscope, 84:766, May '74

1405. One of the main problems in middle ear surgery (tympanoplasty) is assuring that the repositioned ossicles or cartilage struts remain in a fixed position. In an experimental study (squirrel monkeys and cats) the tissue adhesive isobutyl 2-cyangacrylate (coapt) showed that it was:
A. non-toxic
B. relatively easy to use in the middle ear
C. appeared to attach firmly to middle ear structures
D. non-inflammatory
E. toxic with severe inflammatory response
REF. Kaufman RS: The Laryngoscope, 84:793, May '74

1406. One of the main problems in middle ear surgery including stapedectomies and tympanoplasties is the formation of adhesions. The anti-inflammatory effects of glucocorticoids used topically in the middle ear has an anti-inflammatory effect that is:
A. detrimental
B. beneficial
C. no effect
D. controls middle ear inflammatory response to tissue adhesive
E. reduces middle ear inflammatory response to tissue adhesive
REF. Kaufman RS: The Laryngoscope, 84:793, May '74

1407. Among the most active anti-inflammatory glucocorticoids is dexamethasone (decadron) having the advantages of being:
A. water-soluble
B. 25 - 30 times as potent as hydrocortisone
C. very little sodium-retaining property
D. very effective as a topical application
E. anti-inflammatory effects appear to depend upon direct local action of the drug
REF. Kaufman RS: The Laryngoscope, 84:793, May '74

1408. Tubomyringotomy was first introduced in the treatment of serous otitis media by:
A. Beverly Armstrong (20th Century)
B. Astley Cooper (1801)
C. Peter Degravers (1788)
D. Julius Busson (1748)
E. J. A. Saissy (1829)
F. A. Politzer (1860's)
G. probably unknown
REF. Alberti PW: The Laryngoscope, 84:805, May'74

1409. To ascertain vestibular dysfunction, the tests indicated in electronystagmography is in most instances:
A. gaze nystagmus
B. tracing a pendulum
C. spontaneous nystagmus
D. positional nystagmus
E. rotation on a torsion swing
REF. Spector M: The Laryngoscope, 84:816, May'74

1410. Chronic use of marijuana appears to have which of the following effects?
A. decrease in motor performance after immediate use
B. decrease in mental performance after immediate use
C. decrease in maximum amplitude on torsion swing (vestibular tests)
D. increase in incidence of nystagmus in two or more supine positions (vestibular tests)
E. decrease in speed of slow component on caloric tests (vestibular tests)
REF. Spector M: The Laryngoscope, 84:816, May'74

1411. Heavy marijuana users show:
A. no auditory changes
B. sensorineural loss in the higher frequencies
C. no electroencephalography significant effects
D. no acute effects on vestibular system
E. definite positive changes in heavy marijuana users (vestibular)
REF. Spector M: The Laryngoscope, 84:816, May'74

1412. An experimental study with adult squirrel monkeys indicate that prolonged and heavy exposure to lead produces:
A. minimal damage to the labyrinth
B. minimal damage to the cochlea
C. may be a reduction in the duration and intensity of induced nystagmus
D. segmental demyelination of VIIIth nerve fibers
E. axonal degeneration of VIIIth nerve fibers
REF. Wilpizeski C: The Laryngoscope, 84:821, May'74

1413. Unilateral nasal obstruction should alert the physician to:
A. foreign body
B. deviated septum or spurs
C. choanal polyp
D. nasopharyngeal disease
E. benign or malignant tumors
REF. Meyers D, Myers EN: The Laryngoscope, 84:833, May'74

1414. In the management of the "puffy eye" due to sinus disease which of the following signs indicate early inflammatory reaction?
A. edema and redness of eyelids
B. pain
C. febrile course
D. x-ray evidence of sinus disease
E. purulent nasal discharge
REF. Welsh LW, Welsh JJ: The Laryngoscope, 84:848, May'74

1415. In the management of the "puffy eye" due to sinus disease which of the following signs indicate orbital cellulitis?
A. unilateral involvement
B. proptosis
C. chemosis

D. edema of eyelids
E. limitation of extra ocular movements due to orbital congestion and edema
REF. Welsh LW, Welsh JJ: The Laryngoscope, 84:848, May'74

1416. In the management of the "puffy eye" due to sinus disease which of the following signs indicate cavernous sinus thrombosis?
A. bilateral involvement or rapid progression of signs from one eye to the other
B. proptosis, chemosis, edema of eyelids
C. limitation of EOM (extra ocular movements) due to involvement of III, IV, and VI nerves
D. meningitis or meningeal irritation
E. residual III, IV and VI palsies after successful treatment
REF. Welsh LW, Welsh JJ: The Laryngoscope, 84:848, May'74

1417. Most of the patients with orbital complications of sinus disease are in age in years:
A. under 20
B. 21 - 30
C. 31 - 40
D. 41 - 50
E. over 51
REF. Welsh LW, Welsh JJ: The Laryngoscope, 84:848, May'74

1418. Predisposing factors leading to orbital infection from sinus disease are:
A. viral upper respiratory infection during flu epidemics
B. external injury with bacterial invasion
C. surgical trauma, particularly frontal, with bacterial invasion
D. swimming pool contamination as a sequelae to foot entry from a diving board allowing a rush of water into the nose and through the nasofrontal duct into the sinus
E. septal deflection
REF. Welsh LW, Welsh JJ: The Laryngoscope, 84:848, May'74

1419. After failure of aggressive medical therapy, the criteria for surgery in orbital complications of sinus disease are:
A. persistent toxicity, fever, headache
B. continued edema, proptosis and chemosis
C. orbital abscess
D. sinus empyema
E. intra-cranial extension
REF. Welsh LW, Welsh JJ: The Laryngoscope, 84:848, May'74

1420. Factors indicating probable medical failure in orbital complications due to sinus disease are:
A. nature of offending organism cannot be identified before extensive progression of the disease has occurred
B. patients with repeated nasal polypectomy or intranasal ethmoidectomy with trauma and stenosis of the naso-frontal duct area
C. antecedent injury to the sinus ostia (auto accidents, etc.) or inadequately repaired or overlooked fracture of anterior frontal sinus wall
D. polyps or tumor blocking nasofrontal duct
E. patients with metabolic problems - diabetes, immunodeficiency diseases, immune state altered by therapy creating immune suppression or intolerance to infection - sarcoidosis, lymphoma, Wegener's granuloma
F. indifferent or negligent patient
REF. Welsh LW, Welsh JJ: The Laryngoscope, 84:848, May'74

1421. Osteoblastoma of the middle ear is:
A. benign
B. malignant
C. lesion of young people (usually age incidence between six and twelve years)

D. uncommon
E. synonyms are osteogenic fibroma, giant osteoid osteoma
F. synonyms are osteoid osteoma, giant cell tumor, osteogenic sarcoma
REF. Ronis ML, Obando M, Bucko MI, Liebman EP: The Laryngoscope, 84:857, May'74

1422. Although treatment varies depending upon the problems that arise, experience indicates that in undescended thyroid glands the following methods of therapy should be considered:
A. observation
B. suppressive doses of thyroid
C. isotope suppression
D. surgical excision
E. autotransplantation
REF. Wertz ML: The Laryngoscope, 84:507, Apr'74

1423. The fetal primordia of the thyroid gland develops:
A. as a downward growth from the floor of the primitive pharynx, initially anteriorly in the midline and then extends downward as a long tube (the thyroglossal duct)
B. thyroglossal duct follows the descent of the heart and aortic arch
C. the thyroglossal duct is bi-lobed and eventually reaches in front of the trachea and thyroid cartilage
D. thyroglossal duct in front of the trachea and thyroid cartilage coalesce with two lateral outgrowths from the fourth pharyngeal pouch (ultimobranchial bodies)
E. D is usually completed by the 10th fetal week
REF. Wertz ML: The Laryngoscope, 84:507, Apr'74

1424. Midline ectopic thyroid tissue has been found in:
A. base of tongue (lingual)
B. sublingual
C. subhyoid
D. lingual and subhyoid
E. diaphragm
REF. Wertz ML: The Laryngoscope, 84:507, Apr'74

1425. In evaluating a patient presenting a midline neck mass, which of the following should be considered most seriously in the differential diagnosis?
A. thyroglossal duct cyst
B. epidermal inclusion cyst
C. lymph node (benign or malignant)
D. lipoma
E. sebaceous cyst
F. ectopic thyroid gland
G. amyloid
H. angioma
I. adenoma
J. chondroma
REF. Wertz ML: The Laryngoscope, 84:507, Apr'74

1426. All of the following should be considered in the differential diagnosis in evaluating a patient with a midline lingual mass except:
A. lingual thyroid
B. epidermal inclusion cyst
C. angioma
D. amyloid
E. adenoma
F. cyst
G. sebaceous cyst
H. chondroma
I. fibroma
J. gumma
K. hypertrophy of the lingual tonsil
L. lymphangioma
M. papilloma
N. epithelioma
O. lymphosarcoma
REF. Wertz ML: The Laryngoscope, 84:507, Apr'74

1427. A thyroglossal duct cyst has which of the following features?
A. contains little or no functioning thyroid tissue
B. surgery is indicated because of disfiguration
C. surgery is indicated because of tendency toward recurrent inflammation
D. carcinomatous changes occur in approximately 4-6 percent
E. scintogram or scintiscan with radio-iodine indicated
REF. Wertz ML: The Laryngoscope, 84:507, Apr'74

1428. Undescended thyroid glands (ectopic thyroid glands) have which of the following features?
A. usually represents the only functioning thyroid tissue
B. carcinoma may be present (may be associated with prolonged excessive thyroid stimulating hormone (TSH) stimulation in a quantitatively deficient gland)
C. surgery always indicated
D. surgery never indicated
E. suppressive doses of thyroid in a euthyroid patient when significant functional or cosmetic change is indicated
REF. Wertz ML: The Laryngoscope, 84:507, Apr'74

1429. The management of undescended lingual and subhyoid ectopic thyroid tissue may consist of which of the following surgical procedures?
A. total removal
B. autogenous transplantation from subhyoid to lateral neck
C. B with excision of lingual thyroid
D. subhyoid transplantation to abdominal muscles
E. lingual transplantation to pectoralis muscle and abdomen with delayed transplant to liver
F. lingual transplantation (wafers) to abdomen
G. lingual transplantation wafers to neck musculature
H. lingual transplantation to neck as pedicle graft and wafers to abdomen
REF. Wertz ML: The Laryngoscope, 84:507, Apr'74

1430. Sudden pain in an ectopic thyroid gland indicates:
A. carcinomatous changes
B. sudden hypertrophy with extension into surrounding tissues
C. infection (bacterial)
D. thyroiditis (Hashimoto's disease)
E. severe hemorrhage
REF. Wertz ML: The Laryngoscope, 84:507, Apr'74

1431. Mucous membrane lesions associated with systemic lupus erythematosus (S. L. E.) and laryngeal manifestations necessitating tracheotomy are:
A. acute epiglottitis
B. acute laryngitis with mucosal ulceration, hemorrhagic bullae, perichondritis and diffuse edema
C. cricoarytenoid arthritis
D. cord tumor
E. vocal cord paralysis
REF. Toomey JM, Snyder GG, Maenza RM, Rothfield NF: The Laryngoscope, 84:522, Apr'74. Minchina RA, Fastovsky WA, Antonoua NA: Zhurnal Ushykth, 12:67, '71. Babich IF; Taranov: Vestnik Otorinolaryngol, 32:88, '70. Chatelanat F, Rauch S: Revue de Laryngol, Otologie-Rhinol, 80:233, '59

1432. In the differential diagnosis of a parotid growth with radiographic findings of calcification, which of the following should be considered?
A. mixed tumor
B. hemangioma
C. tuberculosis (lymph nodes)
D. lymph nodes involved with medullary thyroid carcinoma
E. pilomatrixoma (calcifying epithelioma of Malherbe)
REF. Krausen AS, Ansel DG, Mays BR: The Laryngoscope, 84:528, Apr'74

1433. In the rhinoplasty patient postoperative swelling can influence the cosmetic result and frustrate both the patient and the surgeon. There is a statistically significant difference and less postoperative edema if the patient's head is elevated:
A. maximally at 90°
B. 45°
C. 30°
D. 15°
E. level with body
REF. Stucker FJ: The Laryngoscope, 84:536, Apr'74

1434. All of the following malignancies occur in the submaxillary gland and are best removed by radical surgery. Which one of the following malignant tumors of the submaxillary gland has shown encouraging responses to irradiation?
A. cylindromas
B. adenocarcinomas
C. malignant mixed tumors
D. mucoepidermoid
E. squamous cell carcinoma
REF. Lowe JT, Farmer JC: The Laryngoscope, 84:542, Apr'74

1435. The most common cause of epistaxis is:
A. idiopathic bleeding from Little's area
B. cardiovascular causes (arteriosclerosis, hypertension, cardiac failure)
C. tumor
D. Osler's disease
E. uremia
REF. Juselius H: J Laryngol Otol, 88:317, Apr'74

1436. The most common cause of severe epistaxis in patients requiring arterial ligation is:
A. puncture maxillary antrum
B. tumor
C. liver disease (cirrhosis)
D. cardiovascular
E. infection
REF. Juselius H: J Laryngol & Otol, 88:317, Apr'74

1437. Although all of the following procedures are necessary at times, which one of the following arterial ligations is most commonly done in severe uncontrolled epistaxis?
A. internal maxillary artery
B. external carotid artery
C. external carotid plus ethmoidal
D. ethmoidal
E. ethmoidal plus internal maxillary plus external carotid
REF. Juselius H: J Laryngol & Otol, 88:317, Apr'74

1438. Ligation of the internal maxillary artery is preferable to ligation of the external carotid artery because:
A. point of ligation is as close as possible to the bleeding-point (good surgical principle)
B. recurrence of epistaxis due to anastomoses less likely to occur
C. procedure easy to perform
D. safely done with local anesthesia
E. operating microscope facilitates the operation
REF. Juselius H: J Laryngol & Otol, 88:317, Apr'74

1439. Recurrent laryngeal nerve paralysis in association with thyroid disease:
A. always indicates malignancy of the thyroid
B. does not necessarily indicate malignancy
REF. Worgan D, Saunders S, Jones J: J Laryngol & Otol, 88:375, Apr'74

1440. Which of the following conditions can cause recurrent laryngeal nerve paralysis:
A. simple goitre
B. left atrium in mitral stenosis
C. aneurysm of the aorta
D. infection
E. substernal goitre at the thoracic inlet
REF. Worgan D, Saunders S, Jones J: J Laryngol & Otol, 88:375, Apr'74

1441. In the differential diagnosis of a peritonsillar abscess, which of the following conditions should be considered (and in any suspicious cases needle aspiration should precede incision and drainage)?
A. internal carotid artery aneurysm
B. A with tonsillitis and/or pharyngitis
C. A with coexistant peritonsillar abscess
D. benign or malignant tumors
E. carotid body tumor with tonsillitis and/or pharyngitis
REF. Henry RC: J Laryngol & Otol, 88:379, Apr'74

1442. Which of the following are indications for revision stapedectomy or at least re-exploration of the middle ear?
A. postural vertigo, not improving (perilymph leak or fistula)
B. fluctuating deafness
C. late conductive deafness (opposite ear better)
D. late conductive deafness (opposite ear worse)
E. sudden conductive hearing loss (possible prosthetic failure)
REF. Shah N: J Laryngol & Otol, 88:379, Apr'74

1443. Although all of the following occur, the most common cause of post-stapedectomy conductive hearing loss is:
A. fixed malleus
B. eccentric strut
C. "short" piston
D. further otosclerosis
E. displaced prosthesis (usually due to necrosis of the lenticular process)
REF. Dawes JDK, Curry AR: J Laryngol & Otol, 88:379, Apr'74

1444. Hypersalivation (drooling) is comparatively rare but sometimes occurs as a problem in cerebral palsy and mentally retarded persons. Drooling has been successfully treated by:
A. atropine
B. atropine-like derivatives
C. tympanotomy with division of the chorda tympani nerve in the middle ear
D. C with extirpation of the submandibular gland on the other side
E. bilateral excision of both submandibular glands
REF. Diamant H, Kumlien A: J Laryngol & Otol, 88:379, Apr'74

1445. In patients with sudden idiopathic sensorineural hearing loss, which of the following procedures may make the patients' condition worse?
A. valsalva maneuver or eustachian tube inflation
B. diagnostic myringotomies
C. caloric irrigations during the first week-may do all other vestibular tests by electronystagmography (ENG)
D. a routine audiogram when severe sensorineural loss exists
E. complete audiological survey-including speech tests, tone decay, loudness balance, Békésy audiograms, SISI, impedance tympanometry
REF. Simmons FB: The Laryngoscope, 83:1221, Aug'73

1446. Temporary threshold shifts in hearing even in a normal ear can be caused by tones in decibels (db) above:
A. 25
B. 33
C. 57
D. 61
E. 85
REF. Simmons FB: The Laryngoscope, 83:1221, Aug'73

1447. Which of the following may cause sudden sensori-neural hearing loss?
A. virus infections (localized in the ear, more than one cranial nerve-encephalitis)
B. blood disorders-spasm, infarcts, hemorrhage, macroglobulinemia, polycythemia

C. bacterial infections-meningitis from the middle ear
D. membrane breaks-round or oval windows
E. Ménière's disease
REF. Simmons FB: The Laryngoscope, 83:1221, Aug'73

1448. Which of the following may cause sudden sensori-neural hearing loss?
A. collagen disorders
B. acoustic tumors
C. head trauma
D. syphilis
E. chemical toxins
REF. Simmons FB: The Laryngoscope, 83:1221, Aug'73

1449. When the interval is three days or less between the onset of symptoms and the first audiogram (and treatment started) in patients with sudden idiopathic sensori-neural hearing loss, the percent of patients recovering their hearing is:
A. 11
B. 18
C. 33
D. 68
E. 97
REF. Simmons FB: The Laryngoscope, 83:1221, Aug'73

1450. When the interval is seven days or more between the onset of symptoms and the first audiogram (and treatment started) in patients with sudden idiopathic sensori-neural hearing loss, the percent of patients recovering their hearing is:
A. 11
B. 18
C. 33
D. 68
E. 97
REF. Simmons FB: The Laryngoscope, 83:1221, Aug'73

1451. Treatment for sudden idiopathic sensori-neural hearing loss is a matter of considerable controversy. Which of the following may be helpful?
A. bed rest
B. steroids
C. intravenous histamine
D. nicotinic acid and other oral vasodilators
E. intravenous xylocaine
F. antibiotics
REF. Simmons FB: The Laryngoscope, 83:1221, Aug'73

1452. Facial paralysis complicating stapes surgery is uncommon in the hands of the experienced otologic surgeon. Paralysis at the end of a stapedectomy is most likely due to:
A. related to the injected local anesthetic and will resolve completely within a few hours
B. prolapse of facial nerve through a dehiscent undersurface of the tympanic facial canal
C. retrograde edema from a slightly traumatized, stretched or severed chorda tympani extending into the fallopian canal
D. otitis media in the presence of a dehiscent nerve
E. surgical trauma or footplate damage to a dehiscent undersurface of the tympanic facial canal
F. local anesthetic in the middle ear in the presence of a dehiscent facial nerve
G. temperature change in a dehiscent nerve
REF. Althaus SR, House HP: The Laryngoscope, 83:1234, Aug'73

1453. Facial nerve paralysis occurring several days after an otherwise successful stapedectomy is most likely due to:
A. related to the injected local anesthetic or local anesthetic in the middle ear cavity in the presence of a dehiscent facial nerve canal

B. spontaneous prolapse of the facial nerve through a dehiscent undersurface of the tympanic facial nerve canal (attachment of the oval window replacement membrane to the perineurium of the dehiscent facial can pull the latter down over the oval window)
C. retrograde edema from a traumatized or severed chorda tympani extending into the fallopian canal
D. otitis media in the presence of a dehiscent nerve
E. temperature changes in a dehiscent nerve
F. surgical trauma or damage to a dehiscent undersurface of the tympanic facial canal

REF. Althaus SR, House HP: The Laryngoscope, 83:1234, Aug'73

1454. The inferior or vestibular surface of the facial nerve canal over the oval window may be dehiscent in the following percent of temporal bones and is not visible to the surgeon at the time of surgery:
A. 5 - 10
B. 15 - 20
C. 25 - 35
D. 40 - 50
E. 60 - 70

REF. Althaus SR, House HP: The Laryngoscope, 83:1234, Aug'73

1455. Facial paralysis may be due to:
A. otitis media
B. otitis externa
C. stapes surgery
D. Bell's palsy
E. acoustic neuroma

REF. Althaus SR, House HP: The Laryngoscope, 83:1234, Aug'73. Sadé J: Ann Otol, 74:94, '65

1456. Bilateral congenital choanal atresia carries a high risk of brain damage due to hypoxia. Diagnosis must be made in the delivery room and temporary measures which can prevent respiratory arrest are:
A. insertion of an oral airway to break the tongue-to-palate seal
B. insertion of a gavage tube
C. trocar or curved female urethral sounds passed along the floor of the nostril staying against the septum and forcing through the atresia followed by gradual dilatation
D. a teflon catheter is passed through one side and returned through the other after cutting a small oval section at the end of the U-shape tube and suturing the tube together with silk 5 mm. anterior to the columella and retained in place at least four to six weeks or longer
E. tracheotomy

REF. Weseman CM: The Laryngoscope, 83:1160, July'73

1457. Pathogenesis of orbital complications in acute sinusitis is due to:
A. dissemination of infection through the venous structures of the orbit
B. absence of valve mechanism in the ophthalmic veins
C. continuity of the ethmoid and ophthalmic veins through the ethmoid labyrinth
D. fragile barriers of the lamina papyracea
E. bony destruction of the floor of the frontal sinus

REF. Welsh LW, Welsh JJ: The Laryngoscope, 84:848, May'74 . Chandler JR et al.: The Laryngoscope, 80:1414, 1970

1458. The postoperative results of tympanoplasty were investigated to determine the relation between the histological changes of antral mucous membrane and postoperative results. The histologic changes in the mucous membrane of the antrum were classified into the following types and the postoperative result was worse in:
A. edematous
B. cell infiltrating
C. fibrous
D. cystiformation
E. cholesterine granuloma
F. cholesteatoma

REF. Baba K: Jap Jour Otol, 76:833, Jul-Dec'73

1459. The development of middle ears in human embryos collected from Japanese cases of artificial abortion were studied and which of the following appear true?
A. primordia of the malleus and incus form an indistinct structure within the condensation of cells connected with Meckel's cartilage
B. malleus and incus are derived from the same origin at approximately the same period, whereas the stapes is derived from a different origin at a later stage
C. vestibular side of the stapedial footplate and margin of the vestibular fenestra develop from the otic capsule, whereas the stapes crura and the tympanic side of the footplate are from a different origin, i. e., Reichert's cartilage
D. stapes crura are derived earlier than the stapedial footplate
E. incudo-stapedial joint is not formed until the 11th week
REF. Kondo Y: Jap Jour Otol 76:929, Jul-Dec '73

1460. In the development of the middle ear in Japanese embryos, the stapedial artery becomes smaller and usually finally disappears in the following week:
A. 4th
B. 8th
C. 11th
D. 16th
E. 18th
REF. Kondo Y: Jap Jour Otol, 76:940, Jul-Dec '73

1461. Compared with whip-lash injury, head trauma is more frequently accompanied by which of the following?
A. auditory disturbance alone
B. tinnitus with disturbance of equilibrium
C. tinnitus alone
D. abnormality in righting reflex
E. perverted nystagmus and optokinetic inversion
REF. Sakashita K: Jap Jour Otol, 76:944, Jul-Dec '73

1462. Compared with head trauma, whip-lash injury is more frequently accompanied by which of the following?
A. auditory disturbance alone
B. tinnitus with disturbance of equilibrium
C. tinnitus alone
D. abnormality in the righting reflex
E. perverted nystagmus and optokinetic inversion
REF. Sakashita K: Jap Jour Otol, 76:944, Jul-Dec '73

1463. Which of the following should be considered in patients with disturbances of equilibrium and auditory disorders following trauma?
A. head injury
B. whip-lash injury
C. abnormality of the cervical spine
D. insufficiency of the vertebral artery
E. post-traumatic hydrocephalus with normal CSF pressure
REF. Sakashita K: Jap Jour Otol, 76:944, Jul-Dec '73

1464. Vestibular function tests and histopathological studies on patients with Ménière's disease following trans-oval-window sacculotomies indicate:
A. inner ear damage is a serous labyrinthitis
B. postoperative functional disturbances did not correlate to the histopathological findings in the temporal bones
C. more cochlear damage than vestibular
D. more vestibular damage than cochlear
E. inner ear damage is a purulent labyrinthitis
REF. Honda H: Jap Jour Otol, 76:1323, Jul-Dec '73

1465. Profound sensorineural deafness of sudden onset during exposure to intense occupational noise have been found in employees:
A. operating pneumatic drills or iron hammers
B. shortly after exposure to use of noise-making machines (but may have been exposed same machines for many years)
C. unilateral usually but may be bilateral
D. U-shaped or flat type audiograms usually- but rarely may be high-frequency
E. positive loudness recruitment but negative temporary threshold shift
F. vestibular disorders occasionally
REF. Suga F: Jap Jour Otol, 76:1373, Jul-Dec'73

1466. Pupillary reactions following olfactory stimuli were studied using an electro-scanning pupillometer. Odorous papers 1.0 x 20 cm in size were soaked with 1. di-camphor, 2. y-undecalactone, 3. iso-valeric acid, 4. cyclotent, 5. scatol and sniffed for 3-4 seconds. The results showed:
A. olfactory threshold could be detected either by subjective sensation or by pupillary reaction in most cases (88 percent)
B. pupillary reactions could be examined in an ascending method using di-camphor and y-undecalactone for the olfactory stimulus
C. pupillary reactions were prominent at the concentration of subjective threshold
D. pupillary reactions were slight or no reaction at the over-threshold concentration of these substances. (No pupillary reaction was observed in anosmia)
E. three types of pupillary reactions were noted: enlargement of the diameter of the pupil (mydriatic-usual in most cases), hippus, and dilation following constriction of the pupil
REF. Nishida H, Kumagami H, Jinnouchi H: Jap Jour Otol, 76:1449, Jul-Dec'73

1467. It is well known that in a normal voice the laryngostroboscopic pattern shows smooth vibrations which should be continuous, regular and symmetrical. Stroboscopic microsurgery aims chiefly at:
A. treatment of the laryngeal lesions morphologically
B. study of laryngostroboscopic pattern of the larynx preoperatively through the operating microscope by patients phonating under neuroleptanalgesic anesthesia
C. B during the operative procedure to determine the end-point of surgery
D. B postoperatively showing objectively (and confirmed clinically) a remarkable improvement in the voice
E. first development of functional microsurgery of the larynx
REF. Saito S, Suzuki Y, Fukuda H, Ogata K, Kitahara S, Akitaya T, Kokawa N, Ono H: Jap Jour Otol, 76:989, Jul-Dec'73

1468. Which of the following findings are present in patients of any age with voice changes caused by anabolic steroids in a dose over 400 mg monthly?
A. indirect laryngoscopy shows normal vocal cords
B. A shows edema of vocal cords
C. in steroid-treated cases, the muscle fibers show marked hypertrophy (autopsy histologic studies)
D. C show no change in the vocal cord muscle fibers
E. steroids cause vocal changes by abnormal tension of the vocal cords due to hypertrophy of the muscle fibers
REF. Kato T: Jap Jour Otol, 76:1073, Jul-Dec'73

1469. Hoarseness or dysphonia in children is common and usually:
A. found more frequently in boys than in girls (4:1)
B. more common in children living in urban than residental areas
C. laryngoscopic findings are normal

D. C with corditis edematosa
E. C with corditis nodosa or nodules
REF. Maekawa H, Ito M. Watanabe T, Moon YI: Jap Jour Otol, 76:1459, Jul-Dec'73

1470. Bilateral facial paralysis is most likely due to:
A. trauma
B. Bell's palsy
C. Heerford's syndrome
D. polyneuritis
E. systemic diseases
REF. Tamaki H, Sugiyama S, Nomura A, Hazama H: Jap Jour Otol, 76:921, Jul-Dec'73

1471. A patient with paralytic dysphagia with paralysis of the left levator veli palatini, middle pharyngeal constrictor and intrinsic laryngeal muscles with an intact cricopharyngeus muscle has which of the following characteristics?
A. esophagram shows barium remains in the hypopharynx with the larynx closed and elevated
B. A with larynx open, barium in the hypopharynx spills into the trachea resulting in severe aspiration
C. cricopharyngeal myotomy helps swallowing
D. nasal leakage and time consuming swallowing occurs
E. pharyngeal flap construct ed on the paretic side after cricopharyngeal myotomy results in improved deglutition
REF. Hirano M, Kunitake H, Mihashi S: Jap Jour Otol, 76:1067, Jul-Dec'73

1472. In an electromyographic study conducted for the purpose of describing oral and nasal articulatory gestures and patterns of velopharyngeal activity which accompany vowel difference and voicing distinction among stop consonants, peroral insertions of bipolar hooked-wire electrodes were introduced into the levator palatini, superior pharyngeal constrictor, palatopharyngeus and palatoglossus. It was revealed that the primary muscle of velopharyngeal closure for enunciation is:
A. palatoglossus
B. palatopharyngeus
C. superior pharyngeal constrictor
D. levator palatini
REF. Hirose H: Jap Jour Otol, 76:1349, Jul-Dec'73

1473. The functions of facial muscles studied in cases of traumatic facial paralysis in those patients who had decompression operations carried out at least two years before revealed:
A. decompression operation is effective for the restoration of function of each muscle
B. frontal muscle shows poorer recovery than the orbicularis oris and oculi muscles
C. smiling is satisfactory
D. closing the eyes is satisfactory
E. pouting is satisfactory
REF. Morimitsu T: Jap Jour Otol, 76:1472, Jul-Dec'73

1474. Guidelines for the use of prophylactic antibiotics in intranasal surgery are not well established. Which of the following infections have followed nasal surgery and indicate prophylactic antibiotic coverage is needed?
A. bacteremia
B. septal abscess
C. bacterial meningitis
D. Staphylococcus aureus endocarditis
E. none of the above
REF. Coursey DL: Arch Otolaryngol, 99:454, June'74

1475. Bacteremia has followed which of the following procedures?
A. tonsillectomy
B. oral surgery
C. posterior nasal pack placement
D. all of the above
E. none of the above
REF. Coursey DL: Arch Otolaryngol, 99:454, June'74

1476. Which of the following drugs appear to decrease or have no significant effect on cochlear blood flow?
A. niacin
B. nicotinyl alcohol
C. atropine sulfate
D. scopolamine hydrobromide
E. neostigmine methylsulfate
F. edrophonium chloride
REF. Snow JB, Suga F: Arch Otolaryngol, 97:365, May'73

1477. Vasodilators have been used for years for the treatment of patients with Ménière's disease and for some forms of sensorineural deafness attributed to circulatory disorders of the inner ear. Which of the following drugs appear to increase cochlear blood flow although experimental observations have been conflicting?
A. papaverine hydrochloride
B. dipyridamole (persantine)
C. bradykinin
D. kallidin
E. histamine phosphate
F. betahistine hydrochloride (serc)
G. hydralazine hydrochloride
H. hypertonic solutions of glucose and sodium bicarbonate
I. inhalation of carbon dioxide
J. inhalation of amyl nitrite
REF. Snow JB, Suga F: Arch Otolaryngol, 97:365, May'73

1478. In a patient with a history of exertion, and sudden sensori-neural hearing loss with lack of vestibular signs (vertigo), the following diagnosis should be seriously but cautiously considered:
A. rupture of Reissner's membrane
B. rupture of wall of the saccule
C. round window membrane rupture
D. oval window rupture
E. either oval or round window, or both, rupture with fistulas and perilymphatic leakage
REF. Pullen FW: (Discussion: Harris IL:) Trans Am Acad Ophthalmol Otolaryngol, 76:1444, Nov-Dec '72

1479. In a patient with a history of exertion and sudden sensori-neural hearing loss without vertigo, which of the following should be considered in the differential diagnosis if exploratory tympanotomy does not reveal any perilymphatic fistulas at either the round or oval windows?
A. rupture of Reissner's membrane
B. rupture of the wall of the saccule
C. round window membrane rupture
D. rupture oval window
E. C and/or D
REF. Pullen FW: (Discussion: Harris I:) Trans Am Acad Ophthalmol Otolaryngol, 76:1444, Nov-Dec'72

1480. In a patient with a history of exertion, and sudden sensori-neural hearing loss without vertigo, management should consist of:
A. bedrest four or five days-avoiding any activity likely to raise intracochlear pressure
B. avoiding valsalva or politizer maneuvers (particularly hazardous in scuba or skin divers)
C. avoiding blowing of the nose or coughing and alcohol
D. avoiding high intensity sounds
E. exploratory tympanotomy for oval or round window fistulas (or both) with closure with gelfoam, fat, or perichondrium graft from the tragus
REF. Pullen FW: (Discussion: Harris I:)Trans Am Acad Ophthalmol Otolaryng, 76:1444, Nov-Dec'72

1481. Internal trauma to the larynx is usually suspected when (excluding tumors):
A. history of dysphonia following aspiration of a foreign body, chemical or iatrogenic
B. voice change
C. stridor

D. failure of extubation
E. tracheotomy for acute laryngeal obstruction
REF. Holinger PH, Schild JA: Trans Amer Laryng Assoc, 93:46, Apr'72

1482. In external trauma to the larynx, the most significant sign is probably:
A. crepitation with x-ray evidence of subcutaneous mediastinal or pericardial emphysema
B. lateral x-ray changes
C. xeroradiogram changes
D. abnormal anteroposterior planograms of the larynx and trachea
E. abnormal laryngograms or tracheograms
REF. Holinger PH, Schild JA: Trans Amer Laryng Assoc,93:46, Apr'72

1483. Decannulation should be performed as early as possible to avoid late sequelae such as the following:
A. granulations
B. infections
C. tracheomalacia
D. stenosis including subglottic
E. peristomal scar tissue formation
REF. Baker DC, Savetsky L: Trans Amer Laryng Assoc, 93:46, Apr'72

1484. The earliest age when arytenoidectomies or arytenoidopexies can be performed is:
A. 3
B. 4
C. 5
D. at puberty
E. anytime after puberty
REF. Fearon B, Cotton R:(Discussion: Priest RE, Montgomery WW, Atkins JP, Baluyot S, Miller AH, Birck HG, Holinger PH) Trans Amer Laryng Assoc 93:57, Apr'72

1485. In order to prevent decannulation problems in infants, which of the following are recommended in performing the tracheostomy?
A. tracheostomy opening below the thyroid isthmus in the fourth to sixth tracheal ring
B. incision through the thyroid isthmus with tracheostomy opening in the second to fourth tracheal ring
C. incision in the trachea can be vertical, cruciate, or removal of a window but should go through lower one-half of the upper ring and upper one-half of the lower ring and should not fully transect the cartilage of the whole ring
D. tube should be proper sized and fixed firmly to the neck to avoid motion and tracheal irritation
E. x-ray study of the position of the tube should be performed early
REF. Baker DC, Savetsky L: Trans Amer Laryng Assoc, 93:46, Apr'72

1486. When is repeated bouginage effective for laryngeal, subglottic and tracheal stenosis?
A. no standard procedure
B. always
C. sometimes
D. only together with skin graft on stents
E. only together with mucosal graft on stents
REF. Fearon B, Cotton R: (Discussion: Priest RE, Montgomery WW, Atkins JP, Baluyot S, Miller AH, Birck HG, Holinger PH) Trans Amer Laryng Assoc, 93:57, Apr'72

1487. To avoid decannulation problems in infants, which of the following is inaccurate?
A. accurate tracheostomy tube fixed firmly to infant's neck to avoid motion and position checked by x-ray study
B. clearing of underlying condition-unsuccessful decannulation may mean subglottic stenosis or edema, vocal cord paralysis, etc.

C. use smaller sized tubes, fenestrated tubes or corking to allow glottic breathing
D. nasotracheal tube should never be allowed to remain in place longer than four days
E. excessive secretions requiring constant suctioning is never a contraindication to decannulation
REF. Baker DC, Savetsky L: Trans Amer Laryng Assoc, 93:46, Apr'72

1488. The laryngeal keel is reserved for operation for:
A. subglottic edema or stenosis
B. extensive papilloma of the larynx
C. bilateral abduction cord paralysis
D. arytenoid fixation
E. simple fusion of the vocal cords or internal larynx
REF. Fearon B, Cotton R: (Discussion: Holinger PH) Trans Amer Laryng Assoc, 93:57, Apr'72

1489. Vertigo in Ménière's disease occurs in well-defined episodes and a definite spell is characterized by all of the following with one incorrect statement which is:
A. prostrating, often with nausea or vomiting
B. persists for prolonged time (20 min. to no more than 24 hours)
C. patient fully oriented and conscious during the spell
D. before a definite spell, hearing in affected ear may decrease, remain same or actually increase with increase in a subjective but variable tinnitus
E. between definite spells there are no adjunctive spells such as motion intolerance, positional vertigo, falling attacks and momentary ataxia
REF. Alford BR, Barber HO, Pennington C, Pulec JL, Schuknecht HF, Tabor JR, McCabe BF: Trans Am Acad Ophthalmol Otolaryngol, 76:1462, '72

1490. During an attack of vertigo, Ménière's disease with nystagmus is:
A. vestibular and always present
B. end-organ variety-fine rapid, quick-slow, in a single definite direction (quick component)
C. horizontal or horizontal rotatory
D. no nystagmus between spells (eyes open)
E. may be nystagmus between spells (eyes closed)
REF. Alford BR, Barber HO, Pennington C, Pulec JL, Schuknecht HF, Tabor JR, McCabe BF: Trans Am Acad Ophthalmol Otolaryngol, 76:1462, Nov-Dec'72

1491. Ménière's disease affects both inner ears in the following percent of patients:
A. 5-10
B. 10-20
C. 30-40
D. 50-60
E. 70-80
REF. Alford BR, Barber HO, Pennington C, Pulec JL, Schuknecht HF, Tabor JR, McCabe BF: Trans Am Acad Ophthalmol Otolaryng, 76:1462, Nov-Dec'72

1492. Which of the following is considered identical with Ménière's disease and all such appellations should be discarded in usage?
A. Ménière's syndrome
B. Ménière's symptom complex
C. Ménière's disorder
D. atypical Ménière's disease
E. positional vertigo
REF. Alford BR, Barber HO, Pennington C, Pulec JL, Schuknecht, HF, Tabor JR, McCabe BF: Trans Am Acad Ophthalmol Otolaryngol, 76:1462, Nov-Dec'72

1493. Ménière's disease has all of the following characteristics except:
A. disease of membranous inner ear
B. deafness is characteristic
C. vertigo is characteristic
D. tinnitus is always present
E. pathologic hydropic distention of the endolymphatic system
REF. Alford BR, Pennington C, Pulec JL, Schuknecht HF, Tabor JR, McCabe BF: Trans Amer Acad Ophthalmol Otolaryngol, 76:1462, Nov-Dec '72

1494. Early in Ménière's disease the deafness is sensori-neural, fluctuating, usually unilateral and progressive with lessening recovery between episodes. Early in Ménière's which of the following tests indicate cochlear, organ of corti, hair cell dysfunction (cochlear deafness)?
A. loudness recruitment
B. decreased speech discrimination
C. lack of tone decay
D. High SISI score
E. diplacusis and distortion
REF. Alford BR, Pulec JL, Schuknecht HF, Tabor JR, McCabe BF: Trans Am Acad Ophthalmol Otolaryngol, 76:1462, Nov-Dec '72

1495. Ménière's disease can occur in:
A. cochlear endolymph alone (cochlear Ménière's disease)
B. labyrinth endolymph alone (vestibular Ménière's disease)
C. both cochlear and vestibular endolymph
D. cochlear perilymph
E. vestibular perilymph
REF. Alford BR, Barber HO, Pennington C, Pulec JL, Schuknecht HF, Tabor JR, McCabe BF: Trans Am Acad Ophthalmol Otolaryngol, 76:1462, Nov-Dec '72

1496. In severe late Ménière's disease, there is which of the following?
A. loudness recruitment with decreased speech discrimination
B. lack of tone decay with high SISI score
C. diplacusis and distortion
D. all of the above
E. none of the above
REF. Alford BR, Pulec JL, Schuknecht HF, Tabor JR, McCabe BF: Trans Am Acad Ophthalmol Otolaryngol, 76:1462, Nov-Dec '72

1497. Audiometric configuration in early Ménière's disease is in most instances:
A. up-sloping with recovery
B. flat with recovery
C. down-sloping with recovery
D. down-sloping without recovery
E. flat without recovery
REF. Alford BR, Pulec JL, Schuknecht HF, Tabor JR, McCabe BF: Trans Am Acad Ophthalmol Otolaryngol, 76:1462, Nov-Dec '72

1498. Audiometric configuration in late Ménière's disease is in most instances:
A. up-sloping with recovery
B. flat with recovery
C. down-sloping with recovery
D. down-sloping without recovery
E. flat without recovery
REF. Alford BR, Pulec JL, Schuknecht HF, Tabor JR, McCabe BF: Trans Am Acad Ophthalmol Otolaryngol, 76:1462, Nov-Dec '72

1499. In Ménière's disease over an extended period of time, there is:
A. more marked variation in the discrimination scores
B. more marked variation in the pure-tone thresholds
C. A and B fluctuate simultaneously at the same rate in the same direction

D. with treatment, discrimination scores can improve without any improvement in the pure-tone thresholds-there can be improved use of amplification
E. with treatment, discrimination scores cannot improve without pure-tone threshold improvement
REF. Clemis JD: Trans Am Acad Ophthalmol Otolaryngol, 76:1444, Nov-Dec'72. Clemis JD, Carver WF: Arch Otolaryng, 86:614, '67

1500. In the malpractice suit problem, which of the following are objectionable from a medical viewpoint?
A. there is actually comparatively little real malpractice by well-trained and competent surgeons, but a great tidal wave of suits
B. awards won in so-called malpractice suits are tax-free
C. ignorance in medical matters by jury members
D. fee-splitting by lawyers being considered legal and ethical and the contingent fee-system where the physician has no recourse to recover time (money), and reputation when he successfully defends himself against an alleged malpractice suit
E. all of the above
REF. Shambaugh GE: Trans Amer Soc Ophthal Otolaryng Allergy, 12:1, Sept'71

The author has taken precautions to thoroughly check all questions and answers. However, in a volume of this size, some possible inaccuracies may appear. When in doubt, consult your references. What may appear to be an inaccuracy at first, may be just a difference of opinion between authors.

THE PUBLISHERS

SECTION I

1. E
2. A
3. E
4. B
5. C
6. D
7. E
8. A, B, C
9. A, C, E
10. C, D, E
11. A thru E
12. A thru E
13. A
14. A
15. A, B, C
16. B, E
17. A
18. D
19. A, C, D
20. A, B, D, E
21. A
22. C
23. E
24. B
25. B, C, D
26. C
27. B, A
28. D
29. A thru E
30. C, D
31. A, B
32. A thru E
33. A
34. A, B, D, E
35. C, D, E
36. F
37. A thru E
38. A thru E
39. A thru E
40. A
41. E
42. B
43. C
44. A
45. A thru E
46. A, B, C, D
47. A
48. A, B
49. E
50. A
51. E
52. A, B, C, D
53. E
54. C
55. A
56. A, B, C
57. D, E
58. A, B, C
59. D
60. A thru E
61. A, B, C, D
62. A, B, C, E
63. E
64. A thru E
65. A thru E
66. A, C
67. B
68. D
69. C
70. A thru E
71. C, D, E
72. A, B, C
73. B, C, D, E
74. E
75. A thru E
76. C
77. C, E
78. D
79. B, C, D, E
80. A thru E
81. E, F (some C)
82. A thru E
83. A, B, C
84. B, D
85. A, B
86. E
87. A, B, E
88. C, D, E
89. E
90. A, B, D
91. A
92. A thru E
93. D (perhaps A, B)
94. C
95. D
96. A, B, C, D
97. B, C, D
98. A, B (C?)
99. A thru E
100. B
101. D
102. D
103. A thru F
104. A thru E
105. A thru E
106. A, B, D, F
107. A, E (B?)
108. A thru E
109. A thru E
110. A, B, D, E
111. A, B, C
112. C
113. D
114. D
115. A
116. A
117. E
118. A, B, C, D
119. A thru E
120. A thru E
121. A thru J
122. A thru E
123. A thru D
124. A thru E
125. A thru E
126. A, C, D
127. A, C, D, E
128. A, B, E
129. A thru E
130. A thru E
131. 1. B
  2. J
  3. H
  4. A
  5. E
  6. D
  7. G
  8. I
  9. F
  10. C
132. A thru E
133. B, D, E
134. B, C, D, E
135. B, C, E
136. A, C, E
137. A thru E
138. A, B, C (D?)
139. A thru H
140. A thru E
141. E
142. E
143. C, E
144. A, B, C, D (especially A)
145. C
146. A thru H
147. A, B
148. A thru E
149. A
150. A thru E
151. C, D, E
152. A, B, C, E
153. A, B, C, D
154. A
155. C
156. D
157. A, B, C
158. D
159. B, C, D, E
160. D
161. A
162. A, C, E
163. B, D, E
164. A, B, C, D
165. A thru E
166. A thru E
167. A thru E
168. A thru E
169. A thru D
170. A thru G
171. A, B, C, D
172. A thru E
173. A thru E
174. A thru E
175. A3, B4, C2, B1
176. A thru E
177. B
178. E
179. D
180. A
181. C
182. D
183. D
184. E
185. A
186. E
187. B
188. C
189. C
190. A, C, D, E
191. A thru F
192. E
193. A, B
194. B, D, E
195. A2, B5, C4, D1, E6, F3
196. B, D

197. A, C, E
198. A
199. A, E
200. A
201. C
202. A thru E
203. A thru F
204. A thru E
205. A, B
206. E
207. A
208. D
209. A thru E
210. B
211. B
212. A, B, E
213. B, C, D, E
214. C
215. C
216. A thru E
217. A thru E
218. A thru E
219. A, B, D, E
220. A
221. D
222. A thru D
223. A
224. A, D
225. E
226. A thru E
227. B, D, E
228. A thru E
229. A thru E
230. D
231. D, E
232. A, B, D
233. A thru H
234. A, C, D, E, F
235. A thru E
236. A thru E
237. A thru E
238. A
239. A thru E
240. A thru K
241. C
242. E
243. E
244. B, C, D, E
245. A thru E
246. A
247. E
248. A, C
249. C, D
250. B, D
251. A. 3
B. 1
C. 2
D. 4
252. E
253. A thru E
254. A, B, D, E
255. A thru E
256. E
257. A thru E
258. B, C, D, E
259. E
260. D, E
261. C
262. A thru E
263. A thru H
264. D
265. A thru E
266. A, E
267. A thru E
268. B, C, D, E
269. A thru E
270. A thru E
271. A
272. A, B, C
273. A thru E
274. A, B, D, E
275. B, C, D, E
276. C, D, E
277. A thru E
278. D
279. C, D, E
280. A, B, C, D
281. A, B, D, E
282. A, D, E
283. A thru E
284. A, C, E
285. B, C, D, E
286. A thru E
287. A thru E
288. A thru E
289. E
290. A
291. B, C, D
292. A thru E
293. A, B, C, E
294. E
295. B
296. A
297. C
298. E
299. A, B, C, D
300. A, B, C, D
301. A, F
302. A thru E
303. C, D, E
304. B, D, E
305. A, D, E
306. A thru E
307. E
308. A thru E
309. A, B, E
310. D, E, F, G
311. A
312. G, H, I
313. A, E
314. B, C, E
315. A, C, D, E, F
316. D
317. E
318. B
319. A, C, D, E, F
320. A. 2, B. 2, C. 1&2, D. 1&2, E. 2, F. 1, G. 1, H. 2
321. A, D, E
322. E
323. A thru E
324. E
325. B
326. E
327. A, B, E
328. A
329. A thru E
330. A thru F
331. C, D
332. A, B, C, D
333. A thru G
334. A, D, E
335. B, C, D, E
336. C, E
337. E
338. A
339. E
340. E
341. A thru E
342. A
343. D
344. A thru E
345. E
346. 1. E, 2. A, 3. B
347. 1. A, 2. E
348. 1. B, 2. D, 3. E, 4. F 5. A, 6. C, 7. G
349. 1. D, 2. A, 3. B, 4. C, 5. E, F
350. D
351. B
352. 1. A, D, 2. D, 3. B, C, 4. A, 5. C
353. A, B
354. A thru E
355. E
356. A, B, C, D
357. 1. D, A, 2. A, 3. C, B, 4. B
358. B, C, D
359. A thru E
360. A thru H
361. E
362. E
363. B, C, F
364. C, D
365. A thru D
366. A, B, C, D
367. D
368. D
369. A thru H
370. B, C
371. A, B, C, D
372. E
373. A thru K
374. E
375. A
376. B
377. C
378. B
379. D
380. E
381. A
382. D
383. B
384. A
385. E
386. E
387. A thru F
388. A, B, D, E
389. A, C, D, F, G
390. D
391. A thru E
392. A, D, E
393. B
394. C
395. C, D, E
396. A, B, C, D
397. A, B, C, E
398. A, C, D, E
399. A, D
400. C, D, E
401. A, E
402. A, B, D
403. D
404. E
405. B, C, D, F
406. A, B, C, D
407. A thru E
408. A thru F
409. A, B, C
410. E
411. A, C, E
412. B, C
413. C
414. A
415. A, E
416. D
417. A, E
418. A, B, C, E
419. A, D, E
420. E
421. D
422. B, C, D, E
423. 1. B, 2. C, 3. E
424. F
425. A thru H
426. A, B, C, D
427. A, C
428. A, B, C, E
429. A thru E
430. A, C, D, E
431. A, B, D

432. B, C, D, E
433. A, D, E
434. E
435. C
436. A thru E
437. A, C, D
438. A, D, E
439. B
440. D
441. A, C, E
442. A thru E
443. D
444. D
445. A thru E
446. A, B, C, E, G
447. C, E
448. A, D, E
449. A thru E
450. A thru D
451. A thru E
452. B
453. A thru E
454. A
455. D
456. A thru E
457. E
458. A thru E
459. A thru G
460. E
461. E, H
462. A thru E
463. E, F
464. D
465. A, B, C
466. C, E
467. A, B
468. B, C, D
469. B, C, E
470. A, B, D, E
471. D, E
472. A
473. A thru E
474. E
475. A, B, C, E
476. A. 3, B. 1, C. 4, D. 2
477. A, B, F
478. A, B, C, E
479. B, C.
480. A thru F
481. A thru J
482. D, E
483. A thru K
484. A, C, D, E, G, H, I
485. A, C, D
486. A, B, C
487. A thru E
488. E
489. 1. B, 2. A, 3. C, D. 4
490. A
491. 1. D, 2. E, 3. A, 4. B, 5. C
492. E
493. B, C, D
494. A thru E
495. A thru E
496. E
497. A thru G
498. 1. F, 2. C, 3. B, 4. E, 5. G, 6. D, 7. A
499. A thru E
500. A thru E
501. A, B, C, D
502. A, D
503. A thru E
504. A
505. C, D, E

<u>SECT. II</u>

506. C
507. E
508. D
509. A
510. A
511. A, B, D, E
512. D, E
513. D, E
514. E
515. E
516. D
517. A thru E
518. A, B
519. C
520. A thru E
521. A, B, C
522. A, C, D, E
523. A
524. B, C
525. D, E
526. E
527. B, C
528. A, B, C, D
529. A, B, C
530. D
531. A thru E
532. A
533. A thru E
534. A thru E
535. C
536. A
537. C
538. A, B, C, D
539. A, B, E
540. A
541. C
542. D
543. A, C, D, E
544. A.
545. B, C, D, E
546. A thru E
547. B, C, D
548. A, E
549. C
550. C, D, E
551. D
552. E
553. E
554. B
555. A, B, C, D
556. A
557. A, B, C
558. E
559. A, B, C, D
560. D
561. A
562. A, B, C
563. A, B, D, E
564. A, B, C, D
565. A thru E
566. A thru F
567. I
568. E
569. A thru E
570. E
571. A thru D
572. D
573. D
574. A
575. A thru E
576. A, B, D, E
577. A thru E
578. E, F
579. A, B, C, D
580. A thru H
581. A, E
582. A
583. A, B, C, D
584. D
585. A thru E
586. A, B, C, D, F
587. A thru J
588. A, B, C, D
589. B
590. A thru I
591. A thru E
592. E
593. A, B, C, E
594. A, B, C, D, F
595. B
596. A thru F
597. B, C, E
598. A
599. A, C, D
600. A
601. A thru E
602. E
603. A, C, D, E
604. B
605. A
606. E
607. A, B, D, E
608. A thru E
609. C, D
610. E
611. A thru E
612. E
613. A thru E
614. 1. B, 2. G, 3. D, 4. C, 5. F, 6. E, 7. A
615. D
616. H
617. A thru E
618. E
619. A thru D
620. G but consider all
621. C
622. A, B, C
623. B, C, D
624. E
625. D, E, I, J, K
626. A thru J
627. A, B, G
628. B, D
629. G
630. E
631. E
632. B
633. A, C, E
634. A, B, E
635. A thru E
636. A, D, E, F
637. D
638. All except G
639. A thru E
640. A thru E
641. A thru E
642. A
643. A thru E
644. E
645. A thru F
646. D, E
647. C
648. E
649. E
650. A, D
651. F
652. B
653. C

<u>SECT. III</u>

654. E
655. A
656. E
657. E
658. C
659. E

660. E
661. D
662. A thru E
663. E
664. A thru E
665. A
666. E
667. B
668. A
669. A
670. E
671. A thru E
672. E
673. E
674. A
675. A thru E
676. A, B
677. B, D, E
678. A thru E
679. D, E
680. A thru E
681. A thru E
682. A, C, D, E
683. B, D
684. A thru E
685. D
686. B, D
687. C, D, F
688. A thru E
689. E
690. B
691. A thru E
692. A thru D
693. C, D, E
694. E
695. A thru F
696. B, D
697. A, B, D
698. B, D
699. B
700. B, C, E
701. A, B, D, E, G, H, I
702. E
703. E
704. B
705. C
706. B
707. D
708. B
709. E
710. E
711. B, C, D, E
712. A
713. A, B
714. A, B, C, D
715. A thru E
716. F
717. A
718. D
719. A
720. A thru O P unknown
721. A, B, E
722. E
723. B
724. E
725. A thru E
726. A, C, D, E
727. A
728. B, C, E
729. B
730. E
731. D
732. A
733. A, B, C, D
734. B, D, E
735. E
736. A thru E
737. A, E
738. A thru E
739. B
740. A, E
741. C
742. B
743. A, E
744. A, B
745. E
746. A thru E
747. A thru E
748. A thru E
749. C
750. A, B, C
751. D
752. A thru E
753. A, E
754. C
755. A, D, E
756. E
757. A thru E
758. A, C, D, E
759. E
760. A thru D
761. A
762. C
763. A, B, D
764. A, B, D

SECT. IV

765. A, B, C, E
766. A
767. A, E
768. C
769. A, B, C, D
770. A, B, C
771. A thru E
772. E
773. A thru E
774. A, B, C
775. E
776. A thru E
777. B
778. A, B, C, E
779. C, D
780. D
781. A
782. C
783. E
784. C
785. E
786. A thru F
787. E
788. D
789. D, E
790. A thru E
791. A thru E
792. A thru E
793. A thru F
794. A thru F
795. C, D
796. A thru E
797. A thru E
798. E
799. A
800. A
801. A thru E
802. A thru E
803. E
804. E
805. A thru E
806. B
807. A thru E
808. B, C, D, E
809. A.1, A.2, A.3, B.4, B.5, B.6
810. A, B, C, E
811. A, B, C
812. A, B, C, D
813. B, C
814. B
815. D
816. A thru E
817. C, D, E
818. E
819. A, B, C
820. K
821. A, B, C
822. A, B, C, D
823. A, E
824. E
825. E
826. A thru E
827. A
828. E
829. B, C, E
830. E
831. E
832. A
833. A thru E
834. E
835. B, C, D, E
836. E
837. A, B, C, D
838. A thru E
839. E
840. C
841. A
842. B
843. D
844. D
845. E
846. E
847. C
848. B
849. A, C, D, E
850. A
851. A, B, C, D
852. A
853. A thru E
854. C, D, E
855. B, E
856. A thru E
857. A, B, C, D
858. C
859. E
860. E
861. E
862. A, B, C
863. A thru E
864. A thru E
865. A thru E
866. A.1, B.2
867. D
868. B.1 thru B.8
869. A thru E
870. C, D, E
871. A, B, C, D
872. A thru E
873. C
874. C
875. A, B, D, E
876. A thru E
877. B, C, D, E
878. E
879. E
880. A, D, E
881. A, C, D, E
882. A, C, D, E
883. A thru E
884. A thru E
885. A thru E
886. A thru E
887. B, D, E
888. B
889. A, B, C
890. D
891. E
892. B
893. A, B, D
894. C
895. D
896. D, E
897. E

898. A thru I
899. A thru E
900. D, E
901. A thru E
902. B, D, E, F, G
903. A, C, D, E, G, H
904. B
905. A, B, C, E, F
906. E
907. A thru E
908. A thru E
909. A
910. A thru D
911. E
912. E
913. E
914. A thru E
915. A thru E
916. E
917. A, B, C, E
918. A. 1, B. 2, C. 3, 4
919. A thru E
920. A thru O
921. A thru E
922. A, C, E
923. E
924. A, B, C
925. B
926. A, C, E
927. C, D
928. A thru H
929. B, C, D, E
930. A, B, E
931. A, B, D, E
932. E
933. A thru F
934. B
935. A thru E
936. A, E
937. A thru G
938. A thru E
939. C
940. A, C, D
941. A thru E
942. A, B, C, E
943. D, E
944. B, C
945. E
946. E
947. A, C, E
948. A thru E
949. A thru E
950. B
951. E
952. E
953. A thru E
954. B, C, D, E
955. C
956. B, E
957. E
958. A, C, D, E
959. E
960. A, B, D, E
961. A, E
962. A, B, C
963. A, C, E
964. C
965. C, D
966. A thru E
967. A, B, C
968. E
969. A thru E
970. B or C
971. A thru E
972. C, E
973. A thru E
974. A, C, E, F, G
975. A, D, E
976. E, F
977. C
978. E
979. A thru E
980. E
981. E
982. C
983. A, C, D
984. A thru J
985. A
986. A, C, D, E
987. A, B, C, D
988. A. 4, 5, 6, B. 3, C. 1, 2, D. 1, 2
989. B, C, D, E
990. A thru E
991. A, C, E
992. E
993. A, B, C, D
994. A, C, E
995. C, D, E
996. A, B, C
997. A, B, C, E
998. C
999. B
1000. A thru E
1001. A, B, C, D
1002. A thru F
1003. A thru F
1004. A, D, E, F
1005. B
1006. C, A, D, B
1007. D
1008. D, E
1009. E
1010. D, E
1011. E
1012. A, C, E
1013. B, C, D
1014. C, D, E
1015. A thru E
1016. A thru G
1017. A
1018. F
1019. A, E
1020. A thru E
1021. D
1022. A, B, D, E
1023. B
1024. A thru E
1025. A thru E
1026. A thru F
1027. A, B, C, E, F
1028. A, B, C, E
1029. A thru E
1030. A
1031. A thru E
1032. C, E
1033. D
1034. B, C, D, E
1035. A thru F
1036. D
1037. B, C, D, E
1038. C
1039. A thru F
1040. A thru E
1041. F
1042. A thru E
1043. A, C, E
1044. E
1045. A, B, C, D, F
1046. A, E, F
1047. A, B, D, E, F, G
1048. A, B, C, D
1049. H
1050. E
1051. A thru E
1052. A thru G
1053. A, B, C, E
1054. A, E
1055. A thru E
1056. A thru F
1057. A thru E
1058. A thru E
1059. A, C, D, E, F, G
1060. A thru F
1061. A, B, C, F
1062. B, C, D, E
1063. E
1064. C, D, E, F
1065. A thru E
1066. E
1067. D
1068. E
1069. A thru E
1070. C, E
1071. A, B, C, E
1072. A, J
1073. A thru E
1074. B, C, E
1075. A thru E
1076. A, B, C, D, E
1077. A thru E
1078. A, C, D, E
1079. A, B, C, E
1080. A thru H
1081. A thru G
1082. A, C, D
1083. A thru F
1084. B, C, E
1085. D
1086. A, C, D, E
1087. A thru L
1088. E
1089. A, B, D, E

SECT. V

1090. E
1091. D
1092. C
1093. C
1094. E
1095. B, D, E
1096. C
1097. E
1098. C
1099. A
1100. A. 4, B. 1, C. 6, D. 2, E. 5, F. 3
1101. A thru E
1102. A. 1, A. 2, A. 3, A. 4, A. 5, B. 6
1103. A. 2, B. 1
1104. A
1105. D
1106. A. 6, B. 5, B. 2, C. 4, D. 3, E. 1
1107. B
1108. E
1109. A
1110. C
1111. A
1112. A thru D
1113. E
1114. A, B, C, E
1115. B
1116. E
1117. A
1118. E
1119. C, E
1120. A thru E
1121. B, C, D, E
1122. A
1123. A, B, C, D
1124. A, E
1125. B
1126. B

1127. C, D
1128. A
1129. E
1130. D
1131. A
1132. B
1133. B
1134. D, E
1135. A
1136. B, C
1137. D, E
1138. E
1139. A thru E
1140. E
1141. E
1142. A2, B1, C3
1143. B, E
1144. A thru E
1145. E
1146. A, B, C
1147. A1, B2, C3
1148. C, D, E
1149. A thru E
1150. A, B, C, D
1151. A, B, C, D
1152. A, B, D, E
1153. A, B, C, E
1154. A, B, D, E
1155. B, C, D, E
1156. C
1157. E
1158. D
1159. B, E
1160. A, C, D
1161. B, C, D, E
1162. E
1163. A thru E
1164. A, B, C, E
1165. A, B, C, E
1166. A
1167. A, B, E
1168. C, E
1169. C, D, E
1170. B, D, E
1171. E
1172. A thru E
1173. B, C
1174. D
1175. A thru E
1176. G
1177. B
1178. A, B, D, E
1179. A, B, C, E
1180. A thru F
1181. A, C, E
1182. A thru F
1183. A thru E
1184. B, E
1185. A, B, C, D
1186. A thru E
1187. A thru H
1188. A thru E
1189. A, B, E
1190. A thru E
1191. A thru E
1192. A, C, D, E
1193. A, E
1194. A thru E
1195. A, C, D, E
1196. A thru E
1197. A, B, C, E
1198. A thru E
1199. A thru E
1200. D, E
1201. B
1202. A, E
1203. A, B, C, D
1204. A, C, E, F
1205. B, C, E

SECT. VI.

1206. A
1207. D
1208. A, B, E
1209. D
1210. A thru E
1211. A thru E
1212. E
1213. A, C, D, E
1214. A, B, D
1215. A thru E
1216. B
1217. A
1218. D
1219. C
1220. A
1221. B
1222. C
1223. B
1224. A4, B2, C3, D1, E5
1225. B
1226. E
1227. B
1228. B
1229. D
1230. B
1231. E
1232. A
1233. A, B, C
1234. D
1235. C
1236. B
1237. B
1238. C
1239. A
1240. A2, B3, C1, D4
1241. C
1242. A, B, D
1243. C
1244. A
1245. D
1246. D
1247. E
1248. A, E
1249. B
1250. C
1251. E
1252. A
1253. A
1254. D
1255. E
1256. A
1257. A
1258. E
1259. E
1260. D
1261. E
1262. D
1263. A thru E
1264. C
1265. A
1266. E
1267. E
1268. A, B
1269. A, B
1270. A5, B1, C3 D4, E2
1271. A3, B4, C2 D1, E5
1272. A2, B1, C4, D3
1273. B
1274. C
1275. B
1276. C
1277. A
1278. A thru E
1279. D
1280. A thru E
1281. A, B, C, D
1282. B, C, D, E
1283. C
1284. A, B
1285. E
1286. A thru E
1287. A thru E
1288. A thru G
1289. A, B, C, D
1290. A thru E
1291. A
1292. A thru E
1293. A, B, D, E
1294. A, B, C
1295. C
1296. A
1297. C
1298. B, C, E
1299. A thru F
1300. A thru D
1301. A thru E
1302. B
1303. C
1304. A, B, C, D
1305. A, E
1306. A thru E
1307. A
1308. A
1309. E
1310. E
1311. A thru E
1312. A
1313. A, C
1314. D
1315. A
1316. C, D, E
1317. A, D
1318. A4, B2, C1, D5, E3
1319. D
1320. A3, B1, C4, D2
1321. B
1322. A thru E
1323. A thru E
1324. A, B, C, D
1325. A, B
1326. B, C, D, E
1327. A thru E
1328. A thru E
1329. E
1330. D
1331. C
1332. A3, B1, C2
1333. A thru D
1334. A, B, C
1335. A thru E
1336. A, C
1337. B
1338. A thru E
1339. A thru F
1340. A thru E
1341. A thru E
1342. A thru E
1343. A thru P
1344. A thru F
1345. A thru E
1346. C, D, E, F
1347. A thru E
1348. E
1349. A1, B2, C3
1350. A, B, C, D
1351. B, C, D
1352. B, C, D
1353. A thru E
1354. A thru E
1355. D
1356. E

1357. A, B
1358. A, B
1359. E
1360. E
1361. A thru F
1362. A, C, E
1363. A, B
1364. E
1365. A
1366. D
1367. A, B, C
1368. A thru E
1369. D
1370. A thru E
1371. A thru E
1372. E
1373. A thru E
1374. A, D
1375. A thru E
1376. A, B, C, D
1377. A, B
1378. C
1379. B
1380. B
1381. C. E
1382. A
1383. D
1384. E
1385. A
1386. A, C

SECTION VII

1387. B
1388. A, B
1389. D, E
1390. A thru E
1391. B
1392. A, C, E
1393. A thru F
1394. A thru E
1395. A thru E
1396. A
1397. E
1398. E
1399. D
1400. C, D, E
1401. B
1402. D
1403. D
1404. B
1405. B, C, E
1406. A
1407. A thru E
1408. G
1409. A thru E
1410. A thru E
1411. A, C, D, E
1412. A, B, C
1413. A thru E
1414. A thru E
1415. A thru E
1416. A thru E
1417. A
1418. A, B, C, D
1419. A thru E
1420. A thru F
1421. A, C, D, E
1422. A, B, D, E
1423. A thru E
1424. A thru E
1425. A thru F
1426. B, G
1427. A, B, C, E
1428. A, B, E
1429. A thru H
1430. E
1431. A thru E
1432. A thru E
1433. A
1434. D
1435. B
1436. D
1437. B
1438. A thru E
1439. B
1440. A, B, C, E
1441. A thru E
1442. A, B, C, E
1443. E
1444. D
1445. A thru E
1446. E
1447. A thru E
1448. A thru E
1449. D
1450. A
1451. A thru F
1452. A, E, F
1453. B, C, D, E
1454. D
1455. A thru E
1456. A, B (sometimes E)
1457. A thru E
1458. B
1459. A thru E
1460. C
1461. A, B, D, E
1462. C
1463. A thru E
1464. A, B, C, E
1465. A thru F
1466. A thru E
1467. B, C, D, E
1468. A, C, E
1469. A, B, C
1470. A, C, D, E
1471. A thru E
1472. D
1473. A, B
1474. A, B, C, D
1475. D
1476. A, B, C, D
1477. A thru J
1478. A
1479. A and/or B
1480. A thru E
1481. A thru E
1482. A
1483. A thru E
1484. A thru E
1485. A, C, D, E
1486. A
1487. E
1488. E
1489. E
1490. A thru E
1491. B
1492. A, B, C, D
1493. D
1494. A thru E
1495. A, B, C
1496. E
1497. B
1498. D
1499. A, D
1500. E